Arine M. Wieland
PhD RNCS

Third Edition 3 *in* Epidemiology Health Care

Barbara Valanis, RN, DrPH, FAAN
Senior Investigator and Director of Nursing Research
Kaiser Permanente Center for Health Research
Portland, Oregon

D0111791

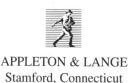

APPLETON & LANGE
Stamford, Connecticut

Copyright © 1999 by Appleton & Lange
A Simon & Schuster Company

Copyright © 1992 by Appleton & Lange
Copyright © 1986 by Appleton-Century-Crofts

www.appletonlange.com

00 01 02 03 / 10 9 8 7 6 5 4 3 2

Prentice Hall International (UK) Limited, *London*
Prentice Hall of Australia Pty. Limited, *Sydney*
Prentice Hall Canada, Inc., *Toronto*
Prentice Hall Hispanoamericana, S.A., *Mexico*
Prentice Hall of India Private Limited, *New Delhi*
Prentice Hall of Japan, Inc., *Tokyo*
Simon & Schuster Asia Pte. Ltd., *Singapore*
Editora Prentice Hall do Brasil Ltda., *Rio de Janeiro*
Prentice Hall, *Upper Saddle River, New Jersey*

Library of Congress Cataloging-in-Publication Data

Valanis, Barbara.
    Epidemiology in health care / Barbara Valanis. — 3rd ed.
        p.   cm.
    Rev. ed. of: Epidemiology in nursing and health care. 2nd ed.
c1992.
    Includes bibliographical references.
    ISBN 0-8385-2227-0 (pbk. : alk. paper)
    1. Epidemiology. 2. Nursing. I. Valanis, Barbara. Epidemiology
in nursing and health care. II. Title.
    [DNLM: 1. Epidemiology. 2. Epidemiologic Methods. 3. Public
Health.   WA 950 V136e 1999]
RA652.V34 1999
614.4—dc21
DNLM/DLC
for Library of Congress   98-15835
                                                           CIP

Acquisitions Editor: Patricia Casey
Editorial Associate: Elisabeth Church Garofalo
Associate Production Editor: Angela Dion
Designer: Janice Barsevich Bielawa
Art Studio: ElectraGraphics, Inc.

ISBN 0-8385-2227-0

9 780838 522271   90000

Table of Contents

Reviewers

Nellie C. Bailey, RN, MA, MS, CS
Associate Dean for Academic Programming
College of Nursing
SUNY State University of New York
Health Science Center at Brooklyn
Brooklyn, New York

Judith A. Barton, RN, PhD
Associate Professor
School of Nursing
University of Colorado Health Sciences Center
Denver, Colorado

Marsha L. Bunker, RN, MSN
Lecturer in Nursing
Department of Nursing
University of Michigan—Flint
Flint, Michigan

Mary Jo Clark, RN, PhD
Associate Dean
Philip Y. Hahn School of Nursing
University of San Diego
San Diego, California

Roberta K. Lee, RN, DrPH, FAAN
Hubert C. Moog Professor of Nursing
Barnes College of Nursing
University of Missouri—St. Louis
St. Louis, Missouri

Rita Morris, RN, PhD
Associate Professor
San Diego State University
San Diego, California

CONTRIBUTORS TO THE SECOND EDITION

The author wishes to thank and acknowledge contributors to the previous edition of this book.

Karen Labuhn, RN, PhD
Associate Professor
Wayne State University
Detroit, Michigan

Linda A. Shortridge-McCauley, RN, PhD
Associate Professor & Scientist
Center for Research on Occupational & Environmental Toxicology
Oregon Health Sciences University
Portland, Oregon

Mary Ann Woodbury, RN, MPH
Epidemiologist
Dow Corning Corporation
Midland, Michigan

Preface

This text provides an introduction to the concepts and methods of epidemiology and to issues in the application of epidemiology to clinical practice, public health, and health administration. Epidemiology is an essential discipline for clinical and community health practice. The importance of this science for the clinician or public health practitioner is demonstrated by the inclusion of epidemiology courses in most medical, nursing, and public health curricula. Epidemiology provides ways of thinking about health and disease and tools for critical appraisal of the medical, nursing, and public health literature. By stimulating a questioning approach to practice, epidemiological thinking can reduce the probability that treatments or interventions inadequately supported by research will be introduced and accepted. Epidemiological thinking can also increase the probability that unusual or associated events, or both, will be promptly recognized.

This book, initially developed for clinicians, aimed to address relevant issues that were not covered adequately in other textbooks. Although a number of other clinical epidemiology books have been published since the release of the first edition of this text, this book remains unique. It provides not only an introduction to methods of epidemiology but also data on major causes of morbidity and mortality through the life cycle, and applications of epidemiology in clinical practice, care management, and public health administration. This third edition retains those elements relevant to student nurses and nurses who work in health institutions or in community health settings. However, its applicability is extended to students and practicing professionals in health administration and other fields of public health, and to those clinicians and other health care providers practicing in managed care settings. This edition has updated all statistical material and related text, added a section on statistical methods, and incorporated examples of applications to managed care wherever appropriate. In addition, exercises have been developed for each chapter and are provided on an interactive disk.

The book is divided into three sections. Section I—Chapters 1 through 7—covers the basic concepts and methods of epidemiology. These chapters include such concepts as natural history of disease, levels of prevention, and causality. General methods including epidemiological measures, study designs, sources of data, statistical approaches, and critical appraisal of epidemiological studies are introduced here. Separate chapters in Section I address the natural history, measurement, and methodological considerations relevant to the study and control of infectious and noninfectious disease. The methods content is equivalent to that of other introductory epidemiological texts in common use, but specialized methodological issues are integrated throughout the remainder of the book where applicable to the topic of discussion, rather than covered in separate methods chapters. For example, issues of sensitivity, specificity, and predictive values are discussed in Chapter 14 on screening for disease. Thus the methods are discussed in the context of use.

Section II—Chapters 8 through 11—presents data on the major causes of morbidity and mortality for four stages of the life cycle: pregnancy and infancy; childhood and adolescence; young and middle-aged adults; and older persons. Section III—Chapters 12 through 16—discusses issues and methods relating to the application of epidemiology to disease control and surveillance activities, screening programs, clinical decision-making, planning and evaluation of health services, and conducting research into the etiology and natural history of disease.

I hope that for some readers the introduction to epidemiological thinking presented in this book will stimulate an interest in pursuing further studies. I also hope for all readers that the strategies of epidemiology present herein will add a new and rewarding dimension to your clinical and administrative practice and serve as a useful reference on an ongoing basis.

Barbara Valanis

Acknowledgments

I wish to thank all faculty and students who have used the previous editions of this book and taken the time to provide feedback on what was useful and what might make the text more helpful. Many of these suggestions (for example, adding a section on statistical methods and exercises for each chapter) have been incorporated into this edition. I would also like to thank Dr. Linda Shortridge-McCauley for providing the class exercises she developed for use with her students to supplement an earlier edition of this book and allowing some of them to be incorporated into this edition. The change in title of the book and its broadened focus are due in great part to the encouragement and support of Dr. Mervyn Susser and Dr. Zena Stein, my friends and mentors. I thank them for suggesting this book be marketed to a wider audience. A big thank you is also owed, once again, to my husband, Kirk Valanis, for his support and patience throughout all the evenings and weekends spent on this revision.

I appreciate the support, encouragement, and even the gentle nagging from Elisabeth Church-Garofalo and Angela Dion at Appleton & Lange. They helped keep me on track during the work on this third edition. Thanks to Lauren Keller for her persistance in persuading me to take on this edition. Stacy Prassas of Spotted Dog Media deserves special thanks for her reworking of the study questions to make them fit the constraints of the computer software.

Finally, to all those colleagues who have molded my beliefs, shared ideas, and been supportive throughout the years, I express my sincere gratitude.

Introduction
and Methods

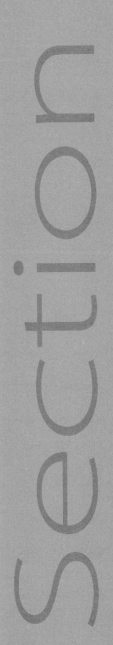

Epidemiology: What Is It About?

he history of a science provides a framework for understanding its form, substance, and methods. This chapter provides a brief history of epidemiology, introduces epidemiological theory, discusses interrelationships of epidemiology with clinical practice, and explores seven basic uses of epidemiology in public health and clinical practice: investigation of disease etiology and natural history; identification of risks; identification of syndromes and classification of disease; differential diagnosis and planning clinical treatment; surveillance of the health status of populations; community diagnosis and planning of health services; and evaluation of health services and public health interventions.

A BRIEF OVERVIEW

Epidemiology is a term derived from the Greek language (epi = upon; demos = people; logos = science). It is a science concerned with health events in human populations. In practical terms, it is the study of how various states of health are distributed in the population and what environmental conditions, lifestyles, or other circumstances are associated with the presence or absence of disease. Epidemiologists are essentially medical detectives concerned with the who, what, where, when, and how of disease causation. By searching to find who does and who does not get sick with a particular disease and determining where the illness is and is not found, under what particular circumstances, epidemiologists narrow down the suspected causal agents. Once an agent is identified, public health officials can take steps to prevent or control the occurrence of the disease.

The process of investigating the disease generates other information useful to public health officials and to medical and nursing clinicians. Epidemiological investigations may provide measures of disease frequency that are useful in assessing the need for specific community health services, for example, rates of occurrence of stroke in different age groups and the expected rate of disability among those having suffered a stroke. These data permit estimation of both the probable number of hospital beds needed and the required staffing for home care and rehabilitation programs. Epidemiologists also generate information about the natural history of a disease—how disease occurs and progresses in the human host. They identify the various signs and symptoms of the condition and the usual patterns of presentation. They may identify physiological changes that, because they occur before presentation of clinical signs and symptoms of the disease, are identifiable only through laboratory tests. Such tests can be used for early case finding so that, where effective treatment is available, it can be instituted to arrest the progression of the disease.

In the process of describing disease patterns, epidemiologists may identify new clinical syndromes, refine disease classifications, or identify factors that are associated with a high risk of developing a particular condition. Such information is useful to physicians in making differential diagnoses and deciding on the most effective treatment. Nurses use such information in physical assessments or in selecting groups for specific health education programs. When a specific causal agent is identified, programs to eliminate the agent from the environment or to protect the human population from the agent can be instituted. Because epidemiology provides these basic data needed for decision making in public health, it is considered one of the basic sciences of public health, just as anatomy, physiology, biochemistry, and genetics constitute basic sciences for medicine and nursing.

COMPONENTS OF EPIDEMIOLOGY

The term *epidemiology* has come to refer both to the particular methods applied in studies of disease causation and to the body of knowledge that arises from such investigations. The collection of epidemiological knowledge is usually termed *substantive epidemiology,* although some authors may refer to it as *descriptive epidemiology.* To avoid confusion, the term "descriptive epidemiology" will be used here for the first phase of epidemiological research. The term "substantive epidemiology" will be used to refer to the cumulative body of knowledge generated through epidemiological research. This comprises the epidemiological descriptions of various diseases and states of health, including their natural history, patterns of occurrence, and factors associated with high risk of developing the condition (risk factors).

DEVELOPMENT OF EPIDEMIOLOGICAL SCIENCE

Three characteristics are generally considered to differentiate one scientific discipline from another. These are the methods by which data are collected, how the body of knowledge is accumulated by the discipline, and how the underlying theory that guides the collection of data is developed. Epidemiological methods, the body of knowledge, and epidemiological theory are each introduced briefly in the following paragraphs and developed further in other chapters.

Evolvement of Methods

For thousands of years people have been trying to explain what causes disease. Supernatural events were often used to explain the occurrence of illness. Hippocrates (460 to 377 BC) attempted to explain disease occurrence on a rational rather than a supernatural basis. In several books, *Airs, Waters and Places, Epidemics I,* and *Epidemics II,* he pointed out that disease is a mass phenomenon, one that affects groups or populations as well as individuals. He differentiated between *endemic disease*, that which tends to be always present at a low level, and *epidemic disease*, the occurrence of a given illness clearly in excess of the normal frequency. Further, he noted that environment and lifestyle are related to the occurrence of disease (Adams, 1886).

Even in Biblical times public health measures were instituted. These were based solely on observations about the occurrence of diseases in populations because the causes were unknown. For example, the practice of isolating persons with a disease such as leprosy was based on the observation that the disease often developed among seemingly healthy individuals who came in contact with those already afflicted with the disease. Many religious laws or practices grew out of similar observations. The Jewish prohibition of eating pork may have developed from the observation that eating pork frequently resulted in illness (trichinosis). Incest laws are thought to have grown out of observations regarding the high occurrence of congenital malformations and other conditions associated with close consanguinity. Most of these measures were based on observations comparing people who got sick with those who did not, and most involved epidemics of disease. During each epidemic, a clear excess of disease seemed to be associated with certain events.

In more recent history, James Lind suspected that scurvy might be related to the limited diet of sailors. In 1747, he conducted a small experiment in which small groups of ill sailors were given different supplements to their standard diet. Those receiving citrus fruits recovered while the others did not (Lind, 1753). Some years later, measures were taken to prevent the use of certain water supplies on the basis of the investigative observations of John Snow (1855) in England. His work in the 1850s led him to suspect contaminated water as the source of cholera outbreaks. Use of quantitative measures of disease frequency, known as rates, enabled him to determine that rates of cholera were much higher among those persons who drank the water than among those who did not. This determination was made well before the actual isolation of the cholera vibrio by Koch (1880). Snow also developed a theory of disease communication and, as early as 1849, promoted frequent hand washing by those attending patients (Winkelstein, 1995).

The use of rates to measure the frequency of disease occurrence provided a scientific basis for the growth of systematic methods to study disease. These systematic methods, when applied to the investigation of disease patterns as they relate to the distribution of potential causal factors, form a basis for the science of epidemiology. Investigations based on these methods have, over the years, provided a substantial amount of data about human health and disease. This accumulation of data provides an epidemiological body of knowledge about what factors are associated with the occurrence and progression of diseases.

The Body of Knowledge

The scope of the body of epidemiological knowledge is broadening with time. The earliest epidemiological investigations focused most frequently on infectious conditions, such as plague, cholera, or typhoid, rather than on noninfectious conditions (stroke, mental retardation), because much of the world was plagued with epidemics of infectious disease accompanied by high mortality. As a result of these early efforts, we now have considerable information about many infectious illnesses.

Common nutritional diseases, such as scurvy and pellagra, were important focuses of epidemiological study early in the 20th century. Chronic illnesses, such as heart disease and cancer, became major causes of mortality and morbidity as infectious and nutritional diseases were controlled. Thus, during the past half century, in particular, epidemiological investigation has expanded to include all diseases, communicable, noncommunicable, acute, or chronic, irrespective of whether their frequency shows short-term epidemic fluctuations. Further, epidemiology today is not limited to the study of diseases or patterns of ill health. It can also focus on other health-related characteristics of populations such as studies of body weight in relation to height and of blood group subtypes in different population groups. By extending its scope to include mental and social conditions in addition to disease, epidemiology has helped behavioral scientists, social workers, community health planners, and, in general, all those concerned with the health and well-being of human populations. It is truly multidisciplinary, providing information to the medical, social, and behavioral sciences, and drawing on these sciences in its research. A strength of epidemiology as a science is its multidisciplinary approach to health problems, because the broader the scope of observation, the greater the chances for uncovering the many factors that contribute to poor health. This recognition has led in recent years to a wider spectrum of professionals who participate in epidemiological research. Although most epidemiologists in the past were physicians and nurses, today the field attracts sociologists, psychologists, anthropologists, environmentalists, and many others.

Epidemiologic Theory

Stallones (1980) pointed out that the theory of a discipline is its most distinctive feature. He proposed the following as the central axiom on which epidemiology is based:

- Axiom: Disease does not distribute randomly in human populations.
- Corollary 1: Nonrandom aggregations of human disease are manifested along axes of measurement of time, of space, of individual personal characteristics, and of certain community characteristics.
- Corollary 2: Variations in the frequency of human disease occur in response to variations in the intensity of exposure to etiologic agents or other more remote causes, or to variations in the susceptibility of individuals to the operation of those causes (Stallones, p. 80).

This axiom recognizes that patterns of disease occurrence or other alterations of states of health in human communities are determined by forces that can be identified and measured and that modification of these forces is the most effective way to prevent disease. A definition of epidemiology should therefore reflect this theoretical basis for the discipline.

In the late 1970s there was considerable discussion among epidemiologists attempting to formulate a single best definition of modern epidemiology (Lilienfeld, 1978; Evans, 1979; Frerichs & Neutra, 1979; Rich, 1979).

The following definition of epidemiology reflects the major components of the modern discipline: *Epidemiology is the study of the distribution of states of health and of the determinants of deviations from health in human populations.* The *purposes of modern epidemiology* are to (1) identify the etiology of deviations from health; (2) provide the data necessary to prevent or control disease through public health intervention; and (3) provide data necessary to maximize the timing and effectiveness of clinical interventions.

EPIDEMIOLOGY AND THE CLINICIAN

Although historically, epidemiological research has often grown out of clinical practice and observation, the focus of epidemiology differs from that of clinical practice. Clinical practice focuses on the health of the individual. The focus of epidemiology is the health of the group to which the individual belongs, whether this group is large or small, representative of a "natural" population (family, school, community, nation), or of a more heterogeneous "aggregate" (club, party). The *clinical* description of a disease differs from its *epidemiological* description insofar as the former relates to an *individual patient* whereas the latter describes a *group of individuals* similarly affected. Here the epidemiologist has to single out, in terms of probabilities, averages, and means, those characteristics that are significantly more common in the diseased population.

Practicing clinicians make use of epidemiological information in their art of diagnosis; they also contribute to epidemiological knowledge of disease through careful observation, examination, and laboratory workup of their patients. In general, epidemiological studies rely heavily on health data that are recorded for purposes other than epidemiological investigation. Thus physicians, nurses, and other health personnel are essential in providing the required data. Further, because these clinical personnel are regularly in contact with patients, they are in a superb position to note patterns of disease occurrence and progression and to raise questions about anything unusual. Understanding epidemiological methods can lead to "thinking epidemiologically" and thus increases the likelihood of appropriate observation which is why most medical schools, nursing schools, and schools of allied health professions now offer some training in epidemiology.

Thinking Epidemiologically

Although the unit of observation in epidemiology is basically a population group, measures of disease frequency are based on the appropriate diagnosis of a disease in each individual patient. Therefore, accurate case definition is essential to the epidemiologist. By relating clinical signs and symptoms of current patients with those of similar cases previously encountered, either in their own experience or as reported in the literature, clinicians and epidemiologists may identify a clustering of similar cases and thus identify and classify new diseases.

Patterns of symptoms often cluster in a particular age group, geographical area, or time period. Recognition of such patterns is the first step in learning what causes a particular disease. The identification in the 1980s of acquired immune deficiency syndrome (AIDS) as a new illness, restricted to certain population groups, required that clinicians be aware that they were seeing the same unusual symptoms in multiple patients within a short time period and the awareness that all these patients had some common characteristics. In this instance, the early cases were among homosexual males. Since that time, other population groups, such as hemophiliacs, intravenous drug users, and heterosexual partners of persons with human immunodeficiency virus (HIV) infection, have also been observed to have a high rate of this condition (Centers for Disease Control, 1987).

Another example of this epidemological thinking is the investigation of Legionnaire's disease. A unique set of symptoms, resulting in high mortality rates, was recognized primarily among attendees of an American Legion convention in Philadelphia in 1976. Later, while reviewing case records from several previous small epidemics of unknown origin, epidemiologists discovered that these epidemics were of the same condition as those seen among those identified with Legionnaire's disease. Comparison of the circumstances surrounding each outbreak led to the hypothesis that the organism may have been disseminated through air conditioning systems (Frazer & McDade, 1979). Despite this long-held hypothesis, Legionnaire's disease continues to be a problem today.

Another instance of epidemiological thinking occurred when several physicians discovered that each of them had recently treated a patient with an unusual cell type (adenocarcinoma) of vaginal cancer. A further unusual factor was that each of the cases occurred in teenaged girls, an unusual age for this type of cancer. These observations led to a search of hospital records to determine whether further cases could be located, and a study to learn what might be common to all the cases followed. The common factor appeared to be fetal exposure to diethylstilbesterol (DES), a drug that at one time was given to women during pregnancy to reduce the occurrence of spontaneous abortion. This case illustrates the importance of complete recording by clinical and laboratory personnel of information on the onset of symptoms and of laboratory data.

Nurses working on an inpatient medical unit of a large urban hospital thought they were seeing an unusually high occurrence of bladder infections among patients with indwelling catheters. When they checked unit records they found that during the most recent 3 months, the rate of new infections was three times that of the previous 3 months. Approximately 3 months before, a new brand of catheter had been purchased to replace a more expensive brand previously used on the unit. Further examination of nursing notes revealed that the frequency with which the new, less expensive catheters became displaced and had to be reinserted was much higher than with the previous brand. As a result, the nurses recommended to the hospital administrator that the more expensive brand be reinstated as the cost in added personnel time, illness, and use of multiple catheters per patient was far greater than the few cents saved per catheter with the new brand. After a return to the original brand, reinsertion rates and rates of bladder infection returned to their previous low levels. This example of epidemiological thinking illustrates the importance of being aware of the usual frequency with which events occur, and the need for adequate records with which to validate one's observation that the perceived frequency of an event did indeed change.

Clinical personnel often make use of epidemiological data in the course of their practice. As previously mentioned, physicians use knowledge of the patterns of disease occurrence to make differential diagnoses. Nursing assessments use knowledge of distribution of symptoms in relation to age to determine whether a particular symptom needs followup or intervention. A blood pressure of 140/90 is probably no cause for alarm in an 80 year old, but most likely requires intervention in a 25 year old. Additionally, epidemiological input is useful to clinical personnel in determining the optimum therapy, the dosage of medication, and the duration of treatment. For example, through the systematic observation of a considerable number of children who have undergone surgery at different ages for repair of congenital heart disease, it is now possible to select the most appropriate age for this intervention. HIV infection is another condition where data on its natural history are key elements of providing care. The association of mortality risk with severe CD4 count supression can be used to help patients make decisions about employment, travel, and other types of activities, while the correlation of current CD4 counts with short to intermediate risk of specific opportunistic infections guides decisions about starting preemptive antibiotic therapy (Volberding, 1996). Furthermore, recent data show that age at infection is a strong predictor of prognosis (Darby et al, 1996). AIDS risk and mortality increase in a stepwise manner from the youngest cohort to the oldest, suggesting a need to modify treatment guidelines initially developed for younger patients; for older patients more agressive therapies should be initiated earlier.

Early detection of disease may contribute to improved prognosis. Identifying risk factors for breast cancer, for example, permits the identification of high-risk women who need more frequent screening to identify a cancer before metastasis and should be cautious in use of drugs, such as long-term estrogen replacement therapy for prevention of heart disease cautiously and under regular medical super-vision as numerous studies have shown them to be associated with an increase in breast cancer risk (Colditz, 1993; Hulka, 1990; Bergkvist, 1989; Persson, 1992; Colditz, 1995). Furthermore, these high-risk women should be taught how to do regular breast self-examinations so they can monitor themselves between mammo-graphic examinations for any occurrence of a lump.

USES OF EPIDEMIOLOGY

Different systems for classifying uses of epidemiology have been devised. A system that classifies uses into seven categories is useful and includes: (1) Investigation of disease etiology; (2) identification of risks; (3) identification of syndromes and clas-sification of disease; (4) differential diagnoses and planning clinical treatment; (5) surveillance of population health status; (6) community diagnosis and planning of health services; and (7) evaluation of health services and public health interven-tions. Each of these is discussed briefly on the following pages.

Investigation of Disease Etiology and Determination of the Natural History of Disease

Because the purpose of epidemiological investigation is to delineate the etiology of disease, thus providing the data needed for control or eradication, etiological studies represent a major use of epidemiological methods. These studies produce informa-tion on the natural history of the disease. *Natural history* refers to the processes nor-mally leading to disease occurrence, before any intervention, and to the course and outcome of the disease process. It includes the description of the disease process from the first forces creating the disease stimulus in the environment or elsewhere, through the time of host-agent interaction, and to the resulting response in humans, including illness, recovery, permanent disability, or death. For disease prevention, the cause(s) of the disease must be identified and the means by which causal agents are transmitted to the human host must be understood. In contrast to epidemiologi-cal studies, which emphasize the prepathogenic or early pathogenic stages of dis-ease in total population groups, research carried out by clinicians, whether physi-cians, nurses, or other health professionals, is largely concerned with patient responses to treatment (physiological and psychological) during the later stages of the natural history and is usually based only on the study of patients who have sought treatment for symptoms of illness.

Although there are epidemiological studies based solely on populations of hos-pitalized cases, the evolution of a complete body of knowledge about the natural his-tory of a disease demands the study of a spectrum of ascertainable cases in a popula-tion, including those cases too mild to have sought or require medical treatment. Without this spectrum of disease severity, it is impossible to understand the natural history. Thus, epidemiological research studies often produce a different picture of the disease than do studies derived only from data on hospitalized patients. As a clas-sic example, data show that half or more of the deaths of middle-aged men from coronary heart disease occur in the initial days of the first clinical attack of coronary thrombosis. Because a substantial portion of these deaths occur in the first hours before the patient reaches the hospital, these cases are never part of clinical research. In addition, many cases of "silent" myocardial infarction (MI) are generally unknown to the clinician (Russek & Zohman, 1951). These data provide important information, however, that can be used for planning early intervention directed toward identification and treatment of the "silent MI" group through identification and monitoring of high-risk individuals. In addition, the data on the high rates of early mortality associated with clinical attacks suggested the need for mobile life squads trained in cardiopulmonary resuscitation with readily available equipment.

Identification of Risks

Risk refers to the *probability of an unfavorable event.* In epidemiology, the term generally refers to the likelihood that people who are without a disease, but who come in contact with certain factors thought to increase disease risk, will acquire the disease. Factors associated with an increased risk of acquiring disease are called *risk factors.* These factors may be part of the physical environment, such as toxins, infectious organisms, radiation, or part of the social environment, such as stressful life events, divorce, or death of a spouse. They may also be behavioral, such as smoking and lack of exercise, or inherited, such as hemoglobin S, which increases risk for infection.

In general, the risk to an individual of developing a particular disease can be estimated only on the basis of the experience of whole populations of individuals. Once this experience is known, the relevant risks can be calculated for persons who are similar to those in that population. Further, population data on disease occurrence can be used for estimating the effect of a public health intervention on disease rates.

A measure called the *relative risk ratio,* estimates how much the risk of acquiring a disease increases with exposure to a particular causal agent or known risk factor. This ratio is derived by comparing the occurrence of disease in a population exposed to the causal agent to the occurrence of disease in a nonexposed population. Thus, a relative risk ratio of 5 implies that the risk of acquiring that disease is five times greater for someone exposed to an etiological agent than for someone not exposed. Relative risk ratios are a useful tool for identifying factors that represent increased risk for development of a disease. Diabetes, obesity, hypertension, and smoking are considered risk factors for cardiovascular disease because populations with these characteristics show several times the rate of that disease as opposed to populations without those conditions or behaviors. Once risk factors are identified, public health programs can be instituted to change high-risk behaviors, such as smoking, and to identify high-risk individuals through comprehensive screening programs that ensure medical treatment to reduce risk. In addition, nurses and other clinicians can counsel high-risk individuals on how they can reduce their risk by adopting healthier lifestyles. Relative risk ratios are discussed in more detail in Chapter 4 on epidemiological and biostatistical methods and measures.

A measure called *attributable risk* estimates the effect on disease occurrence of public health intervention(s) that eliminate exposure to a causal agent. This measure subtracts the rate of disease occurrence (incidence) in the nonexposed population from the rate of disease occurrence (incidence) in the exposed population. If a non-smoking population develops cardiovascular disease at a rate of 350 per 100,000 and a smoking population develops cardiovascular disease at a rate of 685 per 100,000, then 335 cases per 100,000 population are attributable to cigarette smoking and should be preventable through the elimination of cigarette smoking.

Identification of Syndromes and Classification of Disease

This use of epidemiology relates directly to clinical medicine. Broad descriptive clinical and pathological categories often include very different elements. Variations in their statistical distribution and in the ways in which diseases progress or behave in a population (natural history) may make it possible to distinguish elements of one disease from another. Previously, all vascular diseases were classified together. As epidemiological data accumulated, it became clear that cerebrovascular disease and cardiovascular disease were distinct conditions, although both shared the characteristic narrowing or occlusion of a blood vessel as a preceding mechanism. Populations with high rates of cerebrovascular disease, such as the Japanese, had low rates of cardiovascular disease, whereas populations with high rates of cardiovascular disease had lower rates of cerebrovascular disease (Morris, 1975).

Clustering of signs, symptoms, and similarities of natural history allows the identification of syndromes. An historical, but still relevant example, rubella syndrome, was identified as a collection of malformations and functional problems common to offspring of mothers infected with rubella during pregnancy, particularly during the first trimester (Gregg, 1941). A more recent example is the identification of toxic shock syndrome (TSS) as a definable group of symptoms and test results as listed in Table 1–1. Toxic shock syndrome, when first identified, was associated with menstruation and was linked to the use of tampons. Investigations are now in progress on a 1997 outbreak (Centers for Disease Control, 1997).

Differential Diagnoses and Planning Clinical Treatment

Descriptive data, such as age and sex distributions of disease incidence, aid the clinician in understanding the condition and in sorting through multiple possible diagnoses that present with the same or similar symptoms. Such data also facilitate the planning of treatment. Recognizing the association of age with prognosis for long-term breast cancer survival, for example, will likely influence treatment and may also influence followup programs. Breast cancers diagnosed premenopausally tend to be more lethal than postmenopausal breast cancers and thus require more aggressive treatment and closer followup. Mumps may be a mild self-limiting disease in childhood, but in men it can lead to infertility. Public health intervention to reduce susceptibility or to prevent exposure of men who did not acquire mumps during childhood, therefore, is crucial.

Since the 1980s, observations about variability in medical and public health practices have led to attempts to identify "best practices" in order to improve quality and decrease costs. These efforts to assess the best approaches to diagnosis and

TABLE 1–1. TOXIC SHOCK SYNDROME CASE DEFINITION

1. Fever [temperature ≥38.9°C (102°F)].
2. Rash (diffuse, macular, erothematous).
3. Desquamation, 1-2 weeks after onset of illness, particularly of palms and soles.
4. Hypotension (systolic blood pressure ≤90 mm Hg for adults or <5th percentile by age for children <16 years of age, or orthostatic syncope).
5. Involvement of three or more of the following organ systems:
    a. Gastrointestinal (vomiting or diarrhea at onset of illness).
    b. Muscular (severe myalgia or creatine phosphokinase level ≥2 × ULN[a]).
    c. Mucous membrane (vaginal, oropharyngeal, or conjunctival hyperemia).
    d. Renal (BUN[b] or Cr[c] ≥2 × ULN or ≥5 white blood cells per high-power field—in the absence of a urinary tract infection).
    e. Hepatic (total bilirubin, SGOT[d], or SGPT[e] ≥2 × ULN).
    f. Hematologic (platelets ≤100,000/mm^3).
    g. Central nervous system (disorientation or alterations in consciousness without focal neurologic signs when fever and hypotension are absent).
6. Negative results on the following tests, if obtained:
    a. Blood, throat, or cerebrospinal fluid cultures.
    b. Serologic tests for Rocky Mountain spotted fever, leptospirosis, or measles.

[a]Twice upper limits of normal for laboratory.
[b]Blood urea nitrogen level.
[c]Creatinine level.
[d]Serum glutamic oxaloacetic transaminase level.
[e]Serum glutamic pyruvic transaminase level.
(From *Centers for Disease Control. Follow-up on toxic shock syndrome.* Morbidity and Mortality Weekly Report, *1980; 29, 442.*)

treatment began with the Federal Government's U.S. Prevention Services Taskforce (USPSTF) in 1984. The taskforce was charged to develop evidence-based practice guidelines on use of screening tests and other preventive services. The USPSTF used the criteria of "a demonstrated improvement in a meaningful health outcome" to declare a preventive service effective (Woolf et al, 1996). Subsequently, the Agency for Health Care Policy and Research convened a series of expert panels focused on a range of diseases and conditions and charged them to review the epidemiological and clinical trials literature on diagnosis and treatment, then develop evidence-based practice guidelines. Many managed care organizations have initiated their own programs of practice guidelines development. The philosophy underlying all these efforts is that providing clinical guidelines is a way of keeping clinicians current with what the literature shows to be most effective at achieving desired outcomes.

Surveillance of the Health Status of Populations

Surveillance means keeping watch over. Epidemiological descriptions of diseases provide data on who is at high risk of contracting a disease, in which geographical locations it is more likely to occur, and when in time it is most frequently observed. This information alerts health workers to situations that should be monitored for early indication of a disease outbreak so that early detection programs may be set up and intervention promptly instituted. As an example, influenza rates tend to increase during late fall and early winter. Specific types of influenza are likely to recur in 2- to 3-year or 4- to 6-year cycles (Benenson, 1990). Groups at high risk of becoming seriously ill and dying of influenza are infants, young children, and the elderly. By monitoring reports of deaths caused by influenza, cases seen at emergency rooms, or absence from schools or work caused by respiratory illness, public health officials detect the signs of an outbreak early and can take steps to immunize susceptible populations at high risk of complications to prevent occurrence of the illness in these individuals.

In an additional example, the descriptive epidemiology of measles indicates that it occurs most frequently among school-aged children, that rates vary by season with highest rates in the fall, and that there are long-term cycles with increased rates every other year in large communities and at less frequent intervals in smaller communities, where outbreaks tend to be more severe. Measles is transmitted from person to person by close contact; therefore, it tends to occur in locations where children congregate (Benenson, 1990). Armed with this information, the school nurse can be alert to signs and symptoms of measles during the fall and can follow up on absences to determine if measles caused the absence. Numerous absences may indicate a need to review the immunization status of the school population. Although most schools, in theory, require up-to-date immunizations for students to be admitted, all too often monitoring does not occur and followup programs must be instituted to obtain immunizations for the susceptible children.

Monitoring of newly diagnosed cancer cases or birth defects can alert officials to clusters of cases that may suggest clues as to their causes. The example described here illustrates a classic example of how followup of such clusters can identify new causes of disease. The occurrence of several cases of adenocarcinoma of the vagina of young girls was noted by physicians in Boston. They realized that the occurrence of several cases in a short period of time in this age group was a highly unusual event. Their followup investigation identified the probable causal agent as DES, a drug given to the mothers of these patients during their pregnancies (Herbst et al, 1972). As a result, the female offspring of women who took DES have been identified and urged to undergo regular monitoring for the cancer with Papanicolaou (Pap) smears and other examinations to identify problems at their earliest stage.

Community Diagnosis and Planning of Health Services

Epidemiology provides the facts about community health. It describes the nature and relative size of the health problems to be dealt with, as well as how they are distributed in terms of geographical location, age group, socioeconomic group, and so on. This kind of information is the basis for planning the number and types of services required to meet the needs of a particular community. A neighborhood with a high proportion of elderly individuals is likely to have high rates of cardiovascular disease, cancer, and other chronic, debilitating diseases. Particularly if it is a low income neighborhood, elderly residents may lack the financial resources to travel to a distant source of medical care. Thus, health planners need to consider either setting up a satellite clinic in the neighborhood or providing transportation or home services, or both. Maternal-child health services can be planned to meet the needs of a community with a young population and a high birth rate. Family planning facilities, well-child centers, which include immunization services and health education programs aimed at prevention of disease through promotion of good health habits, may be appropriate. A community health assessment provides the basic information needed for allocation of limited resources to meet priority needs.

Evaluation of Health Services and Public Health Interventions

Because many health services are initiated to treat a community problem identified by epidemiological data, these same data, used as a monitoring device, are useful in the evaluation of these services. For example, one means of evaluating the effectiveness of a maternal-child health center established to reduce the rates of morbidity and mortality among mothers and children is to follow closely the morbidity and mortality rates and see if they drop and remain low after the health center begins operation.

In another example, after use of super-absorbent tampons was linked to occurrence of TSS, one brand (Rely) was withdrawn from the market, and later the fiber content of tampons was changed. Massive public education campaigns warned women about the risks of continuous tampon use and how to maximize safety of use, and informed women of the early signs and symptoms of TSS so they could seek medical care early if the illness did occur. The Centers for Disease Control in Atlanta, continued to monitor occurrence of the disease to determine whether these intervention efforts were successful. As can be seen in Figure 1–1, after the

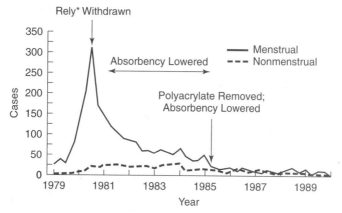

*Use of trade names is for identification only.

Figure 1–1. Reported cases of toxic shock syndrome, meeting definitions by the Centers for Disease Control, by quarter—United States, January 1, 1979–March 31, 1990. (*Adapted from Centers for Disease Control. Reduced incidence of menstrual toxic-shock syndrome—United States, 1980–1990.* Morbidity and Mortality Weekly Reports, *1990; 39(25):421.*)

withdrawal of Rely and with the lowering of absorbency in other brands, rates of TSS in menstruating women dropped dramatically. Monitoring these rates provided feedback on program effectiveness. Specifics of how epidemiology can be used to plan and evaluate health services are discussed in Chapter 16.

REFERENCES

Adams F. (1886) *The genuine works of Hippocrates* (trans. from the Greek). New York: William Word.

Benenson A. S. (Ed.). (1990) *Control of communicable disease in man* (14th ed.). New York: American Public Health Association.

Bergkvist L., Adami H.O., Persson I., Hoover R., Schairer C. (1989) The risk of breast cancer after estrogen and estrogen-progestin replacement. *N Engl J Med, 321*(5),293–297.

Centers for Disease Control. (1987) Human immunodeficiency virus infection in the United States: A review of current knowledge. *Morbidity and Mortality Weekly Reports, 36* (Suppl. 5–6).

Centers for Disease Control. (1997) Toxic Shock Syndrome—United States. *Morbidity and Mortality Weekly Reports, 46,*22.

Colditz G. A., Egan K. M., Stampfer M. J. (1993) Hormone replacement therapy and the risk of breast cancer: results from epidemiologic studies. *Am J Obstet Gynecol, 168,*1473–1480.

Colditz G. A., Hankinson S. E., Hunter D. J., Willett W. C., Manson J. E., Stempfer M. J. (1995) The use of estrogens and progestins and the risk of breast cancer in postmenopausal women. N Engl J Med, *332,*1589–93.

Darby S. C., Ewart D. W., Giangrande P. L., Spooner R. J. D., Rizza C. R. For the UK Haemophilia Centre Directors Organisation. (1996) *The Lancet, 347,* 1573–1579.

Evans A. S. (1979) Letter to the editor. *American Journal of Epidemiology, 109,* 379–382.

Frazer D. W., McDade J. E. (1979) Legionellosis. *Scientific American, 241,* 82–99.

Frerichs R. R., Neutra R. (1979) Letter to the editor. *American Journal of Epidemiology, 108,* 74–75.

Gregg N. M. (1941) Congenital cataract following German Measles in the mother. *Transactions of the Ophthalmologic Society Australia. 3,* 35.

Herbst A. L., Kurman R. J., Scully R. E. (1972) Vaginal and cervical abnormalities after exposure to stilbesterol *in utero. Obstetrics and Gynecology, 40,* 287–298.

Hulka B. S. (1990) Hormone replacement therapy and the risk of breast cancer. *California Cancer Journal Clinics 40*(5),289–296.

Koch R. (1880) *Investigations into the etiology of traumatic infective diseases,* trans. W. Watson Cheyne. London: The New Sydenham Society.

Lilienfeld A. D. (1978) Definitions of epidemiology. *American Journal of Epidemiology, 107,* 87–90.

Lind J. (1753) *A treatise of the scurvy.* Edinburgh: Kincaird and Donaldson. (Reprinted in C. P. Steward, D. Guthrie [Eds.]. (1953) *Lind's treatise on scurvy.* Edinburgh: University Press.)

Morris J. N. (1975) *Uses of epidemiology.* New York: Churchill and Livingston.

Persson I., Yuen J., Bergkvist L., Adami H. O., Hoover R., Schairer C. (1992) Combined estrogen-progestogen replacement and breast cancer risk [Letter to the editor]. *The Lancet, 340*(8826):1044.

Rich H. (1979) Letter to the editor. *American Journal of Epidemiology, 109,* 102.

Russek H. I., Zohman B. L. (1951) Chances for survival in acute myocardial infection. *Journal of the American Medical Association, 156,* 765.

Snow J. (1855) *On the mode of communication of cholera* (2nd ed.). London: Churchill. (Reprinted in *Snow on cholera.* (1936) New York: Commonwealth Fund.)

Stallones R. A. (1980) To advance epidemiology. *Annual Review of Public Health, 1,* 69–82.

Volberding P. A. (1996) Age as a predictor of progression in HIV infection [Letter to the editor]. *The Lancet, 347,* 1569.

Winkelstein W. (1995) A new perspective on John Snow's Communicable disease theory. *American Journal of Epidemiology,* (suppl.): *142*(9), 53–59.

Woolf S. H., DiGuiseppi C. G., Atkens D., Kamerow D. B. (1996) Developing evidence-based clinical practice guidelines. Lessons learned by the U.S. Preventive Services Task Force. *Annual Reviews of Public Health, 17,* 511–538.

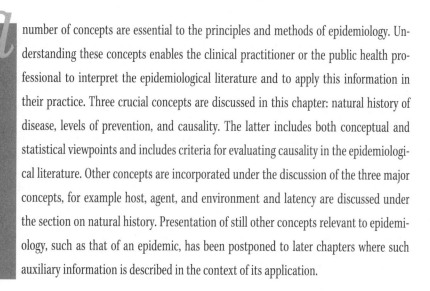

Some Useful Concepts in Epidemiology

number of concepts are essential to the principles and methods of epidemiology. Understanding these concepts enables the clinical practitioner or the public health professional to interpret the epidemiological literature and to apply this information in their practice. Three crucial concepts are discussed in this chapter: natural history of disease, levels of prevention, and causality. The latter includes both conceptual and statistical viewpoints and includes criteria for evaluating causality in the epidemiological literature. Other concepts are incorporated under the discussion of the three major concepts, for example host, agent, and environment and latency are discussed under the section on natural history. Presentation of still other concepts relevant to epidemiology, such as that of an epidemic, has been postponed to later chapters where such auxiliary information is described in the context of its application.

NATURAL HISTORY OF DISEASE

Natural history of disease is the process by which diseases occur and progress in the human host. This process involves the interaction of three different kinds of factors: the causative agent(s), a susceptible host (human), and the environment. As long as a state of equilibrium exists between host, agent, and environment, a state of health is maintained. A disequilibrium, such as an increase in the amount of the agent resulting from a change in environmental conditions, increases the likelihood that a susceptible host will be exposed. An increase in host susceptibility because of lack of sleep, malnutrition, excessive stress, aging, or a variety of other factors also increases the risk of disease. Changes in the environment contribute to changes in host susceptibility as well as to the conditions for viability of the agent.

The Agent

An *agent* is a factor whose presence causes a disease or one whose absence causes disease. An example of the former is *Salmonella,* which causes salmonellosis; an example of the latter is lack of vitamin D, which leads to rickets. Categories of agents include physical, chemical, nutrient, biological, genetic, and psychological agents. *Physical agents* include mechanical forces or frictions that may produce injury or atmospheric conditions such as extremes of temperature and excessive radiation. *Chemical agents* are those that affect human physiology through chemical action and include substances such as dusts, gases, vapors, fumes, or liquids. *Nutrient agents* are chemical in nature but refer specifically to basic components of the diet. Agents transmitted from parent to child through the genes are *genetic agents. Psychological agents* are those stresses in the environment, such as social circumstances, that affect physiology by psychosomatic means. The category of *biological agents* encompasses all living organisms, including insects, worms, protozoa, fungi, bacteria, rickettsia, and viruses. Biological agents are infectious in nature.

Certain characteristics of agents affect their ability to produce disease in the host. For infectious agents, the characteristics are infectivity, pathogenicity, and virulence. These characteristics are measured by the infection or attack rate, pathogenicity rate, and case fatality rate, respectively. These rates provide a means of population surveillance, allowing public health officials to assess the nature of the problem they are confronting and to plan appropriate intervention. Characteristics of infectious agents and these rates are discussed further in Chapter 6.

Important characteristics of noninfectious agents include concentration and toxicity for chemical agents, size, shape, and intensity for physical agents, chronicity or suddenness for psychological agents, and homo- or heterozygocity of genetic material for genetic agents. These are discussed in relation to noninfectious diseases in Chapter 7.

The Environment

Environment refers to all external conditions and influences affecting the life of living things. Physical, biological, and socioeconomic environments provide *reservoirs,* places where agents can reside or reproduce, or both, and modes of transmission for transporting agents from the reservoir to a human host. The *physical environment* includes the geological structure of an area and the availability of resources, such as water and flora, that influence the number and variety of animal reservoirs and certain insects that function as vectors to carry an agent from the reservoir to the host. Weather, climate, and season are important influences in the physical environment.

The *socioeconomic environment* contributes to the types of infectious agents in a locality because social and economic conditions relate both to the extent of environmental sanitation practices, such as disposal of garbage and excreta, and to the availability of medical facilities for immunization and medical care. The socioeconomic environment may also influence noninfectious agents. More psychological stressors may be found in poorer socioeconomic environments than in more affluent ones. Poor socioeconomic neighborhoods are more likely to be located near industrial plants, which may produce dangerous chemicals or emit physical particles of agents such as asbestos or coal tar.

Finally, there is the *biologic environment,* which includes living plants and animals that may serve as either the *reservoir* or the *vector* (living carrier that transports an infectious agent from an infected individual or its wastes to a susceptible individual or its food or immediate surroundings). Brucellosis is a disease in which animals, particularly cattle, swine, sheep, goats, horses, and reindeer, serve as reservoirs for human infection. The disease is transmitted from these animals to humans by contact with tissues, blood, urine, vaginal discharges, aborted fetuses or placentas, or by ingestion of milk or dairy products from infected animals. Special animal inspection and disposal procedures and education of farmers, animal handlers, and slaughterhouse workers help to control the spread of this disease among these groups (Benenson, 1990). Pasteurization of milk is an effective control measure for protecting the general population. In the case of plague, wild rodents are the usual reservoir, although infective fleas serve as the mode of transmission of the disease to humans (Benenson, 1990).

The Host

A *host* is the individual human in whom an agent produces disease. Disease can occur only in a host who is susceptible. Lack of susceptibility may be due to immunity or to inherent resistance. *Immunity* is the resistance on the part of a host to a specific infectious agent. Immunity can be humoral (antibodies in the blood) or cellular (specific to each type of cell), and of short-term or long-term duration. The role of immunity varies with the type of infectious agent. Immunity is discussed further in Chapter 6.

In contrast to immunity, the term *inherent resistance* refers to the ability to resist disease independently of antibodies or of specifically developed tissue response. Inherent resistance commonly rests in the anatomical or physiological characteristics of the host; it may be genetic or acquired, permanent or temporary. The concept of inherent resistance is useful in understanding host resistance both to infectious agents as well as to other types of agents. Factors such as general health status or nutrition, for example, may affect resistance to disease. Someone in good health who maintains good nutrition and a regular schedule of rest and exercise may be exposed to the common cold virus and resist infection even though the person is not immune to the organism. Similarly, this same individual, if exposed to psychological stress, may resist ulcers better than would someone in poorer general health.

The Disease Process

Occurrence of disease in a human host is not a single event at one point in time. Rather it is a process occurring over a period of time—the *natural history of the disease*. This natural history may be divided into two periods: prepathogenesis and pathogenesis. Stages in prepathogenesis are susceptibility and adaptation. Pathogenesis can also be broken down into two stages: early pathogenesis and clinical disease (Fig. 2–1). These stages are discussed in the following paragraphs. The subsequent section in this chapter, "Levels of Prevention," describes how the events that occur at each stage of a disease process can be used as a basis for determining intervention measures.

Prepathogenesis.   Exposure of the host to an agent occurs during the stage of *susceptibility*. In this first stage of prepathogenesis disease has not yet developed, although the groundwork has been laid through presence of factors that favor its occurrence. For example, poor eating habits and fatigue resulting from lack of sleep, often present among college students during exam week, represent risk factors that favor the occurrence of the common cold. If exposure to an agent occurs at this time, a response will take place. Initial responses reflect the normal adaptation response of the cell or functional system (eg, the immune system). If these adaptation responses are successful, then no disease occurs and the process is arrested in the second stage of prepathogenesis, *adaptation.*

In the case of infectious agents, exposure is followed by an *incubation period,* a time when the organism multiplies to sufficient numbers to produce a host reaction and clinical symptoms. This time period is relatively short, usually hours to months. For diseases caused by noninfectious agents, however, this time period

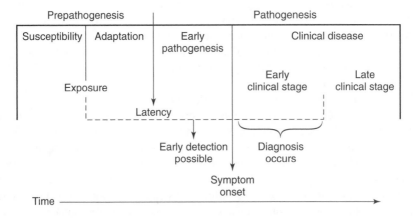

Figure 2–1. The natural history of disease.

from exposure to onset of symptoms, called the *induction period* or *latency period,* is often years to decades, although shorter induction periods may occur. Accidents resulting from a severe psychological stressor may occur shortly after initial exposure to the stressor. Elevated blood pressure, as a consequence of psychological stress, may require years of exposure to the stress. One of the shorter known latency periods for cancer is the 5-year latency period for leukemia in children exposed to radiation. Lung cancer resulting from asbestos exposure may have a latency period of 40 years between exposure and detection of the disease. Some chemical agents cause almost instantaneous, acute episodes of poisoning. The end of the incubation or induction period is the point of disease detection, whether by screening or by appearance of clinical signs and symptoms, although the time of clinically observable illness has conventionally been used.

Pathogenesis.   The next stage in the natural history of a disease is the stage of *presymptomatic disease,* sometimes called *early pathogenesis.* At this stage, the individual has no symptoms indicating the presence of illness. Adaptation, however, has been unsuccessful and pathogenic changes have begun. This happens during the incubation or latency period. These changes, which may be detectable by sophisticated laboratory tests, are called subclinical because they are below the level of the *clinical horizon,* an imaginary line dividing the point where there are detectable signs and symptoms from that where there are not. Premalignant changes or early malignant tissue changes in the cervix, for example, may be detected by a Papanicolaou (Pap) smear long before a woman experiences symptoms and before signs are visible to a gynecologist on visual examination. Such tests that can detect disease during the preclinical stage of early pathogenesis are used for screening to detect disease earlier than it would normally be discovered through the clinical presentation of symptoms.

The end of the incubation or induction period is the point of disease detection. This is stage four in the natural history, *clinical disease.* Clinical disease is defined as disease that is detectable because of symptoms experienced by the patient or signs apparent to a clinician during a physical examination. By this stage, sufficient anatomical or functional changes have occurred to produce recognizable signs and symptoms. This stage includes a range of disease severity from early clinical disease to that so advanced that death is inevitable. Possible outcomes, once a patient has entered this stage, may be complete recovery, residual defect that produces some degree of disability, or death. In an attempt to further understand this stage, clinicians and researchers have developed classification schemes for degrees of disease severity, including the staging systems used for malignancies, and the functional and therapeutic classifications used for cardiac disease.

Another difference between diseases caused by infectious agents and those caused by noninfectious agents or by still unidentified agents, is the likelihood for the latter to be conditions of a chronic nature. Most, but not all, diseases with infectious causes are of relatively short duration. The patient is usually ill for a period ranging from a few days to several months and generally recovers without any residual disability or, if the illness was severe, may die from the illness. The patient who has recovered rarely requires long-term follow up, although there are exceptions. Rheumatic heart disease, which results from a staphylococcal infection, is a disease caused by an infectious agent that is chronic in nature. The herpes virus may produce a single acute infection or may become chronic with repeated outbreaks of the infection following periods of remission. In the case of noninfectious agents, residual disability requiring prolonged medical treatment and rehabilitation programs is common. Patients with cardiovascular disease, for example, are likely to require ongoing supervision with prescribed medications, control of diet, and indefinite modifications of lifestyle.

LEVELS OF PREVENTION

The natural history of a disease provides the basis for planning intervention. Because a disease evolves over time and pathological change becomes less reversible as the disease process continues, the ultimate aim of intervention programs is to halt or reverse the process of pathological change as early as possible, thus preventing further damage. Three levels of prevention—primary, secondary, and tertiary—based on the stages of disease natural history, have proved useful (Table 2–1). The goal of intervention at each of the three levels is to prevent the pathogenic process from evolving further.

Primary prevention is aimed at intervening before pathological changes have begun, during the natural history stage of susceptibility. Primary prevention seeks to keep the agent away from contact with the host or to eliminate or reduce host susceptibility. These aims are accomplished through two types of activities: general health promotion and specific protection. *General health promotion* includes all activities that optimize the environment and favor healthy living. Thus, efforts to improve the physical environment, whether that of outdoors, home, school, or work, would be included. Health education aimed at educating the population about good nutrition, hygiene, the need for rest and recreation, preparation for retirement, or the harmful effects of smoking or drug use is a form of general health promotion. *Specific protection* refers to measures aimed at protecting individuals against specific agents. These measures include immunization against specific disease, such as diphtheria or polio, and removal of harmful agents from the environment, through processes such as sewage treatment, pasteurization of milk, or chlorination of water.

Since 1900, the effects of primary prevention can be seen in the dramatic reduction in the proportion of total mortality that results from infectious diseases (Fig. 2–2). This reduction in infectious disease mortality is largely a result of environmental manipulation and immunization programs, particularly among infants, young children, young women, and the elderly, and has led to a larger total population and to the advent of chronic disease as a major public health concern.

As fewer people die of infectious disease, more live to older ages where chronic diseases are common. Also, industrialization and changes in lifestyle have increased exposure to potential causal agents of noninfectious disease. These epidemiological transitions are discussed at length in Chapter 5. Recent advances, such as the ability to detect genes associated with higher risk for cancer, eg, the BRCA1

TABLE 2–1. NATURAL HISTORY OF DISEASE AND APPLICATION OF PREVENTIVE MEASURES

PERIOD	STAGE	EVENTS	LEVEL OF APPLICATION OF PREVENTIVE MEASURES	SPECIFIC INTERVENTIONS
Prepathogenesis	Susceptibility	1. Interrelations of various host, agent, and environmental factors bring host and agent(s) together 2. Disease-provoking stimulus is produced in the known host	Primary prevention	Health promotion (health education, nutrition counseling, adequate housing, personal hygiene, etc.) Specific protection (immunizations, sanitation, removing occupational and environmental hazards, use of specific nutrients, etc.)
	Adaptation	1. Adaptive processes are initiated		
Pathogenesis	Presymptomatic disease			
	A. Early pathogenesis	1. Interaction of host and stimulus continues after failure of adaptive response 2. Stimulus or agent becomes established (if infectious agent, increases by multiplication) 3. Beginning tissue and physiological changes		
	B. Discernible early lesions	1. Clinical recognition of disease is possible through laboratory or other tests that detect early physiological changes 2. Patient develops early symptoms that go unrecognized	Secondary prevention	Early diagnosis and prompt treatment (screening, case finding, selective examination)
	C. Clinical disease	1. Acute illness 2. Disability 3. Defect 4. Chronic state 5. Death	Tertiary prevention	Disability limitation (treatment to arrest disease process) Rehabilitation retraining for maximum use of remaining capacities, facilitating reentry to the family unit and to the workplace

(*Adapted from Leavell H. R. & Clark D. W.* Preventive medicine for the doctor in his community. *New York: McGraw-Hill, 1958.*)

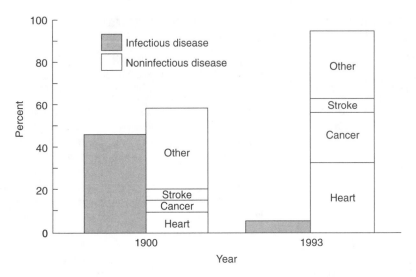

Figure 2–2. Proportional distribution of deaths from infectious and major noninfectious diseases, United States, 1900 and 1993.

gene for breast cancer, have raised hopes that primary prevention of cancer may be possible if individuals identified as high risk will change behaviors to reduce their chances of developing disease (Lerman et al, 1997). The efficacy of low fat diet in preventing breast cancer is currently being tested in a large clinical trial of post-menopausal women—the Women's Health Initiative, known as WHI (Roussouw et al, 1995). Conclusions from this study may lead to a standard recommendation that women identified as high risk for breast cancer should reduce the amount of fat in their diet. In addition, tamoxifen was tested in a clinical trial to determine whether it can prevent development of breast cancer in high risk women (Elias et al, 1994; Nayfield, 1995). Results released at a news conference but not yet published were favorable; tamoxifen may become a regular, primary preventive measure for controlling this disease among women at high risk.

Secondary prevention seeks to detect disease early, treat promptly, and cure disease at its earliest stage or, when cure is not possible, to slow its progression, prevent complications, and limit disability. Secondary prevention is therefore focused primarily on the stage of presymptomatic disease or on the very early stage of clinical disease. Screening is the most common form of secondary prevention. Many screening tests can detect early physiological indicators of disease before the individual has any symptom of illness. Examples include the Pap smear for cervical cancer, hearing tests for hearing impairment, the skin test for tuberculosis, and the phenylalanine test for phenylketonuria (PKU) in infants. Such screening programs have become very popular in recent years as improved technology has led to a proliferation of available test procedures. Detection and treatment of conditions at the stage allowed by screening tests provide benefits ranging from prevention of mental retardation in children with PKU by maintaining a special diet until adulthood, through preservation of life for cancer patients whose disease is detected while in an early stage, when it is curable. In the case of communicable diseases, early detection and treatment benefit not only those who are detected and treated; the screening programs provide primary prevention for other persons in proximity to affected individuals because they will no longer be exposing others to the infectious agent. For example, the VDRL can screen for syphilis and identify infected individuals who are treatable. Once treated, they cannot transmit the disease to others. Further discussion of epidemiological issues in the planning, implementation, and evaluation of screening programs is presented in Chapter 14.

Tertiary prevention includes limitation of disability and rehabilitation of those persons for whom residual damage already exists. Treatment activities are focused on the middle to later phases of clinical disease, when irreversible pathological damage produces disability. Exercise therapy to preserve muscle tone, restore motion, and prevent contractures in stroke patients is a form of tertiary prevention because it limits disability and begins the process of rehabilitation by maximizing the individual's residual capacities. Psychosocial and vocational services are usually part of a rehabilitation program as well.

Comparison of Prevention for Infectious and Noninfectious Diseases

Prevention of Infectious Diseases. Primary prevention for the control of infectious (communicable) disease uses measures aimed at (1) preventing the spread of the infectious agent from those environments that harbor it to individuals who are susceptible and who may be exposed, and (2) increasing host resistance. The former can be achieved by modifying or eliminating the environment in which the infectious agent lives or by interfering with the means of transmission to the human host, the latter by increasing host immunity. Immunization programs and general health maintenance efforts are used to increase host immunity. Control is facilitated by surveillance programs that quickly identify new cases and follow up with isolation methods to prevent exposure of susceptibles or institute specific treatments to limit the period of communicability and progression of pathology (secondary prevention). Tertiary prevention plays a smaller role in infectious disease programs than in noninfectious programs because infectious disease less often results in long-term disability.

Prevention of Noninfectious Diseases. In the case of infectious diseases, illness can be prevented if the infectious agent is destroyed or otherwise removed from the environment, or if specific protection is instituted through vaccination programs. These programs are effective because the infectious agent is necessary to produce the disease. For chronic conditions caused by noninfectious agents, however, there is usually no single agent responsible for its occurrence. Emphysema, for example, may result from smoking, air pollution, genetic susceptibility, or a variety of other agents. Each and every agent must be eliminated to prevent occurrence of the disease. For this reason, measures aimed at specific protection through removal of hazardous substances from the workplace or other environment often will reduce occurrence of the disease associated with exposure but will not eliminate it. Isocyanates, for example, have been implicated as a cause of asthma. Because they are only one of many causes, however, elimination of isocyonate in the workplace may dramatically reduce the occurrence of attacks among the worker population, but will not eliminate the disease entirely, even among those workers.

Synergistic effects of two or more agents are frequently seen in instances of causation by noninfectious agents. For example, nonsmoking workers exposed to asbestos have an increase of about eight times in the risk of dying from lung cancer when compared with nonsmoking, nonexposed individuals. Workers who smoke and are exposed to asbestos, however, are estimated to have 92 times the risk of the nonsmoking, nonexposed individuals (Kleinfeld et al, 1967). This is of concern because control efforts often must settle for minimizing rather than eliminating exposure to workplace agents. It is possible that if exposures to harmful environmental agents can be kept low, then the latency period before onset of symptoms would be so long that the average individual would not develop problems until old age. The synergistic effect of other agents could mean that substantial risk remains even with low level exposures. Because synergism may shorten latency periods, producing illness in the prime of life even at low exposure levels, the reduction of behavioral risks such as smoking is crucial.

Because of these factors, efforts aimed at primary prevention of chronic, noninfectious conditions such as heart disease must focus, for example, on maternal diet during pregnancy, diet of the child during early life, regular exercise, and education programs regarding the hazards of smoking. Although success cannot be guaranteed, prospects for success are greatest if intervention occurs early in life, before physiological risk factors such as obesity and elevated cholesterol levels are permitted to develop. Since these physiological states involve cellular changes that are steps in the development of disease, risk factor reduction is already secondary prevention.

CAUSALITY

A Statistical Approach to Causality

As commonly used, the term *cause* is understood to mean a stimulus that produces an effect or outcome. In epidemiology, cause deals with the production of an effect or outcome effected by a change in the host-agent-environment balance. A cause can be any of a large number of characteristics relating to time, place, person, or events. A health condition is likely to have multiple causes. Because an epidemiologist must rely on statistical measures of association to investigate and present causal relationships between a stimulus and an outcome, it is important to understand ways in which events or circumstances may be related in statistical terms. One *operational definition of cause* for such statistical investigations is a factor whose frequency varies with that of the health condition of interest. An increase or decrease in the amount or frequency of the causal factor produces a parallel increase or decrease in the frequency of the health condition.

Statistical Relationships. The first question to be addressed is "does a statistical relationship exist between two factors?" Stated another way, the first step in investigating statistical relationships between two factors or events is to determine whether any relationship (association) that does exist can be expected to occur by chance alone or whether the two factors occur together with a frequency greater than would be expected by chance. This is determined by applying one of a variety of statistical tests for independence or association, such as the chi-square test or a correlation coefficient. If such a test is statistically significant, then the two factors are not independent—they do have a statistical relationship that is not explained by chance alone.

A table presents rates of developing complications after mastectomy for women with and without anxious personalities. A chi-square test on these data is statistically significant at $p < 0.05$. This implies that at least 95 times out of 100, one would not expect to find such differences in complication rates between the two personality types by chance alone. Thus, the two factors—personality and complication rates—are not independent; they have a significant statistical association. The presence of a statistically significant association does not mean, however, that personality type causes complications. Determination of a statistically significant association is only the first step in assessing whether a relationship is causal. A strong statistical association between two factors or events, however, may suggest the possibility of a causal association.

Note that statistical associations are determined for categories or groups and not for individual instances. In the previous example, although groups of women with anxious personalities are more likely to have complications after mastectomy than are women not undergoing mastectomy, it is not possible to say that any individual with an anxious personality will have complications, although if the association is causal, an individual with an anxious personality will be more likely to have complications than an individual without.

Causal Relationships. Once it has been determined that two factors are not independent (ie, that they have a statistically significant association), the next step is to determine whether the relationship is causal. Statistically significant (nonindependent) factors may be causally or noncausally related. A *noncausal relationship* can be statistically significant because the hypothetical causal factor varies systematically with the actual causal variable. When uncontrolled, its effect cannot be distinguished from that of a causal variable with which it is highly correlated. Paternal age, for example, shows a statistically significant relationship with infant birth weight. This association occurs because paternal age is highly correlated with maternal age, the actual causal variable; most husbands and wives are close in age, so the two vary together. In this instance, it is difficult to derive any logical biological explanation for why a father's age should affect the birth weight of a child, so a researcher finding this association would suggest that it is not causal and would search for an explanation for the association. It is possible in the process of epidemiological investigation to identify such factors or variables through appropriate analysis. However, it is important for clinical practitioners to bear in mind when reading the epidemiological literature that in the early stages of epidemiological investigation of a problem, published reports may not yet have identified such non-causal relationships. Guidelines to facilitate the process of interpreting the epidemiological literature in regard to the validity of causal evidence are presented later in this chapter.

Causal relationships may be of two types: direct and indirect. It is important to distinguish between direct and indirect relationships to understand the natural history of a disease. *Direct causal associations* are those in which a factor causes a disease with no other factor intervening.

Causal factor → Outcome

An example of a direct cause would be the tubercule bacillus or any other infectious organism.

Tubercule bacillus → Tuberculosis

Apparent directness depends on the limitations of current knowledge; what is considered a direct association may be identified as indirect when information arising from further studies of a causal mechanism reveals a new, more direct cause for the association. An historical example is the association of certain water sources with the outbreaks of cholera observed by Dr. John Snow in England in 1853 (Snow, 1855). Subsequent intervention to ban the identified sources of water greatly reduced the incidence of cholera. We now know that it was not the water itself, but rather the cholera vibrio in the water that was the direct cause of the cholera epidemics.

For public health practitioners interested in reducing or eliminating onset of disease, the distinction between direct and indirect cause is often not crucial. The available information may be a sufficient basis for initiating intervention, as in the example of cholera where restricting access to the suspect water supplies controlled the spread of the disease. Because clinicians more often deal with patients having signs or symptoms of disease already present, for them the distinction is more crucial. Toxic shock syndrome (TSS) provides a useful example. A direct cause of this condition is suspected to be the staphylococcal organism. Tampons are an indirect (contributing) cause. Public health officials were able to intervene even before the staphylococcal organism was identified as the direct cause. Education programs were aimed at eliminating use of tampons or changing the way tampons were used to reduce the risk of developing toxic shock; specifically, it was suggested that women avoid super absorbent tampons, change tampons frequently using good hygienic practices, and avoid leaving tampons in overnight (Centers for Disease Control, 1980). Clinicians, however, needed to know that the organism was the cause of the symptoms to treat patients appropriately with antibiotics. Knowledge of the role of tampons, however, is also useful to clinicians who need to counsel toxic shock patients regarding the risks of resuming tampon use in order to prevent future episodes.

In *indirect causal associations,* a third variable, an intervening variable, occupies an intermediate stage between the cause and effect. If, in the model below, A is causally related to D (A is the cause and D the effect), but only through the interposition of one or several linked factors such as B and C, the association between A and D is one of an indirect causal relationship.

$$A \to B \to C \to D$$

One example of an indirect causal association is the relationship of cigarette smoke to chronic bronchitis. Breathing air polluted by cigarette or other smoke (A) causes damage to the respiratory epithelium (B); this damage increases the susceptibility of the epithelium to infection (C); which results in chronic bronchitis (D). In this example, knowledge about B and C is not essential to primary prevention of chronic bronchitis; eliminating the inhalation of cigarette smoke may greatly reduce the frequency of occurrence of chronic bronchitis. For purposes of secondary and tertiary prevention, however, understanding B and C is important. Awareness of the role of epithelial damage on the development of chronic bronchitis offers an opportunity to test for early epithelial changes in high-risk individuals. Although it may not be possible to reverse the damage, counseling these individuals as to their risk for bronchitis and the role smoking may play may at least encourage them to reduce their use of cigarettes. Furthermore, individuals with epithelial damage are more susceptible to infection. They should be advised to avoid close contact with individuals known to have acute respiratory infections and to seek early treatment to avoid further damage in the event that they develop an infection.

In the previous example of TSS, tampons are an indirect cause of the disease. The direct cause is staphylococcal organisms in the vagina. The tampons are a contributing cause in that they create an ideal environment for proliferation of the organism (Centers for Disease Control, 1980). From the standpoint of primary prevention, the disease could be prevented by eliminating tampon use or changing the way in which they are used. Theoretically, it could also be prevented by treating women who are vaginal carriers of staphylococcal organisms with antibiotics, but this is less practical because of the expense and difficulty of identifying carriers and the possibility that the organism will recur again after treatment. From the standpoint of treatment (tertiary prevention), however, knowing that *Staphylococcus* is the direct cause is useful because the physician can treat the disease with antibiotics to eliminate the source of the infection.

The Concept of Multiple Cause

Thus far, for simplicity of presentation, we have discussed causality as if each disease had a single cause, although this is certainly not the case. Historically, since early epidemiology focused on outbreaks of diseases with infectious origins, the idea of single cause was quite workable for control of the disease. Cholera outbreaks could be controlled by eliminating the source of the cholera vibrio. Diphtheria could be eliminated through vaccination programs. Scarlet fever could be kept from spreading by imposing a quarantine on all exposed individuals. These measures were effective because infectious agents were necessary to produce the disease. Therefore, elimination or isolation of the agent and elimination of host susceptibility through vaccination were effective measures.

With the advent of chronic diseases of noninfectious origin as major causes of morbidity and mortality, however, modern epidemiology has been forced to move from the single cause conceptualization of causality to one that recognizes the presence of multiple causes in any biological phenomenon, including infectious conditions. *Staphylococcus,* for instance, was identified as *the* cause of TSS because this organism must be present for the disease to occur. This does not mean that it will always cause a clinically recognizable disease. Circumstances do exist when an organism is present and no disease occurs. The host has to be susceptible to the organism; susceptibility reflects previous exposure to the organism, immune response, and so on. If the host is not susceptible, no disease occurs. The environment is also important because the likelihood of exposure to an organism may vary greatly in different geographical areas; if temperature and moisture conditions are not ideal for proliferation of an organism, exposure is less likely.

With diseases caused by noninfectious agents, the single cause model has limited usefulness because there is no single factor or agent that must be present to cause the disease. For example, even though smoking is recognized as a major cause of lung cancer, nonsmokers and individuals who have never been exposed to the cigarette smoke of others do get lung cancer. Clearly, there must be other substances that cause the disease. Nonsmokers exposed to asbestos may develop lung cancer. Furthermore, smokers who are exposed to substances such as asbestos are more likely to develop lung cancer than smokers not exposed to asbestos. Exposure to multiple causal factors may have an additive or multiplicative effect.

In a different example, automobile accidents may result from numerous factors, including speeding, faulty equipment, heavy traffic, poor visibility, driver inexperience, or drinking and driving. Any of these factors could cause an accident. All are amenable to intervention, as through public education, better engineering design, and better vehicle maintenance. Several of these factors together increase the risk of an accident. Such interrelationships between a multitude of factors, some known and some unknown, but all bearing ultimately on the cause of the disease, constitute the *web of causation.* It is, fortunately, not necessary to understand completely the intricacy of relationships between factors to institute adequate preventive measures.

Using our earlier definition of cause, numerous factors such as smoking, obesity, blood cholesterol level, and stress are causes of heart attack. The more of these factors present in an individual, the greater the risk of infarction. Because presence of these factors increases the risk for contracting a disease, we call them *risk factors.* Although we may not understand how these factors work or how they interact with each other, we can intervene and reduce the risk of heart attack by persuading individuals to give up smoking, lose weight, exercise regularly, or change their diet to reduce cholesterol.

Establishing Causality

Preliminary evidence of causality is provided through demonstration in multiple studies of statistical association between a factor and occurrence of a disease. The ultimate determination of the causality of an observed association is reached through an epidemiological experiment or a clinical trial. For factors whose presence appears to cause a disease, a factor is considered causal when reducing the amount or frequency of the suspected cause reduces the frequency of the effect, in this case, the illness of interest. If treating hypertensives to keep their blood pressure low reduces the frequency of stroke compared with the frequency of stroke in an equivalent, untreated group of hypertensives, hypertension would be considered a cause of stroke. Such experimental evidence of causality gives us an alternative *operational definition of a cause*. A factor is a cause when a reduction in the frequency of the factor produces a reduction in the frequency of occurrence of the related disease. In instances where the absence of a factor is associated with a higher frequency of disease and presence of the factor is associated with a lower frequency of disease, causality can be established by conducting a randomized clinical trial. A recent example of this was a series of trials conducted to confirm the protective role of beta-carotene in preventing lung cancer. An extensive epidemiological literature review as well as *in vivo* and *in vitro* laboratory studies and experiments with animals suggested a causal role for beta-carotene (an antioxidant) in preventing cancer occurrence. Three randomized clinical trials were conducted, two with high-risk populations and one with male physicians. The latter found no benefit while the first two indicated possible harm in the form of increased rates of lung cancer resulting from administration of beta-carotene (The Alpha-tocopherol, Beta-carotene Cancer Prevention Study Group, 1994; Omenn et al, 1996; Hennekens et al, 1996).

Criteria for Evaluating Causality in the Literature

Studies reported in the literature may show conflicting results. An epidemiological experiment is not always feasible or desirable. In these instances, criteria based on available epidemiological data are needed for making decisions regarding intervention. Five criteria often accepted for assessing causality in such instances were used in the 1964 Surgeon General's Report (U.S. Department of Health, Education, and Welfare, 1964) for assessing the causal relationship between smoking and a variety of health outcomes. The five criteria are: (1) correctness of temporality; (2) strength of the association; (3) specificity of the association; (4) consistency of the association; and (5) biological plausibility.

Correctness of temporality requires evidence that exposure to the causal factor did, in fact, occur before initiation of the disease process. For diseases such as cancer, definitive proof that the exposure occurred before the first cell transformations may be difficult to obtain because there is a long period of latency during which cell replication and growth continues. This period may be as long as 20 to 40 years after the initial exposure to a causal agent before the tumor is diagnosed. Suppose someone with lung cancer has been smoking for 10 years. Did smoking initiate the disease process or did it speed up growth of a tumor that was already initiated by another agent? The answer cannot be definitely established, but it is much more likely that smoking is causal if a patient smoked for 10 years before diagnosis than if the patient smoked for only 18 months. Clearly, however, if it can be shown that exposure did not occur before the disease, the relationship cannot be causal despite a strong statistical association.

Strength of the association is usually measured by a statistic called the *relative risk ratio* or alternatively, the *odds ratio*. In general, the larger the ratio, the stronger the association and the greater the likelihood that the association is causal. Another aspect of strength of the association is *dose effect*. The strength of association should be stronger at higher doses, or levels of exposure, than at lower doses or levels.

Specificity of the association refers to the uniqueness of the relationship between the putative causal factor and the disease occurrence. The terms *necessary* and *sufficient* can be used to clarify this concept. If the disease can occur without the presence of a particular agent, the agent is not necessary. Lung cancer can occur in nonsmokers; TSS, however, cannot occur without exposure to *Staphylococcus*. Sufficient refers to whether the agent is always able to produce the outcome. Although asbestos fibers are necessary to produce asbestosis, the fibers may not be sufficient; it is possible to be exposed to asbestos and not develop asbestosis. Prolonged exposure to flame is always sufficient to produce a burn, although severity may vary. Fire is not necessary to produce a burn, however, because burns may result from chemical exposures as well. A highly specific, therefore unique, association exists when an agent is both necessary for disease occurrence and sufficient, by itself, to produce the disease. Such a specific relationship would be definitively causal. The closer an agent comes to meeting these criteria, the greater the likelihood of causality. As discussed in the next chapter, however, meeting both the necessary and sufficient criteria simultaneously is incompatible with the concept of multiple causes.

Consistency of the association refers to the findings of various epidemiological studies. There may be conflicting results among reported studies on the association of a specific agent with a specific disease. Some studies may find no association, others an inverse (negative) association. Still others may find a positive association. The strength of the association may vary widely in the studies reporting a positive association. Barring major flaws in study designs, consistent findings of a positive association would be expected if the association is causal.

Biological plausibility, sometimes called *coherence,* implies the presence of a reasonable biological mechanism to explain the physiological process by which an agent could produce the specific disease of interest. Documentation of biological plausibility is dependent on other scientific disciplines such as physiology, microbiology, toxicology, and pharmacology. Causality demands a reasonable biological explanation for the observed association. Exposure of laboratory animals to an agent should, if an appropriate animal system is used, produce effects similar to those seen in humans.

REFERENCES

The Alpha-tocopherol, Beta-carotene (ATBC) Cancer Prevention Study Group. (1994) The effect of vitamin E and beta-carotene on the incidence of lung cancer and other cancers in male smokers. *New England Journal of Medicine, 330,* 1029–1035.

Benenson A. S. (Ed.). (1990) *Control of communicable disease in man* (14th ed.). New York: American Public Health Association.

Centers for Disease Control. (1980) Follow-up on toxic shock syndrome. *Morbidity and Mortality Weekly Reports, 29*(37), 441–445.

Elias E. G., Brown S. D., Buda B. S., Honts S. L. (1994) Breast cancer prevention trial. *Maryland Medical Journal, 43*(3), 249–252.

Hennekens C. H., Buring J. E., Manson J. E., et al. (1996) Lack of effect of long-term supplementation with beta-carotene on the incidence of malignant neoplasms and cardiovascular disease. *New England Journal of Medicine, 334*, 1145–1149.

Kleinfeld M., Messite J., Koozman O. (1967) Mortality experience in a group of asbestos workers. *Archives of Environmental Health, 15*, 176–180.

Lerman C., Biesecker B., Benkendorf J., Kerner J., et al. (1997) Controlled trial of pretest educational approaches to enhance informed decision-making for BRCA1 gene testing. *Journal of the National Cancer Institute, 89*(2), 148–157.

Nayfield S. G. (1995) Tamoxifen's role in chemoprevention of breast cancer: An update. *Journal of Cellular Biochemistry* (suppl.), *22*, 42–50.

Omenn G. S., Goodman G. E., Thornquist M. D., et al. (1996) Effects of a combination of beta-carotene and vitamin A on lung cancer and cardiovascular disease. *New England Journal of Medicine, 334*, 1150–1155.

Roussouw J. E., Finnegan L. P., Harlan W. R., Pinn V. W., Clifford C., McGowan J. A. (1995) The evolution of the Women's Health Initiative: Perspectives from the NIH. *Journal of the American Medical Women's Association, 50*(2), 50–55.

Snow J. (1855) *On the mode of communication of cholera* (2nd ed.). London: Churchill. (Reprinted in *Snow on cholera.* (1936) New York: Commonwealth Fund.)

U.S. Department of Health, Education, and Welfare. (1964) *Smoking and health: Report of the Advisory Committee to the Surgeon General of the Public Health Service* (PHS Publication No. 1103). Washington, D.C.: U.S. Government Printing Office.

3

Rates: A Basic Epidemiological Tool

*i*n order to study patterns of illness and response to intervention, epidemiologists must quantitatively measure risk factors, states of health, and a variety of possible outcomes. Quantitative measures in the form of rates provide indices of health that permit comparison of frequency between different populations, across time, or among individuals with and without particular exposures or risk characteristics. Some rates have primary use in public health monitoring, planning, and evaluation. Other rates are particularly useful for hypothesis generation and testing. This chapter presents the conceptual basis of rates and ennumerates the rates most commonly used as indices of community health, for epidemiological and clinical investigation, and to assess functional status and quality of life. The sources of data used to generate these rates are presented in Chapter 4.

RATES AS MEASURES OF EVENTS

Concept of Rates

In epidemiology, a count or frequency of health events is of limited interest by itself. However, when frequency is used as the numerator of a fraction that expresses a proportion with specification of a relevant time frame, it is of great value and is called a *rate*. The reporting, for example, of three cases of infectious hepatitis without indicating if they occurred among 1,000 students in a school (3/1000 = 0.3%) or among 20 in a dormitory (3/20 = 15%) is of little practical value to the epidemiologist or a public health practitioner, except for the fact that the number of cases of this disease may be useful to estimate the need for additional medical services. The rates, however, can be compared with rates for other times or places to assess trends and identify excesses of disease occurrence or to evaluate progress in control efforts. For example, public health officials have observed that the rates of lung cancer deaths among women have been increasing rapidly since 1965. By 1986 lung cancer overtook breast cancer as the leading cause of cancer mortality for women (Ernster, 1996). It has also been observed that smokers who use oral contraceptives have higher rates of death from heart disease than nonsmokers who use oral contraceptives (Brezinska, 1994). In an attempt to reduce these preventable deaths, public health officials have instituted anti-smoking campaigns primarily directed at young women of reproductive age.

In another example, high rates of measles were observed among high school students by school nurses in Cook County, Illinois, in 1976. Measles are unusual among this age group, as highest rates normally occur among primary school children. When these cases of high school measles were reported to the county health department, an investigation was begun. After investigating the exposure and immunization histories of these cases, it was discovered that they were among the earliest groups vaccinated after the measles vaccine first became available. The students had been vaccinated before reaching 6 months of age. Because residual maternal antibody was still present in their blood, the vaccination did not stimulate active antibody production as intended. Thus, when maternal immunity waned, these persons were susceptible to the disease. As a result, such susceptible individuals were actively sought by county officials so they could be revaccinated before a new epidemic occurred (Kuter, 1978).

Both the increase in rates of lung cancer mortality in women and the increase in rates of measles among the students in Cook County represent epidemics. *Epidemics* are defined as rates of disease significantly higher than the usual frequency. The usual frequency represents the *endemic* level. A third term, *pandemic*, is used to describe epidemics that include large areas of the world—a worldwide epidemic. Figure 3–1 illustrates the endemic fluctuation of rates. The peak in September 1995 represents an epidemic because it is clearly in excess of normal rates.

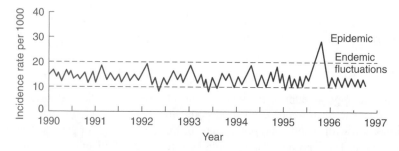

Figure 3–1. Schematic representation of endemic and epidemic rates.

Rates are expressed by a numerator, a denominator, and by specification of person, place, and time. The numerator and denominator of rates may be *general* or *specific*. General rates refer to rates that include the total population, whereas specific rates apply only to the population subgroup specified (eg, all women, children younger than 17 years of age, or black men). Both numerator and denominator have to be similarly restricted by population characteristics (age, sex, and race), place, and time. When the denominator refers to a population that includes the numerator, the relative frequency is expressed as a *rate*. Stated another way, the events represented in the numerator arise from the population at risk in the denominator. For example,

$$\frac{\text{No. of new cases of ovarian cancer in Cincinnati, Ohio, 1997}}{\text{No. of women in Cincinnati, Ohio, 1997}} \times 100,000$$

Because ovarian cancer can only occur among women, only women are included in the denominator. The women in both the numerator and denominator are those living in Cincinnati, Ohio, in 1997. The resulting rate is generally multiplied by some constant value, usually 100,000, so that rates for populations of different sizes can be compared.

By contrast, although any fraction is encompassed by the general term *ratio*, in common usage ratio refers to a fraction where the numerator is not included in the denominator. The annual *fetal death rate* is the number of fetal deaths in a year related to the total number of annual births plus fetal deaths. The annual *fetal death ratio* is the number of fetal deaths in a year in relation to the total number of live births only. In this instance the denominator does not include both the total population of affected and unaffected persons (live births and fetal deaths), but includes only the unaffected. A commonly used ratio is the sex ratio. The numerator is the number of men in a population; the denominator is the number of women in the population.

TYPES OF RATES

The rates most frequently used as indices of community health are listed in Table 3–1. Each of the rates is discussed below.

Death Rates (Mortality Rates)

Mortality rates may be *crude*, pertaining to the total population, or *specific*, pertaining to a population or disease subgroup. The numerator of mortality rates includes all deaths that occurred in the population during a defined period of time, usually 1 year. Because data on mortality are routinely collected by public agencies, these rates are readily available and collected in a standardized way, making them useful both for public health monitoring of populations and for large epidemiological studies investigating risk factors.

Studies of treatment efficacy, which compare the outcomes for several treatments and clinical studies to determine how patients fare, often focus on specified populations of persons with the disease of interest. A commonly used rate for such

TABLE 3–1. RATES MOST FREQUENTLY USED AS INDICES OF COMMUNITY HEALTH

RATES	USUAL POPULATION FACTOR
General Mortality Rates	
Crude death rate $= \dfrac{\text{No. deaths in a year}}{\text{Average (midyear) population}}$	rate per 100,000 population
Cause-specific death rate $= \dfrac{\text{No. deaths in a year}}{\text{Average (midyear) population}}$	rate per 100,000 population
Age-specific death rate $= \dfrac{\text{No. deaths among persons in given age group in a year}}{\text{Average (midyear) population in specified age group}}$	rate per 100,000 population
Proportional mortality rate $= \dfrac{\text{No. deaths from specific cause in specified time period}}{\text{Total deaths in same time period}}$	
Case fatality rate $= \dfrac{\text{No. deaths due to specified disease}}{\text{No. cases of specified disease}}$	% of deaths per 100 cases
Survival rate $= \dfrac{\text{No. cases alive at end of a specified time period}}{\text{No. cases alive at start of period}}$	% alive per 100 cases
Rates Assessing Morbidity	
Incidence $= \dfrac{\text{No. of new cases of disease in place, from time 1 to time 2}}{\text{No. persons in place, midpoint of time period}}$	rate per 100,000 population
Point prevalence $= \dfrac{\text{No. of existing cases in place, at time}}{\text{No. persons in place, at time}}$	rate per 100,000 population
Maternal and Infant Rates	
Maternal (puerperal) mortality rate $= \dfrac{\text{No. deaths from puerperal causes in a year}}{\text{No. of live births in same year}}$	rate per 100,000 live births
Infant mortality rate $= \dfrac{\text{No. infant deaths during year}}{\text{No. of live births in same year}}$	per 1,000 live births
Neonatal mortality rate $= \dfrac{\text{No. deaths in a year of children younger than 28 days of age}}{\text{No. of live births in same year}}$	per 1,000 live births
Fetal death rate $= \dfrac{\text{No. fetal deaths during year}}{\text{No. of live births and fetal deaths in same year}}$	per 1,000 live births and fetal deaths
Perinatal mortality rate $= \dfrac{\text{No. fetal deaths 28 weeks or more and infant deaths younger than 7 days of age during year}}{\text{No. of live births and fetal deaths 28 weeks or more gestation in same year}}$	per 1,000 live births and fetal deaths > 28 weeks gestation

studies and for monitoring virulence of infectious disease agents in epidemic outbreaks, is the *case fatality rate*. This rate uses all cases under study as the denominator and those individuals among these cases who die as the numerator. The rate is expressed as a percentage of all cases. In many efficacy studies, researchers are more interested in those who survive than in those who die and, thus, use survival rates. *Survival rates* usually focus on relatively small groups of cases and are calculated using the number of cases of the disease in the study group as the denominator and the number surviving to a particular point in time as the numerator. Although survival rates are usually specific to a particular population of cases under study, they may be calculated separately for age or gender subgroups. Both case fatality rates and survival rates are shown in Table 3–1.

Crude Versus Specific Rates.   *Crude rates* provide one measure for the experience of the entire population. Crude rates may include in the numerator all deaths from all causes (ie, crude mortality rate for deaths in Ohio in 1997), or deaths due to a single disease or condition (ie, the crude mortality rate for pneumonia shown below, which includes only deaths from pneumonia). This crude rate of deaths from pneumonia, for example, includes deaths among men and women and deaths among young and old. The denominator remains general for both, encompassing the entire population.

$$\frac{\text{No. of deaths from pneumonia in Cincinnati, Ohio, 1997}}{\text{No. of persons in Cincinnati, Ohio, 1997}} \times 100,000$$

Specific rates allow us to assess the experience of subgroups of a population. Sex-specific rates for pneumonia mortality, for example, give us one rate for women and another for men, calculated as:

$$\frac{\text{No. of men who died from pneumonia in Cincinnati, Ohio, 1997}}{\text{No. of men in total population of Cincinnati, Ohio, 1997}} \times 100,000$$

If a similar rate is calculated for women, we can compare the rate for men with that of women. A similar procedure for specific age groups would allow us to compare the experience of younger persons with that of older persons. In this example, were we to look at actual age-specific rates, we would see that the rate of mortality from pneumonia is highest among the elderly.

Crude rates, which provide one rate for the experience of a total population and specific rates for large groups (eg, all men and all women), can present a problem if we wish to compare the population experience of one location with that of another because the distribution of characteristics within the population may vary. For example, suppose we wanted to compare population A and population B. As seen in Table 3–2, the age-specific rates of cardiovascular disease are the same in the two populations (see column 4). The crude rates (column 6) would lead us to believe that the experience of these populations is quite different. This occurs because population B has a large percentage of its members in the older age groups, in which rates of heart disease mortality are high, whereas population A has a heavier concentration of members in the younger age groups, in which rates of heart disease mortality are low. We might observe such a situation when comparing a state with a young population such as Alaska with a state such as Florida, which has a substantial elderly population.

Standardized Rates.   A *"standardized"* or *age-adjusted* rate can be calculated to adjust for differences in age distribution of populations so that comparisons are interpretable. Essentially, age-adjusted rates allow one to answer the question, "Suppose

TABLE 3–2. COMPARISON OF DEATH RATES IN TWO POPULATIONS BY AGE-SPECIFIC RATES, CRUDE RATES, AND ADJUSTED RATES

| AGE (YEARS) | POPULATION NO. | % | ANNUAL AGE-SPECIFIC DEATH RATE (PER 1000) | ANNUAL NO. OF DEATHS | CRUDE DEATH RATE (PER 1000) | ADJUSTED RATE FOR B; A AS STANDARD POPULATION AGE-SPECIFIC RATES | | ADJUSTED RATE FOR A; B AS STANDARD POPULATION AGE-SPECIFIC RATES | |
						$\frac{\text{Pop. B}}{1000} \times$ Pop. A = Expected No. Deaths	Adjusted Rate	$\frac{\text{Pop. A}}{1000} \times$ Pop. B = Expected No. Deaths	Adjusted Rate
Population A									
<25	4000	40	2.0	8				$2.0 \times 1500 = 3$	
25–44	3000	30	4.0	12				$4.0 \times 3500 = 14$	
45–64	2000	20	50.0	100				$50.0 \times 4000 = 200$	
65+	1000	10	100.0	100				$100.0 \times 1000 = 100$	
All ages	10,000	100		220	$\frac{220}{10,000} = 22.0$			317	$\frac{317}{10,000} = 31.7$
Population B									
<25	1500	15	2.0	3		$2.0 \times 4000 = 8$			
25–44	3500	35	4.0	14		$4.0 \times 3000 = 12$			
45–64	4000	40	50.0	200		$50.0 \times 2000 = 100$			
65+	1000	10	100.0	100		$100.0 \times 1000 = 100$			
All Ages	10,000	100		317	$\frac{317}{10,000} = 31.7$	220	$\frac{220}{10,000} = 22.0$		

(From Valanis B. The epidemiological model and community health nursing. In M. Stanhope & J. Lancaster [Eds.]. Community health nursing: Process and practice for promoting health. St. Louis: C. V. Mosby, 1984.)

these populations have the same age distribution, how would their overall experience with this disease compare?" Calculation of these rates uses two pieces of basic information: (1) the actual age-specific rates for each population being compared and (2) a population distribution to which the specific rates are applied. The absolute number obtained will differ depending on the population distribution used. This number, although "fictitious" because of how it is calculated, nonetheless represents a valid way to compare the experiences of these two populations because it is not the absolute level but the relative position that is important. Therefore, it does not matter which population is chosen as the standard. For example, in Table 3–2, if we use the population distribution of population A in calculating the standardized rate for B, we obtain a rate of 22 for population B. Because the age-specific rates for the two populations are the same, this adjusted rate is the same as the crude rate for population A. If the distribution of population B is used for the calculation, we obtain a standardized rate of 31.7 for population A, the same as the crude rate of B. In both cases, we learn that population A and population B have the same rate of heart disease. It should be remembered that these numbers are meaningful only as comparison and mean nothing alone. This leads us to the same conclusion we would have drawn by examining the age-specific rates: these two populations have the same experience for heart disease mortality. You may ask, "Why not just compare the age-specific rates rather than going to so much trouble?" This is a reasonable approach if you are trying to compare only two or three populations. However, if your aim is to compare rates for each of the 50 states, or among 20 neighborhoods in a city, or for 50 different years, you might find the task of making sense of so many age-specific rates overwhelming. Use of a single standardized rate to represent the experience of each unit (state, neighborhood, year) makes the task manageable. In addition to standardization for age, rates can be standardized for differences in racial distribution, gender distribution, and for other characteristics associated with differences in specific rates that are distributed differently in the populations being compared.

Figure 3–2 illustrates the crude and age-adjusted death rates for the United States from 1940 to 1992. Since the average age in the United States has increased over the past 50 years as a result of increasing life spans and a declining birth rate and most of the major causes of death are the chronic degenerative diseases most common among older persons, it is not surprising that the crude death rate for the years 1940 to 1992 does not show a substantial decline. Use of an age-adjusted rate, however, controls for the effect of the increasing age of the population. The age-adjusted rate in Figure 3–2, in sharp contrast to the crude rate, shows the dramatic decline in the death rate during this 52-year period.

Proportional Rates.   Another kind of mortality rate compares the number of deaths from a particular illness, such as cancer, with deaths from all other causes. Such a rate, called a *proportional mortality rate,* is calculated as:

$$\frac{\text{No. of cancer deaths in place in year}}{\text{No. of total deaths from all causes in place, in year}} \times 100 = \begin{array}{c}\text{Percentage of}\\\text{deaths due}\\\text{to cancer}\end{array}$$

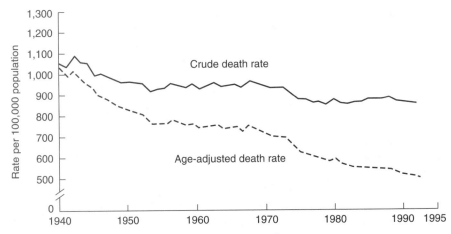

NOTE: Crude death rates on an annual basis per 100,000 population; age-adjusted rates per 100,000 U.S. standard million population.

Figure 3–2. Crude and age-adjusted death rates: United States, 1940–1992. (*Adapted from National Center for Health Statistics, Monthly Vital Statistics Report, 1995; 43[No.6–S].*)

This rate then tells us what percentage of all deaths are due to cancer. Other proportional mortality rates can be derived. If one were interested in what percentage of all cancer deaths are due to breast cancer, the numerator would be the number of breast cancer deaths and the denominator would be the total number of deaths from cancer. In either instance, if the numerator is specific for certain age, sex, or race groups, the denominator has to be likewise restricted to these same groups. For instance, to calculate the proportional mortality rate for coronary heart disease in U.S. white men older than 50 years of age in relation to all deaths from coronary heart disease, the numerator would include all deaths in this restricted group of the general population for a given year; the denominator would be all deaths from coronary heart disease in this segment of the population in that year:

$$\frac{\text{No. of coronary heart disease deaths in U.S. white men over 50 years of age in 1997}}{\text{No. of coronary heart disease deaths in U.S. in 1997}} \times 100$$

Life Expectancy

Life insurance companies commonly use a measure called *life expectancy,* the average number of years an individual is expected to live, in determining their rates. This measure is also used in comparing the health status of international populations. For this latter purpose, life expectancy is generally based on expectation of life at birth; how many years the average individual is expected to live from the time of birth onward. However, expectation of life can be calculated for any age. Life expectancy at age 45, for example, would represent how many more years someone who had reached age 45 could expect to live, on average. Insurance companies use an individual's current age. Life expectancy data for various ethnic and gender subgroups of the U.S. population are shown in Chapter 5.

Maternal and Infant Rates

Some special rates are used in monitoring events useful in determining the health status of mothers and infants. The rate most often used to monitor maternal mortality is the *puerperal mortality rate.* As shown in Table 3–1, this rate is calculated by dividing the number of deaths from pregnancy-related causes (numerator) by the number of live births in the same year. Although really a ratio, rather than a rate because the denominator is not strictly the number of women potentially exposed to death from pregnancy, this ratio is used as a rate; it is much easier to obtain the number of live births than the number of pregnancies, since some pregnancies result in spontaneous miscarriage and do not get recorded.

Infant health is monitored by use of a number of different rates, shown in Table 3–1. Because different adverse events are common at different times during a pregnancy and require specific intervention at a time appropriate to the occurrence of the event, use of rates specific to each stage of fetal and infant development help public health officials to detect changes specific to these stages and to take appropriate action. Therefore, the fetal death rate is useful for detecting events that occur during pregnancy and affect fetal viability. The perinatal period, the last months of pregnancy and the first 7 days after birth are particularly susceptible to factors relating to infant status, for example, effects of a congenital malformation. Thus, mortality during this period is calculated separately from mortality during the first 28 days of life, the neonatal period, resulting in two separate rates: the *perinatal mortality rate* and the *neonatal mortality rate.* Factors such as the trauma of delivery and low birth weight in particular may affect survival during the neonatal period. The *infant mortality rate* is used to reflect the mortality experience of infants throughout their first year of life. Chapter 8 shows these rates over time and in different populations in the United States.

Other rates that reflect maternal and child health include rates of congenital malformations, low birth weight, illegitimacy, proportion of mothers receiving prenatal care, and immunization rates.

Morbidity Rates

The two most commonly used morbidity rates are *incidence* and *prevalence.* Incidence rates provide a picture of new disease occurrence over time, whereas prevalence rates provide a snapshot of all cases present at a point in time. Incidence provides a measure of risk and is useful in etiological studies. Prevalence is a useful measure for assessing current needs for health services. Other methods are used to measure the impact of disease on function and quality of life. These measures of disability are also discussed here.

Incidence Measures.   *Incidence rates* are a measure of all new cases arising in a population at risk during a defined period of time, usually 1 year.

$$\text{Incidence} = \frac{\text{No. of new cases in place during time of observation}}{\text{Population in place at midpoint of time}} \times K$$

For the incidence rate shown above, the denominator uses the population size at the midpoint of the time period. This incidence rate, called a *cumulative incidence*, is the one commonly used for large general population estimates. As with rates discussed earlier, multiplication by a constant, K, facilitates comparing rates.

Other measures of incidence, such as *incidence density*, are modifications of the cumulative incidence rate. Incidence density is a measure often used in cohort studies in which a defined group of persons is followed over time. To account for those who die, are lost to follow up, or have contracted the disease and are therefore not at risk for the whole time period of the study, a measure called *person-years* is used as the denominator of these incidence rates. A person-year represents one person at risk for 1 year. The numerator of the rate is the total number of cases accumulated over the study period.

$$\text{Incidence density} = \frac{\text{Total new cases accumulated during study period}}{\text{Person-years accumulated by study subjects}} \times K$$

This rate, yielded by dividing the numerator by the denominator, can subsequently be divided by the number of followup years to determine an average incidence density.

Incidence represents a measure of the risk for developing a particular disease. Thus, incidence rates are useful in studies of disease etiology. A measure called the *relative risk ratio* is used to compare the risks of developing a disease among a group exposed and one not exposed to a presumptive etiological agent by comparing incidence rates for those exposed to a putative etiological agent with incidence rates for those not exposed.

$$\text{Relative risk ratio} = \frac{\text{Incidence rate in exposed group}}{\text{Incidence rate in nonexposed group}}$$

A relative risk of 1.0 means that the risk is the same for both groups. A risk greater than 1.0 indicates excess risk in the exposed group. Statistical tests and confidence intervals are used to determine whether any increase in risk is greater than would be expected by chance alone. These rates are discussed further in Chapter 4.

Incidence rates are useful for monitoring the occurrence of a disease in defined populations over time. Incidence rates are preferable to mortality rates for this purpose because incidence reflects only diagnosed occurrence of the disease and not additional factors reflected by mortality rates, such as improvements in treatment leading to improved survival. Such monitoring of disease can alert public health personnel to the presence of new hazards in the environment. A sudden increase in a particular congenital malformation, for example, could indicate an environmental hazard that was recently introduced to that geographic area.

Special incidence rates, called *attack rates*, are frequently used in surveillance and control of infectious diseases. Attack rates are calculated when an identifiable population has been exposed to an infectious agent; the rate represents the incidence of illness among that exposed population. An example of this is the incidence of hepatitis B in a classroom of children exposed to a contagious classmate at a day-care center. Changes in attack rates across episodes of the disease over time may indicate a change in the immune status of a population, as with the Cook County measles epidemic discussed earlier, or may be an indication of a more virile strain of organism. These rates are explored further in Chapter 6 which discusses diseases of infectious origin.

Prevalence Measures.   *Prevalence rates* are a measure of the existing number of cases present in a population at a given time. Prevalence rates are expressed as a rate per unit of population, eg, per 100,000. They are particularly useful for diseases of a chronic nature that will require care over a long period of time.

$$\text{Point prevalence} = \frac{\text{No. of existing cases in place at point in time}}{\text{No. of persons in place at midpoint of year}} \times K$$

To evaluate adequacy of existing services and to plan for future needs, public health officials require a measure of the caseload requiring care. Prevalence serves not only as a measure of current caseload; future prevalence can be projected by using incidence, recovery, and mortality rates to estimate changes in prevalence over time as prevalence rates are a function of incidence as well as the duration of the disease. A disease that is chronic in nature and that has low rates of mortality tends to increase the number of persons with the disease in the population if incidence remains the same. Death and recovery are the two most common factors that reduce the case load requiring care. A less common factor is substantial outmigration of individuals from the community.

When unspecified, prevalence usually refers to *point prevalence*. The numerator in a point prevalence rate can be likened to a snapshot of cases present when the picture is taken. The numerator of incidence rates, in contrast, is like a movie of cases taken over a period of time.

A second type of prevalence rate is *period prevalence*. This rate is constructed from prevalence at a point in time, plus incidence cases and recurrences during a succeeding time period (eg, 1 year).

$$\text{Point prevalence} = \frac{\substack{\text{No. of existing cases in place at beginning of period} \\ \text{+ new cases + recurrences during period}}}{\text{Average population of place during period}} \times K$$

This rate is most useful for diseases that are episodic and for which exact date of onset is difficult to determine. It has been used most frequently in the mental health field. A variation of period prevalence, *lifetime prevalence,* is a measure of what proportion of a population has *ever* had a particular disease. This measure is also used primarily in psychiatric epidemiology.

Relation between Incidence and Prevalence.   Prevalence and incidence rates often give very different pictures of the disease status of a population. If two diseases have the same incidence rate but one of these is a chronic disease and the other an acute condition, they will have quite different prevalence rates. Assuming low case fatality rates for both, the chronic disease will show a high rate of prevalence, whereas the acute condition will show a low rate of prevalence because people recover and do not remain prevalent cases. In terms of provision of health services, the initial number of patients requiring treatment (reflected by the incidence rate) is the same for the two conditions. Need for long-term followup services (reflected by the prevalence rate) is quite different.

Measures of Functional Status.   The rates described thus far tell us little about function or quality of life. Because life expectancy has increased dramatically during the 20th century, measures that reflect the impact of disease on survivors become crucial in planning services (Rice, 1992). As resources for health care services become less available and because it is possible with new technology to keep persons alive to older ages, both patients and health care professionals need information on probable functional capability and quality of life for use in decisions about whether to administer life-saving treatments. Level of function is measured in several ways. Insurance companies focus primarily on disability, defined as the inability to engage in gainful employment. However, health officials conceptualize *disability* as any temporary or long-term reduction in a person's activity as a result of acute or chronic illness. The three indices most commonly used by the federal goverment, resulting from the National Health Survey, are *restricted activity days,* days on which a person must cut down on their usual activity for the whole day because of an illness or injury; *work-loss days,* days when a person loses an entire day of work because of illness or injury; and *bed-disability days,* days on which a person spends all or most of the day in bed. Activities of daily living are used as measure of function. Proportion of individuals living alone, proportion in nursing homes or other institutions, and doctors' office visits are also rates used by public health officials in determining population health status. Data on these measures are presented for each life stage in Chapters 8 through 11.

Measures of Risk Factors.   While epidemiological studies often have to devise instruments to measure specific risk factors, there are some measures of risk gathered by the government to measure levels of risk in the overall population. These are usually gathered through surveys. Included among these are measures of drug and alcohol use, smoking, sexual activity, and nutrition. Other indices come from data summarized from records of govenmental agencies, for example, rates of marriage and divorce, unemployment, and crime. Other factors that contribute to health and disease for which measures are also available include housing and income.

REFERENCES

Brezinka V., Padmos I. (1994) Coronary heart disease risk factors in women. *European Heart Journal, 15*(11), 1571–1584.

Ernster V. L. (1976) Female lung cancer. *Annual Review of Public Health, 17*, 97–114.

Kuter B. (1978) *An epidemiologic investigation of a measles epidemic in Cook County, Illinois.* Masters thesis: Columbia University.

Rice D. P. (1992) Data needs for health policy in an aging population (including a survey of data available in the United States of America). *World Health Statistics Quarterly, 45,* 61–67.

4

Epidemiological Methods

*e*pidemiological knowledge evolves from an orderly, sequential process of research beginning with descriptive research, moving to analytical studies, and finally to experimental studies. A few study designs comprise the basis for most epidemiologic analytical studies. Each design has its own particular strengths and weaknesses. Certain methodological issues such as reliability and validity of measurement are pertinent to all designs. This chapter first provides an overview of the process of epidemiological investigation, then presents major study designs, discusses their strengths and weaknesses, and raises general methodological issues related to evaluating the quality of a study. The final section of the chapter discusses basic statistical issues and approaches relevant to epidemiological research.

SEQUENCE OF EPIDEMIOLOGICAL INVESTIGATION

Epidemiological investigations generally proceed in an orderly fashion, beginning with the observation and recording of existing patterns of occurrence for the disease or state of health under study. These observations, recorded as disease rates, are compared for various categories of person, place, and time characteristics. From these recorded observations, one generates a description of which specific characteristics are associated with high versus low frequency of disease occurrence. This first phase of investigation, called *descriptive epidemiology*, suggests hypotheses concerning etiology (causal process).

Description

To illustrate this sequence, suppose that investigators are interested in trying to learn what causes breast cancer. The first step is to obtain the rates of breast cancer for groups of people with different characteristics, in different geographic locations, and at various points in time. Although epidemiologists would prefer to have the rates of newly occurring cases, *incidence rates*, these are not generally available without a special survey or a source of regularly recorded cases such as a disease registry. Therefore, *mortality rates*, the rates of death from the disease, are generally used in early stages of such an investigation. When rates of breast cancer mortality are examined, it is observed that breast cancer is rare among men, and more frequent among whites than nonwhites, among single women than married women, and among those in higher socioeconomic groups than those in lower socioeconomic groups. Breast cancer occurs with increasing frequency in successively older age groups and shows a decreasing frequency as the number of liveborn children increases and as age at first full-term pregnancy decreases. It is also more common among women with early menarche and later menopause. Rates of breast cancer mortality also vary by geographic area. Rates are higher in developed, Western nations than in less developed nations. Rates are lowest in Asian countries such as Japan. Breast cancer mortality was increasing steadily in the early 1900s, but these rates have leveled off during the past 50 years or so, reflecting improvements in early detection and treatment. Now, there is little change in incidence rates for whites, but there continues to be a rise for nonwhites. Such information constitutes an epidemiological description of breast cancer.

Testing Relationships

Hypotheses suggested by the descriptive epidemiology of a condition are tested in the second investigative phase, *analytical epidemiology*. The description of variations in the occurrence of breast cancer described above might suggest looking into the role of hormonal status, because of the association with pregnancy history, the length of active menstruation, and aging. The differences by geographic area and a nation's industrialization status raise questions worth investigating regarding what is different about places with high rates versus low. Is the diet different? What about reproductive patterns?

The observed association of a suspected causal factor with occurrence of a particular disease may be due to other factors, such as *confounding variables*, factors that cause change in the frequency of disease and vary systematically with the hypothetical cause being studied. For example, a study investigating differences in diet between countries with high breast cancer rates compared with countries with low rates might need to control for socioeconomic status or reproductive patterns, since these may differ as well among the countries. When uncontrolled, the effects of confounding variables cannot be distinguished from those of the hypothetical causal variable. Confounding variables may be identified at a later stage of investigation. Suppose that a researcher noted that rates of spontaneous abortion increased with the number of pregnancies. Having more babies might not be the causative factor. The number of pregnancies is related to age of the mother. If physiological aging leads to a decreased capacity for carrying a pregnancy to term, then age would be confounding the original association between parity and spontaneous abortion rates. When the effect is not controlled, parity may appear to be a causal factor. Once age of the mother is controlled, the apparent association with parity may disappear. In this example, parity is noncausally related to risk of spontaneous abortion. Because of this problem, multiple analytical studies of the same hypotheses are usually required to sort out these relationships.

Ecological Versus Relational Analytical Studies.   Analytical studies may be done on either an ecological level or a relational level. *Ecological studies* compare large aggregates of people, usually of a defined geographic area, with another such large population. Ecological studies are generally based on aggregate data collected for other purposes. Data routinely collected by official agencies on water quality or air quality of a particular locality, for example, may be used as a measure of the level of exposure of a population to particular pollutants. These data are then examined in relation to rates of the disease of interest (usually mortality rates) for the resident population of that same locality. For example, cancer rates may be compared for the population of towns with polluted drinking water and towns with pure drinking water to assess whether water pollution is associated with elevated rates of cancer. Per capita data on fat consumption may be compared for countries with high and low rates of colon cancer to investigate a hypothesized causal role of fat consumption in the development of colon cancer.

Because the data used in these studies are already available, such studies are relatively inexpensive and quick to do. These studies often are done early in the process of epidemiological investigation and may be useful in hypothesis generation as well as in stage I hypothesis testing. Such studies, although a useful first step in the analytical phase of investigation, are subject to *ecological fallacy*, the belief that relationships observed among groups can be assumed for individuals. Although there may be a striking relationship between high cancer rates and polluted drinking water in the populations studied, there is not necessarily the same relationship observed on the individual level. Imagine, for example, a study that compared cancer rates for a town with polluted drinking water with cancer rates for a town with pure water and found that cancer rates were higher in the town with the polluted water. It would be fallacious to conclude that the polluted water was the cause of the cases of cancer. It is possible, for example, that most residents of the town with polluted water who developed cancer were men who worked in another town, where they were exposed to carcinogens in the workplace. They actually drank less of the polluted water than did the individuals remaining in the town all day. The study might have detected that the water was an unlikely cause had it examined rates separately for men and women and seen no difference in rates among women between the two towns, but observed differences among men.

Relational studies, in contrast, do relate exposure and disease in the same individuals. For each individual in the study population, data are obtained on the presence or absence of exposure and on the level and time period when the exposure was present; thus, the presence or absence of disease is assessed for each individual. The frequency of joint presence of disease and exposure is then assessed for this group of persons.

Time of disease onset is also important information. Relational studies try to obtain individual information regarding this and other factors that are already known to relate to the disease process or factors that may lead to false inferences if not controlled in study design or analysis. For example, in studies on pregnancy where the outcome of interest may be maternal health status or fetal health, the age of the mother will be important regardless of what exposure is the object of investigation. It is necessary to control for effects of age because it is known to have a strong impact on pregnancy outcomes. Further, if the exposure being studied varies with age, it would appear to be causally related if age were not controlled. In other instances, age may interact with another exposure to produce a synergistic effect. Specific study designs used for analytic epidemiological studies include: cross-sectional, case-control, historical cohort, and prospective cohort designs. These designs are described later in this chapter and the strengths and weaknesses of each are discussed.

Experimentation

When sufficient evidence has accumulated from analytical studies to suggest that a specific factor is causally related to the occurrence of a particular disease, the experimental phase of epidemiological investigation is begun. The experimental phase employs a study design called a *randomized trial*. In contrast to the observational studies previously discussed, the investigator, not the individual, determines through random assignment who is exposed or not exposed to each experimental condition and controls the nature of each experimental condition. Because the investigator has control over who is or is not exposed, as well as the experimental conditions, the problems of causal inference inherent to the analytical studies are not generally present. As a result, data from experimental studies are typically used to prove causal relationships.

Since it would be unethical to expose human subjects to an agent thought to be harmful, in most epidemiological experiments the study sample is chosen from individuals already exposed to the causal agent under study. The suspected causal factor is then taken away from one study group and their disease experience is compared with that of the group that remains exposed to the suspected factor. Subjects are randomly assigned to a study group. For example, if hypertension is thought to be a causal agent for stroke, patients with hypertension may be randomly assigned to a treatment group that is given medication to reduce blood pressure, whereas the remaining subjects receive either no treatment or diet treatment only. The two groups are then followed forward in time and compared for the incidence of stroke.

In some instances, the occurrence of a disease appears to be associated with the absence of a factor and presence of the factor is associated with a lower rate of the disease. An example of this is the association observed in many epidemiological studies of lower cancer rates with diets high in beta-carotene, an antioxidant (Mayne, 1990; Frontham, 1990; Willett, 1990; Omenn, 1995). Because *in vivo* and *in vitro* studies demonstrated the mechanism by which beta-carotene could prevent cancer and randomized trials with rats showed lower rates of developing malignant tumors after exposure to carcinogens if the animals were given beta-carotene, several randomized trials were conducted in humans to confirm that cancers, particularly lung cancer, could be prevented by administration of beta-carotene (The Alpha-tocopheral, Beta-carotene Cancer Prevention Study Group, 1994; Hennekens et al, 1996; Omenn et al, 1996). Unfortunately, the one trial with low-risk individuals showed no difference between those receiving and not receiving beta-carotene (Hennekens et al, 1996), while two trials with persons at high risk (The Alpha-tocopheral, Beta-carotene Cancer Prevention Study Group, 1994; Omenn et al, 1996) showed an excess of lung cancer associated with beta-carotene use.

SOURCES OF DATA

Epidemiological investigations use data from a variety of existing sources, such as census data routinely collected by the government or medical record data maintained by hospitals. In other instances, the data may be generated for a specific study through surveys that include interviews and physical examinations.

Epidemiologists require four types of data:

1. Population statistics for denominators of rates
2. Frequency of health events (morbidity and mortality data)
3. Exposure for hypothesized causal factors or events
4. Linkage data that permit researchers to track individual study subjects over time

Population Statistics

Data from a population census carried out every 10 years in many countries are the main source of population statistics. Census data include a count of the total population and a variety of information about geographic, economic, and personal demographic characteristics of individuals and households. Some of these data provide the denominator for routine health statistics.

Health Events

Data on frequency of health events are of two types: mortality data and morbidity data. Mortality statistics are generally based on the numbers and causes of death listed on death certificates because, in most of the world, registration of deaths is required by law. As a result, these data provide a fairly complete record of the number of deaths. Accuracy of the reported cause of death varies from place to place, but these data are probably adequate indicators of the mortality count for major causes of death. International comparison of mortality has been facilitated by general use of the International Statistical Classification of Diseases, Injuries, and Causes of Death (ICD).

Deaths are one type of vital statistic. *Vital statistics* is a term used for the data collected from ongoing registration of "vital" events relating to births, deaths, and marriages. They include births and adoptions, deaths and fetal deaths, marriages, divorces, legal separations, and annulments. Certification of births, deaths, and fetal deaths are the vital events of most use in epidemiological research. Birth certificates, for example, provide information for the numerator and for the denominator of various rates measuring health aspects of childbirth and infancy. Although in the United States certificates are filed locally, each state and certain large cities hold legal responsibility for registration and reporting of vital events. A standard format for certificates is recommended by the National Center for Health Statistics (NCHS) in conjunction with its Cooperative Health Statistics System (CHSS). Although most states adopt these standard forms, the amount of available information varies because each state may determine the format and context of its own certificate. To facilitate epidemiological research based on mortality data, the NCHS established the National Death Index in 1979. This central, computerized index is compiled by NCHS from tapes provided by the various state vital statistics offices. The NDI allows epidemiologists to trace people who have died through one central source rather than having to contact individual states. Coding of causes of death is standardized by using the International Statistical Classification of Diseases and Related Health Problems, now in the 10th revision (World Health Organization, 1992).

Morbidity data, except for that in notification systems, are not routinely recorded as public records and, therefore, are harder to obtain and may be less accurate than mortality statistics. Two major sources of morbidity data are hospital records and notification systems, such as those that require the reporting of 52 infectious diseases decreed as reportable in all states since 1995 (Centers for Disease Control, 1995). Another type of notification system is the reporting required by disease registries such as cancer registries and birth defects registries. The U.S. Centers for Disease Control systematically collect data on abortions, congenital anomalies, nosocomial infections, and other conditions with preventable components. Special surveys may be conducted when data are not otherwise available. The National Health Survey, established by Congress in 1956, is conducted by NCHS and provides a continual source of information about the health status and needs of the entire country. Components of this survey include the Health Interview Survey (comprised of approximately 40,000 households per year) and the Health and Nutrition Examination Survey. Additional NCHS surveys include the National Hospital Discharge Survey, the National Nursing Home Survey, and the National Family Growth Survey. Summary statistics for a community are frequently available from organizations that routinely use them for health planning purposes. These organizations include health departments, regional planning agencies, hospitals, and a variety of governmental agencies.

Probably the most difficult morbidity data to obtain are outcome data. While diagnostic criteria for defining a case of a disease may vary somewhat from physician to physician, diagnosis is generally available in the medical record and can often be standardized from various sources by additionally using available laboratory or pathology data. Data on outcomes are much more variable in medical records and, therefore, more difficult to make equivalent across sources.

Causal Factors

Data on hypothesized causal factors is sometimes available from existing sources such as hospital records. This source might include data on factors such as age, race, drugs used, smoking history, reproductive history, previous diseases, or occupation. Unfortunately, completeness and accuracy of these records may vary widely. Records kept by employers and unions may be a source of information on toxic exposures experienced by workers. In other cases, the investigator must resort to special surveys using industrial hygiene assessments, interviews, or questionnaires to obtain information on exposure to hypothesized causal agents.

Sources of data that measure frequency, duration, and dosage (intesity) of exposures or health events vary considerably in their accuracy. Clearly, if the information used to measure events is not accurate, erroneous conclusions may result from the study. Therefore, epidemiologists must be concerned with how accurately they can measure the events they are attempting to study.

Linkage Data

The final type of data required by epidemiologists allows an investigator to follow an individual through time. Consider the example of an historical cohort study with the purpose of determining whether a group of workers exposed to benzene in 1945 has a higher rate of cancer of the urinary tract than workers not exposed to benzene. To answer the research question, workers will be followed until 1998 or death, whichever comes first. Death certificates will be required to determine the cause of death of the deceased workers. The National Death Index mentioned previously will help here. For those still alive, physical examinations will be conducted. Many workers may have moved since 1945, so some means of locating them will be required. Sources of data such as social security records, state motor vehicle records, and town registries must be used.

DESIGNS USED IN ANALYTIC EPIDEMIOLOGICAL STUDIES

Four basic types of designs are commonly used in analytic epidemiological studies: (1) *cross-sectional;* (2) *case-control;* (3) *cohort;* and (4) *historical cohort.* Other names used synonymously with these terms, along with the design of each type of study, are listed in Table 4–1. These designs differ in time frame, and therefore in selection of study groups, in required numbers of subjects, in potential sources of data that can be used, and in methods of analysis. The time framework for these studies is illustrated in Figure 4–1.

TABLE 4–1. COMPARISON OF ECOLOGICAL AND RELATIONAL STUDY DESIGNS FOR OBSERVATIONAL STUDIES

LEVEL OF STUDY	TYPES OF STUDIES	OTHER COMMON TERMS FOR STUDY DESIGN	BASIC DESIGN
Ecological	Cross-sectional	Correlational Ecological correlational Ecological survey	Rates of disease frequency for places are correlated with frequency of factors in those places at various points in time
	Case-control	Retrospective	Places with high rates of a disease are compared with places with low rates for levels of factors thought to be related to causing that disease
	Cohort	Prospective Logitudinal	Future rates of disease occurrence are compared for places with current environmental exposures and places known not to have such exposures
	Historical cohort	Retrospective-prospective Nonconcurrent cohort	Rates of disease occurrence are compared for places with known past exposure to an environmental factor and places known not to have such exposures. Tracking of rates begins at the time of exposure and continues to the present
Relational	Cross-sectional	Correlational Prevalence study Prevalence survey Survey study	Current rates of exposure among individuals are correlated with current rates of disease frequency among these same individuals
	Case-control	Retrospective Case comparison	Frequency of prior exposure to the study factor is compared for individuals with the study disease and a group of individuals without the disease, who are similar in regard to other characteristics
	Cohort	Prospective Logitudinal Prospective population	A group of individuals known to be exposed to a factor and a group of similar individuals not exposed are followed into the future and their respective incidence of the disease of interest is compared
	Historical cohort	Retrospective-prospective Nonconcurrent cohort Retrospective cohort Retrospective mortality Retrospective incidence	A group of individuals known to have been exposed to a factor at a time in the past are compared with a group of individuals not exposed and their rates of disease incidence or mortality compared from the time of exposure to the present

(*From Valanis B. The epidemiological model and community health nursing. In M. Stanhope & J. Lancaster [Eds.].* Community health nursing: Process and practice for promoting health. *St. Louis: C. V. Mosby, 1984, p. 162.*)

These designs may be used both in ecological studies based on aggregate data for entire populations and in relational studies in which specific information on exposure and outcome for each individual is available. For relational investigations, cross-sectional and case-control studies are generally used as first steps because they can be done quickly, require small samples, and are relatively inexpensive. Historical cohort and (prospective) cohort studies generally require large samples, longer times to complete, and are expensive; however, they yield measures of incidence or risk. No incidence can be derived from the cross-sectional or case-control studies, making any risk measures obtainable only by indirect means. In terms of strength of design, ecological studies are generally weaker in their ability

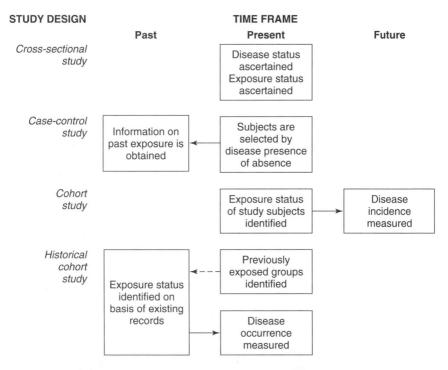

Figure 4–1. The time frame of four epidemiological study designs.

to yield valid inferences about causality than are relational studies. Cohort studies are a stronger design than cross-sectional and case-control designs. The gold standard for causality is an experimental design. Each of these four epidemiological designs and experimental trials are described and discussed in the following sections.

Cross-sectional Studies

Also called *correlational studies,* cross-sectional studies simultaneously ascertain the status of subjects on both the exposure factor and the disease of interest. Consider a study that investigates the relationship of depression (the exposure factor also known as the *independent variable*) to the occurrence of gastric ulcers (disease outcome also known as the *dependent variable*). The study simultaneously obtains for a selected population measures of depression, using depression scales, and presence or absence of gastric ulcer, by physical examinations, history, and tests. This cross-sectional study cannot establish the causal nature of a relationship between depression and gastric ulcers because the design does not allow the investigator to account for the time sequence of events—the major limitation of all cross-sectional studies. It is impossible to know whether depression occurred before the onset of ulcers or ulcers before the onset of depression, or whether the two occurred together.

Case-control Studies

Case-control studies begin by identifying a group of *cases* with the disease of interest and a comparable group of subjects without the disease, called a *control group* or *comparison group*. Attempts are then made to determine the frequency of exposure to the study factor for each group. One case-control study investigated demographic characteristics of mothers, complications related to pregnancy and labor, the method of delivery, and newborn illnesses and injuries as risk factors for neonatal sepsis (Soman et al, 1985). In this study, cases consisted of all 113 instances of sepsis identified on birth certificates in Washington State from 1980 to 1981. Controls were a sample of 347 births randomly selected from the 1981 Washington State birth certificates. Once cases and controls were selected, information as to presence or absence of each risk factor was obtained from each child's birth certificate. Relative frequencies of each factor of interest were compared for cases and controls using the *odds ratio*, a statistic that represents the odds in favor of having the disease with the factor present versus with the factor absent.

Some general rules apply to case-control studies. Because of potential problems in establishing exposure status of subjects, the same sources of data on exposure should be available for the cases and controls; this reduces bias caused by better ascertainment of exposure for one group than for the other. When selecting controls, it is important that controls have the same chance as cases of being exposed to the study factor. This point is elaborated on later in this chapter. Finally, a clear, unambiguous definition of a case is needed to facilitate selection of cases for the study. Optimally, cases should consist of all newly diagnosed *(incident)* cases that have the specified characteristics during the specified period of time in the defined population. Incident cases are preferred to *prevalent* cases (all current cases, both new and old) because use of prevalent cases can introduce bias that is caused by loss from the sample of patients who have a short disease course due to recovery or death. This is particularly a problem when the factor being investigated is related not only to disease onset, but also to the probability of dying or recovering.

Cohort Studies

Cohort designs, whether prospective or historical in type, begin by classifying the study subjects according to their exposure status. Prospective cohort studies follow subjects into the future, monitoring the incidence of the disease of interest for all subjects. The disease incidence or mortality rates for various levels of exposure (eg, high, medium, low, or no exposure) are then compared. If a relationship between exposure and disease occurrence is causal, one would expect to see a significantly higher rate of the disease in those exposed compared with those not exposed. This is measured by the *relative risk ratio*, a statistical measure, discussed later in this chapter. One would also expect to observe a *dose effect* (ie, an increase in disease incidence related to the level or dose of exposure). Perhaps the best known cohort study is the Framingham Study, an investigation of the factors associated with the risk of coronary heart disease (Dawber, 1980; Murabito, 1995). This study, begun in 1949, has provided a rich body of knowledge about the natural history of cardio-vascular disease. A representative sample of 5,209 men and women aged 30 to 59 years selected from the total population of Framingham, Massachusetts, were given a physical examination. The 5,127 individuals determined to be free of coronary heart disease (CHD) were reexamined every other year for evidence of CHD during the 30-plus years of the study. Within the total study cohort of 5,209, subjects were classified as to presence or absence of specific exposure factors of interest (eg, dia-betes, blood pressure, activity, blood cholesterol, and smoking), and incidence of CHD was compared for the subgroups. Much of what we know about risk for CHD has emerged from this study. The study is now following offspring of the original subjects (Shaefer, 1994).

Historical cohort studies differ from prospective cohort studies in that both the exposure and the onset of disease have already occurred. Such studies require the availability of records that permit classification of individuals on the initial exposure and a way of reconstructing the disease history. This study design is frequently used in occupational studies. If one wished to study exposure to benzene in relation to inci-dence of bladder cancer, an historical cohort study would most likely be the design of choice. Because bladder cancer has a relatively low incidence, a large cohort would need to be followed for many years to generate enough cases of bladder cancer for sta-tistical analysis. To complicate matters further, regulation of benzene exposures by the Occupational Safety & Health Administration (OSHA) has led to lower levels of ex-posure among workers in recent years. If there is a causal relationship between ben-zene exposure and bladder cancer, the incidence (or mortality rates) would be lower in groups with low exposure than in groups with high exposure. Thus, a prospective study of current workers would require a larger sample size than an historical cohort study. Associated costs and the length of time before any answers would be available make such a study impractical. An historical cohort study, however, could be conducted if cohorts of workers with a wide variety of exposure doses that occurred in the past can be identified through available records. Suppose a sufficiently large cohort of workers with exposures to benzene between 1950 and 1960 can be identified. All such workers meeting specified eligibility criteria would be entered into the study and tracked until the present to establish their vital status, dead or alive, and if dead, the date, place, and cause of death. This would be done through use of social security records, motor vehi-cle license records, union records, or any other available source of data. A comparison (control) group of unexposed workers could be similarly identified and followed.

Most often, historical cohort studies use general population age- and time-specific mortality rates rather than incidence as a basis for comparison because mor-tality data is more readily available. Using lifetable methods, an expected number of deaths is calculated for the cohort of exposed workers based on the experience of the general population. The observed number of deaths in the cohort is then compared with this expected number. This ratio is known as a *standard mortality ratio;* alterna-tively, a ratio based on proportional rates, the *proportional mortality ratio*, is some-times used. Although a specific comparison group could be identified and this mortal-ity experience reconstructed for comparison with the rate of the benzene workers in the example above, this approach is usually not used because of the expense. When the population mortality experience is used, however, there is a bias toward no difference between the exposed and comparison rates, because of *the healthy worker effect*. This phenomenon reflects the fact that workers are generally healthy to begin with and those who become ill drop out of the worker population; a similar effect does not occur in rates for the general population.

In both types of cohort studies, accurate classification of exposure and disease outcome is essential. This is more easily achieved in the prospective study because the historical design relies on recorded data. Loss to follow up is a potential problem in both of these designs. Efforts must be directed at minimizing such losses and evaluating whether any systematic bias is introduced into the study by those subjects who have dropped out.

Experimental Interventions

Intervention studies are conducted to confirm causal associations and test strategies for intervention using factors identified in epidemiological studies. The interventions may be prophylactic agents or educational/behavior change interventions. There are two types of intervention studies: randomized clinical trials and community trials. The most common form of intervention study is the *randomized clinical trial* which randomizes individuals to receive or not receive an intervention (ie, individuals are assigned by chance to treatment group and the investigator is able to manipulate the study intervention). This type of study tests the efficacy of an intervention. A current example is the Women's Health Initiative (WHI) (Matthews et al, 1997; Rossouw, 1995). Epidemiological evidence has suggested that a high fat diet increases risk of breast cancer and colon cancer among women. Epidemiological studies have also suggested that long-term use of estrogen by postmenopausal women may reduce risks of heart disease mortality and of fractures due to osteoporosis. In addition, calcium and vitamin D appear, in epidemiological studies, to reduce risk of fractures and colon cancer. The WHI includes three randomized clinical trials testing the effects of estrogen, low fat diet, and calcium/vitamin D, respectively, on these diseases in postmenopausal women.

Another type of randomized intervention study tests the effectiveness of the intervention when delivered by the health care system or in the community. These are called *effectiveness trials* or *community trials*. Unlike the efficacy version of the clinical trial which carefully controls the intervention and how it is delivered, the effectiveness trial tests outcomes when the intervention is less precisely controlled. Unlike the highly motivated volunteers in a clinical trial, individuals in the community will have varying degrees of motivation to change behavior. In the WHI low fat diet intervention component of the clinical trial, the intervention is delivered by strict protocol and women who volunteered to participate in the study committed to attend all the intervention sessions and to complete dietary food records and other self-monitoring measures for the duration of the trial (10 to 12 years). This study has reasonably good control over the dietary intake, can determine the extent to which the diet is consumed by the intervention group, and monitors the intake of the control group thus demonstrating the efficacy of the diet in reducing breast cancer incidence and mortality. The women participating in the trial meet tight standards of eligibility. In contrast, an effectiveness trial of a low fat diet, even if it could randomize individuals or clinics to the low fat diet or control conditions and train personnel on dietary protocol, and so forth, would need to depend on physicians, nutritionists, nurses, or other busy professionals in the health care system, rather than project staff, to deliver the intervention. All this would make the intervention likely to be less consistent and the women less motivated to follow through. There would also likely be more variability among the women receiving the intervention than in the efficacy trial. Monitoring of dietary intake would likely be less complete as well. For these reasons, even an efficacious intervention may not be effective as large public health interventions.

Outcomes and extent of behavior change both present measurement problems. An effectiveness trial in a clinic setting might be able to collect data on individuals, but a trial in the community would be able only to sample a proportion of those in the community intervention group to estimate compliance and would use population-based rates to assess outcomes.

CRITERIA FOR EVALUATION OF PUBLISHED STUDIES

Certain methodological criteria must be met if results of a study are to be considered valid. When reading research reports in the literature, you should assess whether the following minimal criteria have been met.

Background and Study Hypothesis

Sufficient information on why the particular issue is being investigated should be presented to convince the reader that there is a need for the study. The background information should provide some indication of which factors are already known to be associated with the occurrence of the particular disease, because these factors need to be controlled in the design or analysis of the study, or both. Hypotheses to be tested should be clearly spelled out in order to provide the basis for developing an appropriate study design.

Equivalence of Subjects in the Two Study Groups

All studies require a comparison group. Usually called a *control group,* this is a group of persons with whom the study group of interest can be compared in regard to frequency of the factor of interest. In case-control studies, all subjects are selected on the basis of presence or absence of the disease, whereas in any form of cohort study they are selected on the basis of presence or absence of exposure. In both instances it is important that the comparison group be similar to the study group (cases of the disease in case-control studies; exposed subjects in cohort studies) for factors other than the study factor. For example, the groups should be of similar socioeconomic status and similar race and gender. The same holds true for ecological studies; there must be equivalence in the two populations being compared. For case-control studies, such equivalence is important to ensure that cases and controls have had an equal chance of being exposed to the study factor. If they have not had an equal chance, then a bias is introduced. For example, in a case-control study to investigate the relationship of estrogen use to occurrence of breast cancer, cases and controls should have equal chances of receiving medical care because the opportunity to have estrogen prescribed is dependent on regular medical care. If cases had more opportunity for medical care than the controls (eg, if the two groups were of different socioeconomic status), then the study would find that estrogen use was more common among breast cancer cases than among controls. This would be due to bias in the study design rather than to a true excess among cases. Similarly, in a cohort study (either historic or prospective), it is crucial that both the study group exposed to the study factor and the nonexposed control group should have equal probability of exposure to other factors that could be related to development of the disease outcome of interest. For example, in a study of the relationship of regular exercise versus no exercise to incidence of chronic obstructive pulmonary disease, both the group exposed to regular exercise and those not exposed to exercise should have similar frequencies of smoking. If one group has a higher percentage of smokers than the other, the effect of smoking on lung function of that group will make it difficult to evaluate the role of amount of exercise when comparing the two groups. If obtaining groups with equivalent smoking status is not possible, and smoking status of study participants is known, then smokers in the regular exercise group could be compared with smokers in the no-exercise group. However, if specific information on smoking is unavailable, the effect cannot be evaluated.

Similar Availability of Information on Study Factors for the Two Study Groups.   If the data required for the study are not likely to be equally available and complete for both groups from the same source, then there is the likelihood that whichever group has a better source of information will show an excess of the factor under study (exposure for case-control studies; presence of disease for cohort studies). Ideally, there should be complete ascertainment of data on both the causal factor(s) of interest and the outcome of interest for both groups.

Accurate Measurement of Study Factors

Important considerations are reliability and validity of measurement (discussed later in this chapter). These measurement issues relate to the criteria for defining what constitutes a "case" of the disease under study, to the measurement of exposures and control factors, and, in studies of treatment efficacy, to measurement of outcomes. If data from multiple hospitals or physician's offices are used, standardization of variable definition will be crucial.

Sample Size, Representativeness, and Power

Presentation of the study design should address the issue of how the size of the study sample was determined, how representative study participants are of the target population, and the statistical power of this sample size to answer the research question. Particularly in studies that did not find the hypothesized relationship between an exposure and a disease, it is important to address whether it is likely that no relationship exists or whether the negative finding was due to inadequate sample size. Knowing the power of the study to detect a specified effect size can help draw inferences about this (see discussion in the statistical methods section on the following pages regarding sample size). Representativeness is important so that the results can be generalized to similar populations in other settings. Providing information on representativeness allows the reader to determine whether the findings are likely to apply to the populations they care for. Cases of a disease chosen for a case-control study, for example, should include a spectrum of mild to severe disease and treated and untreated disease.

Study Processes

There are many opportunities to introduce bias in the process of conducting a study. Several of the crucial areas to assess include appropriateness of exclusion/eligibility criteria, response rates of the targeted baseline sample, completeness of follow up, blinded assessment of outcome, and adequate quality monitoring of data collection and processing.

Analysis

The analytical techniques should be appropriate to the design of the study. A prospective study, for example, should use incidence rates and relative risk measures to capitalize on the strengths of the prospective design, rather than setting up the data for analysis as if they were retrospective in design. Although this seems obvious, there are studies in the literature in which this was not done. Furthermore, confidence limits for risk ratios and other relevant tests should be provided. Presentation of data without such information makes interpretation of results difficult. Finally, the analysis should control for the potential confounding variables that were not controlled by the study design.

Discussion

Quality researchers will compare and contrast the results of their study to the findings of previous studies. Reasons for possible discrepancies in findings should be suggested, including a candid analysis of factors inherent in the design of the current study. Limitations of the study should be specified. The likelihood of associations being causal should be addressed relative to the criteria for assessing causality discussed in Chapter 2. The clinical or public health significance of the findings should also be discussed.

STATISTICAL ISSUES AND METHODS USED IN EPIDEMIOLOGY

The purpose of the following section is to introduce some basic concepts and terms that will help one understand the statistical techniques used in the epidemiological literature. Some of these concepts, such as risk ratios, are further discussed elsewhere in this book. Other statistical terms used specifically in regard to a particular area of epidemiology are discussed only in the chapter dealing with the subject content for which they are relevant, for example sensitivity, specificity, and predictive values are introduced only in Chapter 14 which covers screening.

Sampling

Because studies rarely have data on the entire population, they draw a sample from the target population about which they want to make inferences. To make generalizations about the larger target population from the study sample, one needs to consider how the sample relates to the larger population. *Sampling error* is the term used to refer to the difference between the sample result and the population characteristic the study tries to estimate. If appropriate sampling procedures are used, error can be kept small. Two factors contribute to sampling error: *biased selection* and *random variation*. Biased selection results from selecting an unrepresentative segment of the population and can best be avoided by random selection of subjects, which gives each individual an equal chance of being selected. In additon to eliminating bias, random selection of the study sample enables one to determine the reliability of results, since the only source of sampling error is random variation, which is determined by the heterogeneity of the population and the size of the sample. In studies where it is important to have adequate numbers in population subgroups, a stratified random sample can be used. This is done by stratifying the population on those subgroup variables, for example age or race, and randomly selecting the required number of subjects in each stratum.

Determining Sample Size

Studies are designed to test hypotheses about relationships between an exposure (or intervention) and a health outcome, such as disease incidence or mortality. From a statistical point of view, the statistical analysis of a study is designed to reject the *null hypothesis* when it is false. A null hypothesis states that there is no difference in these relationships among two or more groups being compared and any difference observed is merely the result of chance variation. To decide whether the null hypothesis is accepted or rejected, a statistical test of significance is conducted. This test statistic is compared with a "critical value" obtained from a set of statistical tables. If the test statistic is larger than the critical value, the null hypothesis is rejected and the difference between the groups is called *statistically significant*. A level of statistical significance at which the null hypothesis will be rejected, the P value, is selected by the investigators before beginning the study. Most often, this level is 5% ($P < 0.05$). This level represents the risk of being incorrect in rejecting the null hypothesis, in this case a 5% risk. Thus, if the P value for the statistical test comparing the difference between the two groups is less than $P = 0.05$, the null hypothesis is rejected and the difference between the groups is considered statistically significant, not due to chance alone.

When a study finding is not statistically significant, however, one cannot assume it is just due to chance. A nonsignificant finding could be due to too small a sample size, because with a small sample, sampling error may be quite large. To increase the likelihood that a nonsignificant finding is real, it is important during the design phase to determine the size of sample needed to assure that a real effect will not be missed by sampling error. The needed sample size is based on the following factors: (1) the size of difference one wishes to detect between the study groups (eg, in a case-control study, a relative risk of two in the case group relative to the noncases, or in an intervention study, reducing mortality by 40% in the intervention group compared with that of the control group); (2) frequency of the outcome likely to be present in the control group, ie, the rate of disease incidence or mortality (in prospective studies) or the prevalence of the risk factor (in case-control studies); (3) the significance level chosen (alpha [α], which represents the probability that observed significant results have occurred by chance, called type I error); and (4) the likelihood of failing to detect a significant difference if one exists (beta [β], called type II error), which is often set at 0.2 or 20%. One minus beta is called the *power* of the study. Thus, if beta is 0.2, then $1 - 0.2$ is 0.8 or a power of 80% to reject the null hypothesis when it is false. These four components are entered into published formulae to calculate the sample size needed.

In studies with very large samples, very small differences between groups may be statistically significant. Therefore, it is important to consider the *clinical significance* of the difference. For example, in a large study of an intervention to lower the incidence of low birth weight infants in a population, a difference of 75 g between the intervention group and the control group may be statistically significant. But what is the biological significance of this difference? Is it enough to affect the health and well-being of the infant? Or is a larger difference, say 250 g more meaningful? One would hope that the investigators selected a clinically meaningful difference when designing the study, but this is not always the case. Hence, it is important to evaluate the practical significance of any differences between groups when reading study results.

Issues in Measurement

Techniques are needed to measure, organize, and describe data. A variety of factors determine which techniques are appropriate for any particular data. These factors include accuracy of measurement, level of measurement, inherent variation, study design, and the question being asked of the data. These issues are discussed in the following paragraphs.

Reliability and Validity of Measurements. Two major aspects of measurement are the reliability of the measuring procedure or source of data and the validity of the measurement. *Reliability* is the repeatability of a measurement. Factors that affect repeatability include variations in the attribute being measured, variability in a measuring instrument, and variations between measuring instruments or raters. Blood pressure, for example, is an attribute that varies in an individual. Stress and activity will each result in short-term changes in blood pressure. Furthermore, an instrument such as a sphygmomanometer used to measure blood pressure requires frequent recalibration to ensure that variation in measurement is minimal. Two nurses using the same sphygmomanometer to take the blood pressure of the same patient, one immediately after the other, may obtain different readings. All these factors contribute to a low reliability of blood pressure measurement. To maximize reliability of measurement, the conditions of measurement must be standardized. In this example, measures for all patients should be done under similar conditions, with well-calibrated instruments used by a few nurses who have been trained to do the procedure in the same way.

Validity refers to the accuracy of the measurement. Stated another way, validity is how well the measurement represents reality. A measure must be reliable to be valid, but reliability alone does not produce validity. A measure may be precise but not accurate. For example, the tuberculin test may be used as a screening test for tuberculosis. Even if the reliability of the test administration and test reading is maximized, the test is not a totally accurate or valid test for tuberculosis. Although individuals with tuberculosis should test positive (a true-positive reading and not a false-negative reading), a reading may be positive for reasons other than presence of tuberculosis, such as having been previously vaccinated with bacillus Calmette Guerin (BCG). Thus, some rate of false-positives will be observed. A positive sputum culture for tuberculosis is generally a more valid test for the presence of tuberculosis as long as reliability of testing is maximized. Even in this instance, validity is not 100% because false-negative readings may occur if the specimen was inadequate or was improperly handled. Figure 4–2 illustrates reliability and validity using the concept of a target. Target A indicates a measure that is highly reliable, but invalid, because the center of the target is the actual value. Target B shows a less reliable, but still reasonably valid measure. Were the reliability to decrease, then the validity would also decrease.

Level of Measurement.   Measurement of exposure, disease, and outcome variables can be done at different levels. Statistical techniques for describing and manipulating data differ by level of measurement. Data that are based on categories with no inherent ordering are called *nominal* or *categorical* data. Examples of such measures common in epidemiology are race (white, black, Hispanic, Asian) and gender (male, female). *Ordinal* measures contain some inherent order. For example, a classification such as child, young adult, middle-aged adult, and elderly to represent life stage implies an order. Self-ratings of health as excellent, good, fair, and poor also are ordered. These are ordinal measures. The third level of measures is *interval*

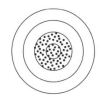

Target A   Target B
Reliable, but not valid   Less reliable, but valid

Figure 4–2. A visual approach to concepts of reliability and validity.

measurement. These measures are ordered and the distance (interval) between one level and the next is equivalent to that between any other two levels. Examples are age measured in years or weight measured in pounds. The difference in time between age 5 and 6 is the same as the difference between age 19 and 20 or age 72 and 73. Such data are also referred to as continuous data. When interval measures are collapsed into categories, for example, grouping age as 0 to 18 years, 19 to 45 years, 46 to 64 years, 65 to 84 years, and 85 years and older, they are treated as ordinal data. If age were collapsed into only two categories, eg ≤ 45, and 46-plus, the data would be treated as nominal (categorical) data. The type of statistical test that can be used in a study depends on the level at which data are measured.

Describing Variability.   All data contain inherent variability. Statistical techniques assist in organizing and describing the variation in a set of measures. Once the measures have been organized and the variability described, appropriate tests for analysis can be selected. Organizing a collection of measurements to derive a picture of which levels are common versus rare can be done by using *frequency distributions*. Table 4–2 shows data on the age distribution of individuals in a study. Column 2 shows how the total of 2,710 subjects is distributed across the 11 age groups shown in column 1. The percentage distribution or *relative frequency* is shown in column 3, calculated by dividing the number in a specific age group by the total, for example, dividing the 440 in the 35 to 39 year age group by 2,710 yields the 15% in column 3. This relative frequency could be used to compare with distributions of other populations that differ in absolute size. The *cumulative percent* adds each age specific frequency to those of the prior age groups and permits statements such as more than half of subjects (53.9%) are age 44 or younger. These techniques for summarizing and describing data are useful for categorical or ordinal data. Interval data can be presented in this manner as well by collapsing the individual ages, eg, 20, 21, 22, 23, 24 into categories as in Table 4–2.

If one wished to express the typical experience of a group, a *measure of central tendency* is used. For categorical data, one would use the *mode*, the most

TABLE 4–2. DISTRIBUTION OF STUDY POPULATION BY AGE

AGE IN YEARS	NUMBER OF SUBJECTS	PERCENT OF TOTAL	CUMULATIVE PERCENT OF TOTAL
20–24	20	0.8	0.8
25–29	150	5.6	6.4
30–34	330	12.4	18.7
35–39	440	15.0	33.7
40–44	540	20.2	53.9
45–49	470	17.6	71.5
50–54	380	14.2	85.8
55–59	160	6.0	91.8
60–64	150	6.5	97.4
65–69	30	1.1	98.5
70 and over	40	1.5	100.0

frequently occurring observation. For ordinal data, either the mode or a measure called the median could be used. The *median* is the level of measurement below which half the observations fall. In Table 4–2, the median is the category of 40 to 44 years. Another measure of central tendency can be used only with interval data. This measure, the *mean*, represents the average value, such as the average age of the sample. If the ages of study subjects were not grouped as in Table 4–2, one could calculate the mean age of the sample by adding the individual ages of all study subjects and dividing by the total number of subjects.

$$\text{Mean} \; = \; \frac{\text{Sum of values for all individuals}}{\text{Number of individuals}}$$

One may also wish to describe the amount of variation. The *range* indicates the difference between the highest and lowest observations and is generally used for interval level measures. Another term is the *standard deviation*, which indicates the average distance of individual values from the mean value for the total sample. Standard deviation is used as a parameter to describe the normal distribution curve. Many naturally occurring phenomena distribute in a bell-shaped curve with values symmetrically distributed around their mean. In the normal curve, 68% of values fall within 1 standard deviation of the mean, 95% of values within 2 standard deviations, and 99.7% within 3 standard deviations. Figure 4–3 shows a normal curve. Since many

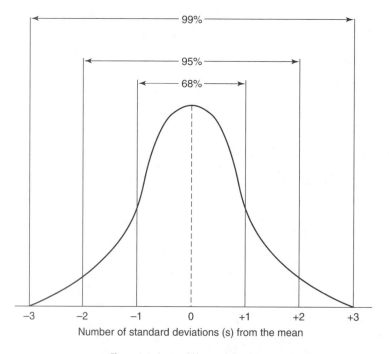

Figure 4–3. A normal (Gaussian) distribution.

biological measures show a normal distribution, the normal curve is often used to determine cutoffs for normal values of laboratory tests. If a distribution follows a normal curve, normal limits are often set as the mean ± 2 standard deviations.

Another measure of variability is the *standard error*. This statistic measures the variability of the mean of the sample, which is used to estimate the true value of the mean for the population from which the sample was drawn. Two or more small samples drawn from a single population are likely to have different means. The average of the sample means would more accurately estimate the true population value than any of the individual sample means. The more samples drawn, the more likely the mean of the samples is to represent that of the overall population. The standard error is used in constructing *confidence intervals*, which allow one to make inferences about the true population parameter (ie, a mean or proportion) in which one is interested. The confidence interval puts bounds on the probable real value of the measure in the population. A 95% confidence interval indicates the range within which the true value has a 95% chance of falling.

Probability

An understanding of probability is needed to appreciate and manipulate the different kinds of rates used in research. A *probability* is a quantitative expression of the likelihood of something occurring. A rate is a probability in that it measures the likelihood that a specified event occurs in a group or that a specific characteristic is possessed by a typical member of a population. A relative frequency or proportion is a rate. The probability of event A is calculated as:

$$\Pr(A) = \frac{\text{Number of times A occurs}}{\text{Total number of times A could occur}}$$

For example, if 36 children in a classroom are exposed to a classmate who has the measles and 12 children subsequently contract measles, the probability of illness (attack rate) was 33% or one third (12 who contract measles divided by 36 exposed). However, some children in the classroom may have been vaccinated against measles and were not susceptible. Contracting the disease is conditional on being susceptible. Thus, the *conditional probability* of contracting measles, if one is susceptible, is calculated as the number of children who were susceptible and became ill divided by the number susceptible.

The probability of a conditional event occurring may be additive or multiplicative. If event A is independent of event B, then the probability of occurrence for an individual can be determined by multiplying the probability of event A times the probability of event B. If A and B are not independent, then the probability is based on the probability of A plus the probability of B.

Testing Associations

Since epidemiology focuses on examining relationships between variables, the techniques of correlation and regression are useful. These techniques specify quantitatively the relationship between the variables. The *correlation coefficient*, usually denoted by *r*, indicates the extent to which two variables are associated and has values between +1.0 and −1.0. A value of zero indicates absence of association. The closer the value of the correlation coefficient to 1.0, the stronger the relationship. Thus, a correlation coefficient of 0.2 indicates a much weaker relationship between factors x and y than does a coefficient of 0.8. A positive correlation indicates that as values of x increase, so do values of y. A negative correlation indicates that as values of x increase, values of y decrease. A positive correlation of 0.65 between blood pressure and stroke indicates that as blood pressure increases, so does the likelihood of a stroke. An example of a negative (inverse) correlation is that between socioeconomic status and childhood mortality. Lower socioeconomic classes have higher rates of mortality than do higher socioeconomic classes.

To rule out the possibility that a correlation is due to chance alone, the *P* value is used to test statistically the probability that a correlation coefficient as large or larger than the observed value would occur for the study sample when no correlation exists in the population. A *Spearman rank order correlation* is used for data with ordinal level measurement and the *product moment correlation* for interval level data. *Bivariate correlations* can be used to examine correlation between two variables with categorical level measurement.

Regression equations are used to develop a predictive model that lets us predict outcome y for a given level of exposure x. The regression equation takes the form $y = \alpha + \beta x$, where α is the value of y when x is zero (intercept) and β = the change in y that results from a change of one unit of x (the slope). The slope shows how much and in which direction y will vary with changes in x. For example, if one were studying the relationship of years of smoking to the incidence of lung cancer and α = 6 cases/1,000 individuals and β = 1.6 cases/1,000, then 1.6 cases/1,000 would be added to the 6 for every additional year of smoking.

Measures of Risk

There are two measures of risk commonly used in epidemiological studies. *Relative risk* is a term for the risk in an exposed group relative to that for the comparison group which has not been exposed. It is a ratio of two rates calculated as:

$$\text{Relative risk} = \frac{\text{Incidence rate among exposed}}{\text{Incidence rate among nonexposed}}$$

For the researcher, relative risk also reflects the strength of an association between an exposure factor and a health outcome, so it is a useful measure in studying disease etiology. A relative risk of 6 is a much stronger association than a relative risk of 1.2. Relative risk is derived directly from cohort studies, since they yield incidence rates for both the exposed and comparison (nonexposed) groups. Case-control studies, because of their retrospective nature, do not yield the incidence rates needed to calculate the relative risk ratio. These studies can estimate an approximation of the relative risk called the *odds ratio* as long as the disease studied has low incidence in the general population and the control group is representative of the general population with respect to the frequency of the exposure attribute. The odds ratio is calculated from a table that displays the data for two categorical variables as shown in Table 4–3.

The odds ratio is calculated as:

$$\text{Odds ratio} = \frac{ad}{bc}$$

where a is the number of individuals with the disease and the exposure, d is the number with neither the disease nor the exposure, b is the number with the exposure and no disease, and c is the number with the disease but no exposure. The odds ratio is interpreted the same as a relative risk ratio in terms of drawing inferences about associations between variables. For both the relative risk ratio and the odds ratio, confidence intervals are used to determine the likely range of the true risk in the population. As an example, if a study shows a 3.0 risk for breast cancer associated with use of estrogen therapy with a 95% confidence interval of 1.8 to 4.6, there is a 95% chance that the real risk for women on estrogen to develop breast cancer is somewhere between 1.8 and 4.6 times that of women not on estrogen.

Relative risk tells the clinician how much increased risk a patient may experience because of a particular exposure, for example smoking, obesity, or lack of exercise. If the relative risk is 4 for a particular exposure, the probability of disease among individuals with the factor is 4 times that of individuals without the factor. This does not translate to risk for any individual; however, it is the average among the population studied with the factor. The relative risk also suggests the impact that eliminating the exposure could have on reducing risk.

Attributable risk is a measure more useful in public health planning than in attributing etiology. It is calculated as: attributable risk = incidence rate for exposed − incidence rate for nonexposed. When multiplied by 100, this indicates the percent reduction in disease incidence that might be achieved by eliminating the exposure in the population. Thus, this measure is helpful to health planners in making decisions about the relative impact of one intervention versus another.

For information on other statistical tests and specialized procedures, such as survival analysis, a statistical text should be consulted.

TABLE 4–3. DATA FROM A CASE-CONTROL STUDY DISPLAYED FOR CALCULATION OF AN ODDS RATIO

EXPOSURE STATUS	DISEASE STATUS		
	Has disease	Doesn't have disease	TOTAL
Exposed	a	b	a + b
Not exposed	c	d	c + d
Total	a + b	b + d	a + b + c + d

REFERENCES

The Alpha-tocopheral, Beta-carotene Cancer Prevention Study Group. (1994) The effect of vitamin E and beta-carotene on the incidence of lung cancer and other cancers in male smokers. *New England Journal of Medicine 330*, 1029–1035.

Dawber T. R. (1980) *The Framingham Study: The epidemiology of atherosclerotic disease.* Cambridge, Massachusetts: Harvard University.

Frontham E. T. (1990) Protective dietary factors and lung cancer. *International Journal of Epidemiology,* (suppl. 1);*19,* 532–542.

Hennekens C. H., Buring J. E., Manson J. E., et al. (1996) Lack of effect of long-term supplementation with beta-carotene on the incidence of malignant neoplasms and cardiovascular disease. *New England Journal of Medicine, 334,* 1145–1149.

Matthews K. A., Shumaker S. A., Bowen D. J., et al. (1997) Women's health initiative. Why now? What is it? What's new? *American Psychologist, 52*(2), 101–116.

Mayne S. T. (1990) Beta-carotene and cancer prevention: What is the evidence? *Connecticut Medical, 54:* 547–551.

Murabito J. (1995) Women and cardiovascular disease: contributions from the Framingham study. *Journal of the American Medical Women's Association, 50*(2), 35–39, 55.

Omenn G. S. (1995) What accounts for the association of vegetables and fruits with lower incidence of cancer and coronary heart disease? *Annals of Epidemiology, 5,* 333–335.

Omenn G. S., Goodman G. E., Thornquist M. D., et al. (1996) Effects of a combination of beta-carotene and vitamin A on lung cancer and cardiovascular disease. *New England Journal of Medicine, 334,* 1150–1155.

Rossouw J. E., Finnegan L. P., Harlan W. R., et al. (1995) The evolution of the Women's Health Initiative: perspectives from the NIH. *Journal of the American Medical Women's Association, 50*(2), 50–55.

Schaefer E. J., Lamon-Fava S., Ordovas J. M., et al. (1994) Factors associated with low and elevated plasma high density lipoprotein cholesterol and apoliproprotein A-1 levels in the Framingham offspring study. *Journal of Lipid Metabolism, 35*(5), 871–882.

Soman M., Green B., Daling, J. (1985) Risk factors for early neonatal sepsis. *American Journal of Epidemiology, 121*(5), 712–719.

Willett W. (1990) Vitamin A and lung cancer. *Nutrition Review 48,* 201–211.

Epidemiological Transitions in Disease Patterns Over Time

his chapter focuses on historical changes in patterns of health and disease. The relationships of the health status of a population to demographic characteristics such as size, density, growth, and distribution are described. In addition, shifts in the health and demographic characteristics in relation to economic and social influences are discussed. Understanding the complex interdependence of the demographic characteristics and health status of populations is necessary for assessing and planning health services because the health status of populations is not static but constantly changing in response to population dynamics. In recent years, worldwide patterns of health and disease have been shaped by both historical forces of change and new ones, such as the international transfer of health risks, which has contributed to health care costs absorbing an increasing share of resources in both developed and less developed countries. Local service delivery agencies are impacted by the shifting demographics of their geographic locale, including the aging of the population through increased longevity and through immigration of elderly retirees or outmigration of younger persons.

HISTORICAL POPULATION CHANGES

Archaeological evidence suggests that at the end of the last glaciation (10,000 BC) humans lived primarily as wanderers, gathering what food could be found. Populations were sparse and scattered. Over the years, as they wandered through changing environments and improved their means of food acquisition, population began to increase, reaching an estimated 10 million total world population by 8000 BC and rising to about 300 million by the advent of the Christian era. This occurred largely because of the development of agriculture, which allowed groups to congregate in one place and to develop a more stable social system. This represented an annual growth rate of 0.06% across a period of 80 centuries. In comparison, modern rates of population growth are phenomenal (Table 5–1), rising from 0.29% between 1650 and 1750 to about 2% through the early 1980s. Since that time, population growth has slowed in most of the industrialized nations. In the period after 1960, population growth in Europe has been less than 1% annually, dropping to a low of 0.3% during the period from 1980 to 1989 (Table 5–2). During this same time, rates of population growth were around 1% or less annually in other developed areas such as the United States, Soviet Union, and Japan. Although there has been a slight decrease of the rate of increase in the less developed regions taken as a whole since 1990, the African population continues to increase at an annual rate approaching 2.5% (U.S. Bureau of the Census, 1984, 1996). A few countries recently torn by civil war are losing population due to emigration and death. Projections for such decreased population include countries previously part of the Soviet Union which had low rates of increase during the 1980s, but are now

TABLE 5–1. WORLD POPULATION FROM 8000 BC TO PRESENT

DATE	POPULATION IN MILLIONS	AVERAGE ANNUAL INCREASE		NO. OF GENERATIONS
		Millions	Percent	
8000 BC	10			
1 AD	300	0.036	0.06	266
1650	545	0.150	0.04	55
1750	728	1.8	0.29	
1800	906	3.5	0.44	
1850	1171	5.3	0.51	
1900	1608	8.7	0.64	13
1950[a]	2493	17.7	0.86	
1980[a]	4654	72.0	2.02	
1990[a]	5282	62.8	1.70	5
2000[b]	6091	65.8	1.40	

[a]Amounts and rates of increase affected by improved collection of data.
[b]Estimated data.
(Data for 8000 BC to 1950 from Broek J., Webb J. A geography of mankind. New York: McGraw-Hill, 1968; 1980 data from U.S. Bureau of the Census. Statistical abstract of the United States. Washington, D.C.: U.S. Government Printing Office, 1984; 1990 data and 2000 projected data from U.S. Bureau of the Census. Statistical abstract of the United States, 1996. Washington, D.C.: U.S. Government Printing Office, 1996.)

TABLE 5–2. WORLD POPULATION GROWTH BY CONTINENT, 1960–1989

REGION	MIDYEAR POPULATION 1960	ANNUAL RATE OF GROWTH (%) 1960– 1965	1965– 1970	1970– 1975	1975– 1980	1980– 1989
Africa	277	2.5	2.6	2.7	2.8	2.9
Asia	1715	2.0	2.5	2.3	1.9	1.9
Latin America	216	2.8	2.7	2.5	2.4	2.1
North America	199	1.5	1.1	1.1	1.0	0.9
Europe	425	0.9	0.7	0.6	0.4	0.3
U.S.S.R.	214	1.5	1.0	0.9	0.8	0.9
Oceania	16	2.1	2.1	1.9	1.3	1.5
World Total	3061	1.9	2.1	2.0	1.8	1.7
more developed regions	945	1.2	0.9	0.9	0.7	0.6
less developed regions	2116	2.2	2.6	2.4	2.1	2.1

(*Adapted from U.S. Bureau of the Census.* Statistical abstract of the United States, 1990 (110th ed.). *Washington, D.C.: U.S. Government Printing Office, 1990.*)

projected to have negative growth for the years 1990 to 2000; for example, Bosnia and Hercegovina (−5.1%) and The Republic of Georgia (−0.6%) (U.S. Bureau of the Census, 1996).

FACTORS AFFECTING POPULATION SIZE AND COMPOSITION

Population growth, in general, is dependent on both birth rates and death rates. Migration is a third factor that may affect the population dynamics of a defined geographic area. Thus, an area with high birth rates, low death rates, and a balance between migration into and out of the area will show an increase in population. With a stable migration situation and death rates equal to or higher than birth rates, the population size will remain the same or decrease. Table 5–3 shows actual and projected rates for these three factors in the United States between 1980 and 2005. Primarily because birth rates remain higher than death rates and there is a net positive migration, the population of the United States continues to increase.

Early world population growth probably was attributable largely to increasing birth rates since mortality remained high. In more recent times, particularly during the last 100 years, death rates for all age groups have dropped dramatically in most of the world, resulting in a concurrent increase in life expectancy. When birth rates remain the same or increase simultaneously with a drop in death rates, a population explosion occurs. This is what we currently observe in parts of Africa and, until the last 25 years, in Asia and Latin America.

Within countries, the rate of population growth is not the same for all subgroups of the population. In the United States, for example, the rate of growth for the white population has been lower than that of the nonwhite population, composed of numerous subgroups, including blacks, Hispanics, Native Americans, Asians, and others.

TABLE 5–3. UNITED STATES POPULATION GROWTH: COMPONENTS OF CHANGE, 1980–1995, AND PROJECTIONS, 1996–2005

| | RATE PER 1000 | MIDYEAR POPULATION | | |
| | | Birth | Death | |
YEAR	Net Growth Rate	Rate Increase	Rate Increase	Net Migration[a]
1980	11.1	16.0	8.6	4.2
1985	9.1	15.8	8.8	2.7
1990	10.3	16.6	8.6	2.3
1995	9.1	15.1	8.9	2.9
2000[b]	8.4	14.2	8.8	3.0
2005[b]	8.0	14.0	8.9	2.9

[a]Covers net international migration and movement of armed forces and federally affiliated citizens and their dependents.
[b]Projected.
(Adapted from Table 4, U.S. Bureau of the Census. Statistical abstract of the United States, 1996 [116th ed.]. Washington, D.C.: U.S. Government Printing Office, 1996.)

In 1982, it was estimated that at the observed rate of growth, by 2025 the white population of the United States would increase 21.2%, an annual average of 0.49%. Estimates for the increase in the nonwhite population during the same time were 65.7%, an annual average of 1.5% (U.S. Bureau of the Census, 1984), with the result that the U.S. nonwhite population would increase from 12.3% in 1982 to 16.9% in 2025. In fact, the percentage of the population that is nonwhite today is even greater than originally projected, as shown in Figure 5–1. This differential growth rate is a function of several factors; one of these being higher birth rates among the nonwhite population. Among blacks and Hispanics, the proportion of married women expecting to have four or more children was higher than among white women—12.0% and 12.9% respectively versus 8.0% for white women. A substantial immigration of Asians, particularly from Thailand, Vietnam, Japan, and Taiwan as well as Hispanics from Mexico, Cuba, and Central and South America since the 1970s has also contributed to a rapid increase in the proportion of the U.S. population that is nonwhite. In 1991 to 1993, of 3,705,400 immigrants, 1,073,500 were from Asia, 189,200 were from South America, and 1,286,500 were from Mexico, accounting for about two thirds of all immigrants. Only 438,900 immigrants to the U.S. were from Europe (U.S. Bureau of the Census, 1996). However, higher death rates among nonwhites, particularly under 45 years of age is also an important factor. Except for Asian-Pacific Islanders, rates of nonwhite deaths are higher than white rates until age 45.

CHANGES IN LIFE EXPECTANCY

In the Middle Ages, the average person had a short and uncertain life expectancy that varied somewhat by social class status. Aristocrats generally fared better than the common folk. Figure 5–2 shows typical survival curves for the people of York, England, during the 16th century. Although early death was common among the

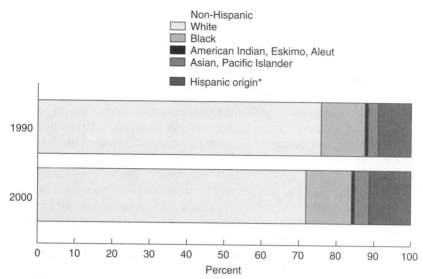

*Persons of Hispanic origin may be of any race.

Figure 5–1. Resident population by race: 1990 and 2000. (*Adapted from U.S. Bureau of the Census. Statistical abstract of the United States, 1996 [116th ed.]. Washington, D.C.: U.S. Government Printing Office, 1996.*)

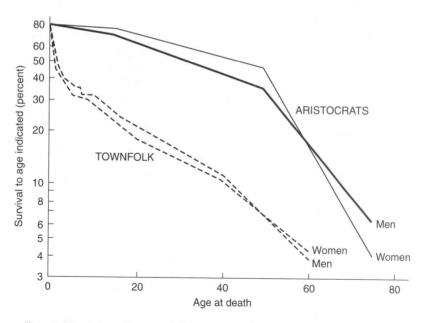

Figure 5–2. Survival curves for York, England, townsfolk and aristocrats in the 16th century. (*Adapted from Cowgill U.M. The people of York: 1538–1812. Scientific American, 1970; 22, 104–112.*)

townsfolk, with just over 10% living to age 40, close to half of the artistocracy lived to that age. The average person was constantly preyed upon by famine and disease, malign forces of nature, and the avarice and brutality of fellow countrymen. Widespread poverty was common. Methods of agriculture were crude and forces of nature such as floods, drought, unseasonable heat or cold, and an unusual number of insects, and other natural hazards of farming, some of which today can be controlled by scientific means, might destroy a peasant's entire crop. As a result, famines, both local and widespread, were common occurrences. Epidemic diseases such as influenza, pneumonia, diarrhea, smallpox, plague, or tuberculosis often accompanied famines, spreading rapidly among a population already weakened by starvation. Even in good years, epidemics were quite common. Poor sanitation and overcrowding facilitated the survival and spread of disease organisms. Poor nutrition increased death rates. Lack of hygiene led to high mortality from simple wound infection, postpartal infection, and infections encountered during infancy. The same situation exists today in many Third World countries. In other instances, special circumstances will produce these conditions in a population that previously did not experience such problems. Examples of special circumstances in this decade include the 1991 epidemic of cholera in Bangladesh that occurred following a typhoon and the high rates of morbidity and mortality experienced by Kurdish refugees after civil unrest in Iraq in the aftermath of the 1991 Gulf War.

In contrast to the Middle Ages and in some Third World countries today, average life expectancy in the United States and in other developed countries is long: 72.7 years for white males born in the United States in 1990 and 79.4 years for white females born at the same time. Before the 1950s, survival was lower for the group of children under 10 years of age because of high mortality among infants and children between the ages of 1 to 6. In contrast, for white women living in the U.S. in 1994, there is an almost constant proportion of the population surviving until age 50. Approximately 79.6% of the total U.S. population born in 1990 will survive to 65 years of age as compared with approximately 41% of the population born in 1901 (U.S. Bureau of the Census, 1996).

As in York, England, in the Middle Ages, however, we continue to observe differences in survival for various population subgroups. In the United States, for example, there are differences in survival at most ages by race, sex, and socioeconomic status. Life expectancy at birth is 64.5 years for a black male born in 1990 compared with 72.7 years for a white male (Fig. 5–3). Comparisons of life expectancy at different ages for whites and nonwhites and men and women are shown in Table 5–4. Women of both races have a longer life expectancy than do men of either race. Researchers have tried to explain these racial discrepancies as relating to socioeconomic (SES) conditions. For causes of death relating to substance use and abuse, evidence that racial differences are explained by differences in SES conditions is fairly strong. For others, such as racial disparities relating to hypertension, SES conditions appear to be only a partial explanation, since race differences persist within SES strata. Rates are higher among those in the lower SES strata than higher strata for all races, regardless of whether SES is measured by education or occupation (Lillie-Blanton et al, 1996). Socioeconomic inequalities in health are also

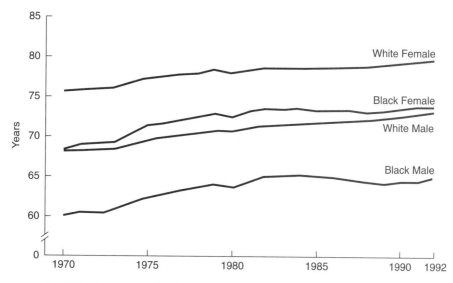

Figure 5–3. Life expectancy at birth by race and sex: United States, 1970–1992. (*Adapted from National Center for Health Statistics,* Health U.S., 1994. *Hyattsville, MD.: Public Health Service, 1995.*)

found in other countries. A study that examined SES variation in morbidity in 11 European countries found associations of SES with perceived general health, long-term disabilities, and chronic conditions (Mackenback et al, 1997). Gender differences in mortality and life expectancy are also not unique to the U.S., but are a worldwide phenomenon. One apparent explanation relates to riskier behaviors among men, including substance abuses such as smoking and violence. Worldwide, there are about two male deaths from violence for every female death (Murray & Lopez, 1997a).

Although life expectancies in Third World countries remain lower than in more industrialized nations, life expectancies, particularly among infants and young children, have been rising quickly in recent years as death rates have dropped. These changes have resulted from improvement in sanitation and living conditions

TABLE 5–4. AVERAGE EXPECTATION OF LIFE IN YEARS BY RACE AND SEX IN THE UNITED STATES, 1990

AGE	WHITES		BLACKS	
	Men	*Women*	*Men*	*Women*
At Birth	72.7	79.4	64.5	73.6
At 1 year	72.3	78.9	65.8	73.8
20	54.0	60.3	46.7	55.3
65	15.2	19.1	13.2	17.2

(*From U.S. Bureau of the Census.* Statistical abstract of the United States, 1996 [116th ed.]. *Washington, D.C.: U.S. Government Printing Office, 1996.*)

and from the introduction of medical technology for prevention and control of disease. Emphasis on prevention and control of infectious disease through environmental hygiene, improved housing and nutrition, vaccination programs, and use of antibiotics for treatment of infection has been a primary factor in permitting populations to live longer.

The rate of transitions in life expectancy has occurred more rapidly in some places than in others. How quickly death rates in a country drop is dependent on whether all these measures are introduced simultaneously, as in Cuba and China, or whether they were introduced gradually. The decrease in mortality in most Western countries occurred gradually over 100 to 200 years because major improvements in sanitation and housing began more than a century ago, before the development of the medical technology of the 20th century, such as vaccines and antibiotics. The transition in mortality and life expectancy was propelled by the social changes of the Industrial Revolution and accompanied by improved family and personal hygiene and improved nutrition. Countries that most recently began their prevention and control efforts have had access to these major technological advances. In most developing nations, the transition in disease mortality began around the 1940s and resulted largely from the introduction of medical technology simultaneously with a period of rapid social change (Omran, 1971; Murray & Lopez, 1997a, 1997b), although in most of these countries the transition in mortality rates is not complete. An example of such a transition is the rapid change in amebiasis in Mexico during the second half of this century (Trevino-Garcia-Manzo et al, 1994); concurrent with social and economic development and improved sanitary conditions, Mexico experienced a steady reduction in both the incidence and mortality of this disease.

EFFECTS OF MORTALITY RATE TRANSITIONS

Transitions in death rates produce several major effects on demographic patterns and social conditions. Four effects are discussed in the following paragraphs.

Change in Major Causes of Death.   Because infectious diseases are more likely to affect the very young, controlling infectious disease has shifted the average age of death to an older age. Degenerative diseases, more common as causes of death in older persons, continue to emerge as major causes of death as age at death increases. Chronic diseases such as heart disease are the most frequent causes of death from middle age onward. Table 5–5 shows the major causes of death in the United States in 1900 and 1995. Although infectious conditions topped the mortality lists in 1900, accounting for more than one-third of deaths, coronary heart disease, cancer, accidents, and stroke are currently the four major causes of death, accounting for nearly 70% of all deaths in the United States.

Similar shifts can be seen in countries that have more recently begun to reduce mortality from infectious disease. China, for example, after nearly 20 years of concentrated effort, has a proportion of deaths caused by heart disease, cancer, and stroke midway between the corresponding 1900 and current U.S. figures.

TABLE 5–5. LEADING CAUSES OF DEATH IN 1900 AND 1995 IN THE UNITED STATES[a]

	1900			1995		
Cause of Death	Deaths per 100,000 Persons	Percentage of all Deaths		Cause of Death	Deaths per 100,000 Persons	Percentage of all Deaths
All Causes	*1719.1*	*100.0*		*All Causes*	*502.9*	*100.0*
Influenza and pneumonia	202.2	11.8		Diseases of the heart	138.2	27.5
Tuberculosis (all forms)	194.4	11.3		Malignant neoplasms	129.8	25.8
Gastritis	142.7	8.3		Accidents	29.2	5.8
Diseases of the heart	137.4	8.0		Cerebrovascular diseases	26.7	5.3
Vascular lesions affecting the nervous system	106.9	6.2		Chronic obstructive lung disease	21.2	4.2
Chronic nephritis	81.0	4.7		Diabetes mellitus	13.2	2.6
Accidents	72.3	4.2		Influenza and pneumonia	13.0	2.6
Malignant neoplasms	64.0	3.7		Human Immunodeficiency Virus infection	11.1	2.2
Certain diseases of early infancy	62.6	3.6		Suicide	11.0	2.2
Diphtheria	40.3	2.3		Homicide	8.8	1.6
All other causes	615.3	35.9		All other causes	101.7	20.2

[a]All rates adjusted to 1940 U.S. population.
(*Data for 1900 adapted from National Center for Health Statistics.* Progress in Health Services, *1961; 10[2]; 1995 data adapted from Table 128, U.S. Bureau of the Census,* Statistical abstract of the United States; 1997 [117th ed.]. *Washington, D.C.; 1997.*)

Table 5–6 shows the top 12 causes of death in the world in 1990. Ischemic heart disease, cerebrovascular disease, and chronic obstructive pulmonary disease are among the top 12 in developed countries and countries in transition, such as China. Worldwide, the top ten causes account for 52% of all deaths (Murray & Lopez, 1997a). However, infections such as lower respiratory infections, tuberculosis, measles, and malaria are more common in developing countries.

At the request of the World Bank and in collaboration with the World Health Organization, the Global Burden of Disease Study, begun in 1992, classified causes of death and disability into three categories: group I causes—communicable diseases, maternal, perinatal, and nutritional disorders; group 2—all noncommunicable diseases; and group 3—all unintentional and intentional injuries. The distribution of these as causes of death in developing and developed countries is shown in Table 5–7. Several instances stand out. First, for every cause of death, rates in developing countries far exceed those in developed countries. However, group 1 causes account for only 6.1% of deaths in developed countries, but 41.9% of deaths in developing countries. Group 2 deaths, in contrast, accounted for 86.2% of all deaths in developed countries, but only 47.4% in developing countries. The contribution of some

TABLE 5–6. RANKINGS FOR THE TOP 12 CAUSES OF DEATH WORLDWIDE IN 1990 AND PROJECTED FOR 2020

RANK	CAUSES IN 1990	CAUSES IN 2020
1	Ischemic heart disease	Ischemic heart disease
2	Cerebrovascular disease	Cerebrovascular disease
3	Lower respiratory infections	Chronic obstructive pulmonary disease
4	Diarrheal diseases	Lower respiratory infections
5	Perinatal disorders	Trachea, bronchus, and lung cancers
6	Chronic obstructive pulmonary disease	Road traffic accidents
7	Tuberculosis	Tuberculosis
8	Measles	Stomach cancer
9	Road traffic accidents	Human immunodeficiency virus
10	Trachea, bronchus, and lung cancers	Self-inflicted injuries
11	Malaria	Diarrheal diseases
12	Cirrhosis of the liver	Cirrhosis of the liver

(*Compiled from Table 1, Murray C.J.L., Lopez A.D.* Alternative projections of mortality and disability by cause 1990–2020: Global Burden of Disease Study. *Lancet, 1997;349,1498–1504.*)

TABLE 5–7. DEATHS ($\times 10^3$) IN DEVELOPED AND DEVELOPING AREAS OF THE WORLD FOR SPECIFIC CAUSES OF DISEASES IN 1990

	DEVELOPED COUNTRIES	DEVELOPING COUNTRIES
All Causes	10,912	39,554
Total Group 1 Causes	667	16,573
Infectious and parasitic diseases	163	9,166
Respiratory infections	389	3,992
Maternal disorders	3	451
Perinatal disorders	82	2,361
Nutritional deficiencies	30	604
Group 2 Disorders	9,411	18,730
Cardiovascular disease	5,245	9,082
Malignant neoplasms	2,413	3,611
Respiratory disorders	424	1,426
Digestive disorders	424	1,426
Neuropsychiatric disorders	274	426
Diabetes mellitus	50	93
Group 3 Disorders	834	4,251
Unintentional injuries	552	2,682
Intentional injuries	282	1,596

(*Compiled from Table 2, Murray C.J.L., Lopez A.D.* Mortality by cause for eight regions of the world: Global Burden of Disease Study. *Lancet, 1997;349,1269–1276.*)

key risk factors to the overall disease picture helps illustrate why these patterns are associated with a particular distribution of diseases. Table 5–8 shows the extent to which ten key risk factors contribute to the burden of illness, expressed as disability-adjusted life years (DALYs). Factors such as malnutrition, poor water, sanitation, and hygiene are major problems in developing regions, while tobacco, alcohol, and other lifestyle factors stand out as major contibutors to ill health in developed nations.

Change in Age Distribution of the Population.   As epidemics of infectious diseases re-cede, fertility improves. In conjunction with improved child survival, an increased number of children will grow to adulthood, moving in waves up through the population and changing the age distribution of the population. Figure 5–4 shows the population pyramids for the United States in 1900 and 1995. The 1900 pyramid is similar to that of the Middle Ages and of many developing countries today, which are currently beginning the transition away from infectious diseases as major causes of death. The pyramid is characterized by a large number of persons in the younger age ranges and a rapid reduction in the proportion of the population in each successive age group. This results in a small number of individuals in the older age groups. The pyramid for 1995 is fairly typical of countries that have completed the transition to death primarily due to chronic, degenerative diseases. This pyramid shows a broadening of population in the middle and older age ranges and a substantial decrease in the very young ages, reflecting the lower birth rates that have resulted from the use of family planning techniques.

Change in the Sex Composition of the Population.   Improvement in the survival of women during the childbearing years leads to a change in the sex composition of the population that becomes more marked as the population ages because men have higher mortality from heart disease and other degenerative diseases at younger ages

TABLE 5–8. PERCENT OF WORLDWIDE DISABILITY-ADJUSTED LIFE YEARS ATTRIBUTABLE TO TEN RISK FACTORS IN DEVELOPED AND DEVELOPING COUNTRIES, 1990

RISK FACTOR	DEVELOPED COUNTRIES	DEVELOPING COUNTRIES	WORLD
Malnutrition	0.0	18.0	15.9
Poor water, sanitation, and hygiene	0.1	7.6	6.8
Unsafe sex	2.1	3.7	3.5
Tobacco	12.1	1.4	2.6
Alcohol	9.6	2.7	3.5
Occupation	4.6	2.5	2.7
Hypertension	4.7	0.9	1.4
Physical activity	4.0	0.6	1.0
Illicit drugs	1.9	0.4	0.6
Air pollution	1.5	0.4	0.5

(*Compiled from Table 5 of Murray C.J.L., Lopez A.D. Global mortality, disability, and the contribution of risk factors: Global Burden of Disease Study. Lancet, 1997; 349;1436–1442.*)

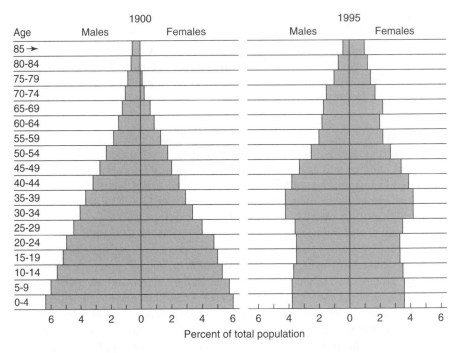

Figure 5–4. U.S. population pyramids, 1900 and 1995. (*Data compiled from U.S. Bureau of the Census. Historical statistics, colonial times to 1978, Series A 23–25, and U.S. Bureau of the Census. Statistical abstract of the United States, 1996, [116th ed.]. Washington, D.C.: U.S. Government Printing Office, 1996.*)

than do women. The male to female ratio among children younger than age 14 in the United States in 1995 was 104.9 to 100.0. By ages 25 to 44, the ratio is 99.2 to 100.0 and continues to drop. For persons aged 65 and older, the ratio is 69.0 to 100.0 (U.S Bureau of the Census, 1996).

Change in the Major Causes of Morbidity.   Although social changes are a major contributing factor in the transition from infectious to chronic diseases, improved health and longevity bring about further social changes and pressures. These include increased efficiency and productivity of the work force, increased economic expectation, the advent of the nuclear family, destruction in group cohesion, and problems of older citizens who face years of life with no productive employment, potentially rising inflation, chronic health problems that may limit mobility, and a lack of family members in close geographic proximity to offer physical care and emotional support. Unfamiliarity with recent and rapid changes in technology, such as voice mail, computerized phone options, and the Internet, make many older folks feel even more isolated, particularly as common impairments experienced by the elderly—those of hearing, sight, and cognition—make coping with this new technology even more difficult. In the presence of these social conditions, major causes of morbidity are often "man-made" diseases, for example, drug or alcohol abuse,

TABLE 5–9. INCIDENCE OF ACUTE CONDITIONS PER 100 PERSONS PER YEAR BY AGE AND CONDITION GROUP:
UNITED STATES, 1994

SEX AND CONDITION GROUP	LESS THAN 5 YEARS	5–17 YEARS	18–24 YEARS	25–44 YEARS	45–64 YEARS	65 YEARS AND OLDER
Infective and parasitic diseases	54.7	41.9	18.5	14.6	7.7	5.2
Common cold	68.5	29.4	26.1	22.4	16.6	12.3
Influenza	37.3	46.3	38.7	37.8	25.9	18.3
Digestive system	10.5	8.3	7.4	4.7	4.1	5.6
Injuries	25.6	26.0	32.7	25.0	17.2	19.6

(*Data compiled from U.S. Bureau of the Census.* Statistical abstract of the United States, 1996 [116th ed.]. *Washington, D.C.: U.S Government Printing Office, 1996.*)

mental illness, accidents, and occupational-related diseases. These morbidities may be divided into acute and chronic illnesses and rates vary by age, race, and sex. Table 5–9 shows U.S. incidence rates of common acute conditions by age. Table 5–10 shows U.S. prevalence for major chronic conditions for the noninstitutionalized population. The major causes of morbidity and mortality for men and women and for various age groups are discussed in Section II of this book in relation to interventions for primary, secondary, and tertiary prevention.

Many of these acute and chronic conditions may be preventable through public health interventions such as sanitation or immunization. Those that are not

TABLE 5–10. PREVALENCE PER 1000 PERSONS OF CHRONIC CONDITIONS WITH HIGHEST PREVALENCE AND HIGHEST
MORTALITY IN THE UNITED STATES CIVILIAN, NONINSTITUTIONALIZED POPULATION, 1990–1992

DISEASES WITH HIGHEST PREVELANCE	PREVALENCE PER 1000	DISEASES WITH HIGHEST MORTALITY	MORTALITY PER 100,000 POPULATION
Deformities or orthopedic impairments	140.6	Ischemic heart disease	241.5
		Senile dementia or organic brain	233.7
Chronic sinusitis	135.6	syndrome	
Arthritis	127.8	Cerebrovascular disease	182.1
High blood pressure	110.0	Arthritis or rheumatism	179.1
Hay fever or allergic rhinitis without	96.7	Essential hypertension	156.4
asthma		Other heart disease	152.3
Deafness and other hearing	93.5	Diabetes mellitus	124.2
impairments		Psychoses other than senile	110.6
Heart disease	82.4	dementia	
Chronic bronchitis	51.8	Congestive heart failure	106.8
Asthma	46.2	Atherosclerosis	74.7
Headache (excluding tension headache)	41.3		

(*Adapted from Table A and Table B, Collins J.G. Prevalence of selected chronic conditions: United States, 1990–1992. National Center for Health Statistics. Vital Health Statistics, 1997; 10[194]. Hyattsville, MD., DHHS Publ. No. [PHS] 97–1522.*)

preventable require medical and nursing intervention. In any event, awareness of which conditions are most common in each age and sex group and of the natural history of the conditions, enables health professionals to function more effectively. This is particularly important within the context of managed care, where population-based planning must provide services ranging from prevention through managing death. Without this information, planning how to deliver needed services within the resources available would be impossible.

OUTLOOK FOR THE FUTURE

Previous epidemiological transitions in populations have been characterized by a substitution of degenerative diseases for infectious diseases and an eventual increase in life expectancy at birth to close to 80 years of age. However, death and disability from these degenerative diseases occurs early in life in countries in the early stages of the epidemiological transition. This can be illustrated with data from the Global Burden of Disease Study (Murray & Lopez, 1997a,b,c). Life expectancy across the regions studied ranged from 48.4 years for males and 51.0 for females in Subsaharan Africa to 73.4 for males and 80.5 for females in established market economies of Europe. A measure of the percentage of life lived with disability adjusted for severity of the disability indicates a range from 15.3 for males and 14.9 for females in Subsaharan Africa to 8.1 for males and 8.3 for females in established market economies. In Latin American countries, which are midway in the transition, life expectancies are on the order of 65.8 for males and 70.3 for females, but both sexes can still expect about 12% of that life to be lived with disability. Thus, in later stages of the transition, not only is life longer, but it is also more disability-free.

Other changes that are likely to accompany the advanced stages of the epidemiological transition are: (1) improvement in survival concentrated among older populations; (2) improvement in survival occurring at the same rate for men and women; and (3) age patterns of morbidity by cause remaining the same, but a progressive shift in the age distribution of deaths for degenerative diseases toward older ages (Olshansky & Ault, 1986).

In the United States, although degenerative diseases remain with us as major causes of death, both the risk of dying and the age of experiencing disability from them is progressively redistributing from younger to older ages (Olshansky & Ault, 1986). These changes will likely have major impact on the size and relative proportion of the population that is in advanced age groups and on the health and vitality of the elderly.

The redistribution of diseases affecting older, rather than younger individuals is due in part to development of new drugs and improved methods of diagnosing and treating degenerative diseases. These factors have slowed the rate of chronic disease progression and reduced case fatality rates. Advances in medical technology have also been accompanied by reduction in the U.S. population of the risk factors for degenerative disease, for example, decline in smoking, more exercise, and better dietary habits that continue to take hold. Further, federal health care programs that began in the 1960s targeted primarily the elderly and poor segments of the population and may have contributed to mortality declines by reducing inequities in access to health care (Gillum et al, 1984).

In 1979, the first Surgeon General's Report on Health Promotion and Disease Prevention, "Healthy People," was issued (U.S. Department of Health, Education, and Welfare, 1979). To improve health of Americans at five major life stages: infancy, childhood, adolescence and young adulthood, middle age, and old age, the report reviewed preventable threats to health and established broad national goals to be achieved by 1990. These goals were expressed as targeted reductions in death rates or disability days. Subsequently, the Public Health Service identified 226 quantitative health promotion and disease prevention objectives for 1990 in "Promoting Health/Preventing Disease: Objectives for the Nation" (U.S. Department of Health and Human Services, 1980; U.S. Department of Health, Education, and Welfare, 1986). These provided a common strategy and frame of reference for state and local government initiatives. By 1988, the United States had made significant progress toward meeting half the objectives (Stoto et al, 1990). The U.S. Public Health Service and the Institute of Medicine later convened a Year 2000 Health Objectives Consortium of more than 300 national professional and voluntary organizations and state and territorial health departments to guide the hearing process for development of goals for the year 2000. More than 800 individuals and organizations submitted testimony toward development of goals for health promotion and disease prevention. Final goals set priorities and focused more on needs of special racial subgroups in order to decrease disparities in health between groups. These final goals were linked to epidemiological and experimental evidence that a method was efficacious and would contribute to achieving each goal (Stoto et al, 1990).

An important question is whether declining mortality at older ages will result in additional years of health or years of frail health. Manton (1982) suggested that acquisition of healthier lifestyles on a population scale may postpone clinical manifestations of chronic diseases and simultaneously slow the process of aging. The extent to which the increasing older population remains healthy has profound implications regarding living arrangements, costs of health care, demand for health care rationing, and the case mix of elderly patients in long-term and acute care facilities. Rice and Feldman (1983) showed that projected changes in the age composition of the U.S. population from 1980 to 2040 will account for 6% of the expected one-half billion increase in annual physician visits, more than half the expected 100% increase in total short stay hospital days, a 350% increase in the total number of nursing home residents, and a $103 billion increase in the health care budget for the population 65 and older (assuming constant 1980 dollars). The extent of impact on the health care industry ultimately depends on the extent to which the aging population remains healthy. We can be sure that this transition will require new ways of thinking about disease, mortality, and how life at advanced ages will be lived.

REFERENCES

Gillum R. F., Folsom A. R., Blackburn, H. (1984) Decline in coronary heart disease mortality: Old questions and new facts. *American Journal of Medicine, 76,* 1055–1065.

Lillie-Blanton M., Parsons P. E., Gayle H., Dievler A. (1996) Racial differences in health: Not just black and white, but shades of gray. *Annual Review Public Health, 17,* 411–418.

Mackenbach J. P., Kunst A. E., Cavelaars A. E., Groenhof F., Geurts J. J. (1997) Socioeconomic inequalities in morbidity and mortality in western Europe. The EU Working Group on Socioeconomic Inequalities in Health. *Lancet, 349*(9066), 1655–1659.

Manton, K. G. (1982) Changing concepts of morbidity and mortality in the elderly population. *Milbank Memorial Fund Quarterly/Health and Society, 60*(2), 183–244.

Murray C. J. L., Lopez A. D. (1997a) Alternative projections of mortality and disability by cause 1990–2020: Global Burden of Disease Study. *Lancet, 349,* 1498–1504.

Murray C. J. L., Lopez A. D. (1997b) Regional patterns of disability-free life expectancy and disability-adjusted life expectancy: Global Burden of Disease Study. *Lancet, 349,* 1347–1352.

Murray C. J. L., Lopez A. D. (1997c) Global mortality, disability, and the contribution of risk factors: Global Burden of Disease Study. *Lancet, 349,* 1436–1442.

Olshansky S. J., Ault B. (1986) The fourth stage of the epidemiologic transition: The age of delayed degenerative disease. *Milbank Memorial Fund Quarterly, 3,* 355–391.

Omran A. R. (1971) The epidemiologic transition: A theory of the epidemiology of population change. *Milbank Memorial Fund Quarterly, 49,* 509–516.

Rice D. P., Feldman J. J. (1983) Living longer in the United States: Demographic changes and health needs of the elderly. *Milbank Memorial Fund Quarterly/Health and Society, 61*(3), 362–369.

Stoto M. A., Behrens R., Rosenmont C. [Eds.]. (1990) *Healthy People 2000. Citizens Chart the Course.* Washington, D.C.: Institute of Medicine, National Academy Press.

Trevino-Garcia-Manzo N., Escandon-Romero C., Escobedo-de-la-Pena J., Hernandez-Ramos J. M., Fierro-Hernandez H. (1994) Amebiasis in the epidemiologic transition in Mexico: Its morbidity and mortality trends in the Mexican Institute of Social Security. *Archives of Medical Research, 25*(4), 393–399.

U.S. Bureau of the Census. (1984) *Statistical abstract of the United States, 1985* (105th ed.). Washington, D.C.: U.S. Government Printing Office.

U.S. Bureau of the Census. (1990) *Statistical abstract of the United States, 1990* (110th ed.). Washington, D.C.: U.S. Government Printing Office.

U.S. Bureau of the Census. (1996) *Statistical abstract of the United States, 1996* (116th ed.). Washington, D.C.: U.S. Government Printing Office.

U.S. Department of Health & Human Services. (1980) *Promoting Health/Preventing Disease: Objectives for the Nation.* Washington, D.C.: U.S. Government Printing Office, November.

U.S. Department of Health, Education, and Welfare. (1979) *Healthy People: The Surgeon Generals Report on Health Promotion and Disease Prevention.* (Pub. No. PHS. 79–55071). Washington, D.C.: U.S. Government Printing Office.

U.S. Department of Health, Education, and Welfare. (1986) *Objectives for the Nation: A Mid-course Review.* Washington, D.C.: U.S. Government Printing Office, November.

Epidemiology and Control
of Diseases
# of Infectious Origin

 lthough epidemiology has its roots in the investigation of outbreaks of infectious disease, during the middle part of this century more effort was expended on developing methods for and conducting studies on the etiology of diseases of noninfectious origin. More recently, the resurgence of infectious disease worldwide has refocused attention on the methods of infectious disease epidemiology. These methods were developed initially for investigating acute outbreaks of infectious disease. As more infectious diseases producing chronic disease were recognized, methodological considerations derived from the study of noninfectious disease were also applied to diseases of infectious origin; thus, separating the two is somewhat artificial. Nonetheless, the methods for dealing with investigation and control of infectious acute epidemics remain an essential part of epidemiology and public health practice. This chapter focuses on traditional methods of investigation and control of infectious diseases and discusses methods for control of infectious disease using the natural history model presented in Chapter 2. Specific examples of the use of the natural history of a disease in determining interventions for primary, secondary, and tertiary prevention are presented. This is followed by a discussion of methods for investigation of an outbreak. Information on diseases common in the United States and worldwide is also presented. Finally, clinical contributions to control of infectious disease are discussed.

HISTORICAL OVERVIEW OF INFECTIOUS DISEASES IN THE WORLD

Epidemiological investigation originated in response to outbreaks of infectious diseases. Study of the outbreaks of diseases, such as plague, cholera, and smallpox in Europe in the 19th century, identified the etiology and mode of transmission of these diseases. Subsequently, measures were instituted for their control. By the mid-20th century, large explosive epidemics of communicable diseases were relatively rare and confined mostly to developing countries in Africa, Asia, and South and Central America. In these developing countries, controllable communicable diseases remain primary public health problems. Member states of the World Health Organization (WHO) from Africa and Asia, for example, list malaria and other parasitic diseases, tuberculosis, malnutrition, diarrheal diseases, leprosy, respiratory diseases other than tuberculosis, venereal diseases, measles, poliomyelitis, and tetanus (particularly neonatal tetanus) as their most important health problems. Changes in global climate, increasing population growth, urbanization, mass migration and movement of refugees and displaced persons, and poverty are all factors that increase the challenge of controlling these diseases.

Smaller outbreaks from a variety of infections continued to occur in limited geographic areas elsewhere in the world. But many developed nations let down their guard. The U.S. Surgeon General, William Stewart, announced in 1967, that the United States could "close the book on infectious disease." This optimistic prediction was based on an expectation that the success of vaccines and antibiotics would expand and conquer infectious disease (Pennisi, 1996). In recent years, however, diseases such as tuberculosis, cholera, and typhus, which had been under control for decades, resurfaced along with acquired immunodeficiency syndrome (AIDS) and new food- and waterborne infections. These accounted for a 58% increase in infectious disease mortality rates between 1980 and 1992 in the United States (Pennisi, 1996) where public health officials are currently concerned with outbreaks of hepatitis, sexually transmitted diseases, salmonellosis, hospital-acquired infections, measles, herpes, tuberculosis, influenza, and other respiratory infections. European public health officials are also on alert as a rising tide of infectious disease around the world—17 million deaths in 1995—has prompted the European Union nations to intensify efforts to coordinate outbreak surveillance (Koenig, 1996a). Ease of travel, mass migration of refugees and displaced persons, and international distribution of food products contribute to spread outbreaks, while emergence of new viral and bacterial strains hinders control efforts. The European surveillance network tracked down 28 outbreaks of Legionairre's disease in

5 years, most contracted by tourists at hotels in warm climates and not diagnosed until they returned home. An outbreak of a rare *Salmonella (S. agona,* phage type 15) among approximately 25 British citizens in 1996 was traced to an Israeli-made corn snack, which also caused outbreaks in Israel and the United States (Koenig, 1996b). Rates of other infectious conditions (eg, malaria) have fluctuated in relation to immigration and veterans of the armed forces returning from endemic areas. Further, changes in the environment have modified the natural history of many diseases and human-produced or artificial factors have changed the susceptibility of the human host to these infections. These factors have resulted from the broader use of immunosuppressive and cytotoxic drugs (eg, in transplantation of organs, for cancer treatment), from nutritional or metabolic deficiencies depressing host resistance (eg, severity of measles in West Africa), and from the increased use of antibiotics that modify the normal flora and make some areas of the body more vulnerable to pathogens. Resistance of diseases to antimicrobials has had a deadly impact on control of such diseases as tuberculosis, malaria, cholera, dysentery, and pneumonia; people with infections remain ill longer and are at greater risk of dying. Also, epidemics are prolonged (WHO, 1996). Familiarity with infectious diseases and methods of control remain important, therefore, in order to prevent future outbreaks.

MECHANISMS OF CAUSATION IN INFECTIOUS DISEASE

The cycle of disease transmission is a concept important to the prepathogenic and earliest pathogenic phase of the disease natural history. This cycle is illustrated in Figure 6–1. Three elements are crucial to maintenance of the transmission cycle: (1) the agent, (2) a susceptible host, and (3) the environment. Furthermore, requirements for maintenance of the transmission cycle include a reservoir, a portal of exit from the reservoir, a means of transport to the susceptible host (mode of transmission), and a portal of entry to the host. Each of these is discussed in the following sections.

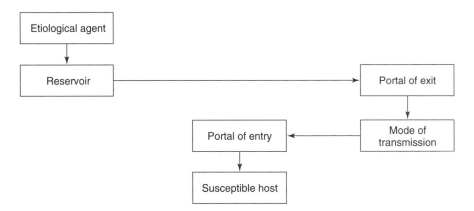

Figure 6–1. The cycle of infectious disease transmission.

The Agent

Infectious agents are invading, living parasites, either plant or animal, including metazoa, protozoa, fungi, bacteria, rickettsia, and virus. Table 6–1 lists some important diseases caused by each of these classes of infectious agents. These agents produce disease in a human host through one of three mechanisms:

1. Production of toxin
2. Invasion and infection
3. Production of an immune response in the host that produces disease

An example of disease that results from a toxin produced by an infectious agent is staphylococcal food poisoning. The food contaminated with *Staphylococ-*

TABLE 6–1. DISEASES CAUSED BY VARIOUS TYPES OF INFECTIOUS AGENTS

TYPE OF AGENT	DISEASE	SPECIFIC AGENT
Metazoa and protozoa	Hookworm	*Filaria*
	Acute amoebic dysentery	*Endamoeba histolytica*
Fungi	Histoplasmosis	*Histoplasma capsulatum*
	Athlete's foot	*Trichophyton rubrum*
Protozoan	Malaria	*Plasmodium*
Bacteria	Strep throat, scarlet fever, rheumatic heart disease	*Streptococcus*
	Syphilis	*Treponema pallidum*
	Tuberculosis	*Mycobacterium tuberculosis*
	Plague	*Yersinia pestus*
	Legionnaire's disease	*Legionella pneumophilia*
Rickettsia	Typhus (classical louseborne)	*Typhus exanthematicus*
	Rocky Mountain spotted fever	*Rickettsia rickettsii*
Viruses	Common cold and other acute upper respiratory infections	Rhinovirus, coronavirus
	Measles	Filterable virus
	Mumps	Paramyxovirus
	Chickenpox	Herpesvirus (varicella zoster)
	Polio	Poliovirus
	Encephalitis	Alphavirus, flavivirus
	Rabies	Rhabdovirus
	Yellow fever	Yellow fever virus
	Infectious hepatitis	IH virus
	Serum hepatitis	SH virus
	AIDS	HIV virus
	Herpes	Herpesvirus

cus produces a medium in which the organism can multiply. The organism produces a toxin and when the food is consumed, the toxin produces illness. This is why symptoms of staphylococcal food poisoning appear soon after the food is consumed. In contrast, *Salmonella* food poisoning does not produce symptoms until 12 to 24 hours after consumption of the food. Because the *Salmonella* produces disease through invasion and infection of the gastrointestinal mucosa, symptomatic response requires some time. One recent disease of concern thought to be an example of the third method of disease production, through the immune response of the host, is AIDS.

Host-related properties of an agent are infectivity, immunogenicity, pathogenicity, and virulence. *Infectivity* is the ability to lodge and multiply in a host, thus the ability to infect a host. The basic laboratory measure of infectivity is the number of infective particles needed to establish an infection. Ideally, epidemiologists would measure infectivity by using an infection rate. However, since measuring the infection rate requires a serological survey, a more useful measure of this property for epidemiologists is the *secondary attack rate.* For contact-transmitted infections, this is the frequency of infection occurrence among susceptible individuals within one incubation period after exposure to a primary case.

Infectivity can be detected through the presence of agent-specific antibodies produced by the host. The ability of an agent to induce such specific response in the host is called *antigenicity* or *immunogenicity.* Thus, when a serological survey of the exposed population can be conducted, an *infection rate (IR)* can be calculated:

$$IR = \frac{\text{No. of persons with antibody response}}{\text{Total no. exposed}}$$

Ideally persons with prior exposure, because they are not susceptible and have measurable antibody response, would be removed from both the numerator and the denominator, but unless baseline serological data on the specific population are available, this is not possible. Estimates of the percentage of the general population with antibody response can provide a guide.

The secondary attack rate and the infection rate permit us to specify infectious diseases according to the relative infectivity of their causal agents. Table 6–2 shows the relative degree of infectivity for some common causal agents. Diseases that have high infectivity, such as measles or chickenpox, may be expected to spread quickly among a susceptible population. Leprosy, in contrast, appears to have low infectivity, requiring up to 30 years of close contact for successful transmission. However, this delay may also reflect a long period of incubation.

Pathogenicity is the ability of an agent to produce disease. Although an agent may successfully infect a host (lodge and multiply and produce an antibody response), it may not induce the signs or symptoms of disease. Whether the disease results from infection depends on such factors as the rapidity and extent to which the agent multiplies in the host, the extent of tissue damage resulting from agent

TABLE 6–2. SOME WELL-KNOWN INFECTIOUS DISEASES ORDERED ACCORDING TO THREE
HOST-RELATED PROPERTIES OF THEIR AGENTS

RELATIVE DEGREE	INFECTIVITY BASIS: SECONDARY ATTACK RATE[a]	PATHOGENICITY BASIS: INFECTED WITH DISEASE Total Infected	VIRULENCE BASIS: SEVERE (EG, FATAL) CASES Total Cases
High	Smallpox Measles Chickenpox Poliomyelitis Ebola	Smallpox Rabies Measles Chickenpox Common cold AIDS Ebola	Rabies Smallpox Tuberculosis Hantavirus Ebola AIDS
Intermediate	Rubella Mumps Common cold	Rubella Mumps	Poliomyelitis
Low	Tuberculosis	Poliomyelitis Tuberculosis	Measles
Very low	Leprosy (?)	Leprosy (?)	Rubella Chickenpox Common cold

[a]Limited to contact-transmitted diseases.

multiplication, and whether the agent produces a toxin. In populations, pathogenicity of an agent is measured by the following rate:

$$\text{Pathogenicity} = \frac{\text{No. infected persons with clinical disease}}{\text{Total no. infected persons}}$$

The rate is specific to the relevant time frame for the current outbreak. The numerator is those persons with detectable signs and symptoms of disease; the denominator is all those with antibodies to the disease organism.

Common childhood diseases, such as measles and chickenpox, are highly pathogenic; nearly all infected individuals show characteristic disease. For polio, however, despite the severity of characteristic disease, infection produces typical paralytic polio only once in about 300 to 1,000 times (Fox et al, 1970).

Virulence refers to the severity of the disease produced and is measured by the case fatality rate when death is the criterion for severity of disease.

$$\text{Case fatality rate} = \frac{\text{No. of fatal cases}}{\text{Total no. of cases}}$$

In other instances, criteria for severity may not be death but rather, severe, permanent sequelae, such as paralysis in the case of polio.

These measures provide a means of population surveillance, allowing public health officials to assess the nature of the problem they are facing to plan for intervention. Given limited fiscal resources, decisions must be made regarding which diseases should receive emphasis. An infectious disease caused by an agent of high infectivity but low pathogenicity and virulence is probably a poorer candidate for such resources than is one with low infectivity but with high pathogenicity or virulence, or both.

The Environment

Environment may be defined as all external conditions and influences affecting the life of an organism. Physical, biological, and socioeconomic environments provide reservoirs and modes of transmission for the agent. Physical environment includes the geological structure of an area and the availability of resources, such as water and flora, that influence the number and variety of animal reservoirs and arthropod vectors. Weather, climate, and season are important influences on these factors.

The socioeconomic environment contributes to the types of infectious agents in a location because social and economic conditions relate to the extent of environmental sanitation, pasteurization of milk, disposal of garbage and excreta, and the availability of medical facilities for immunization and medical care.

Finally, there is the biological environment, which includes other living plants and animals that may serve as either the reservoir or as the vector for transmission of an infectious agent.

Reservoirs.   Because the agent is a living organism, it requires a place to live and multiply. The habitat of the agent is called the *reservoir*. It may be any human, animal, arthropod, plant, soil, or inanimate matter that provides an environment for survival or reproduction. The reservoir is therefore intimately related to the transmission cycle of the agent in nature. In the simplest cycle, the reservoir is the human body. For the majority of infectious diseases to which humans are subject, such as viral and bacterial respiratory infections, most staphylococcal and streptococcal infections, or venereal diseases, humans are both the host and the reservoir. Human reservoirs are individuals who have been infected. They may be acute clinical cases or they may be one of the four types of carriers. A *"carrier"* is any person or animal that harbors a particular infectious agent but does not have discernible clinical disease and serves as a potential source of infection. When acute clinical cases are the reservoir and source of the infectious agent, disease control can be affected by isolating the individual until the period when he or she is infectious to other individuals has passed, thus preventing spread of the infection. This approach to control is effective only when the infectious period follows observable symptoms. Such an approach is ineffective for controlling the spread of infection in diseases that have a stage in the natural history that includes an *incubating carrier.* This type of carrier is an individual who has been exposed to the disease organism before developing observable symptoms. By the time symptoms appear, the individual may have exposed many other persons to the infectious organism. This situation is present for many childhood infections, such as measles and chickenpox.

Other types of carriers are inapparent carriers, convalescent carriers, and chronic carriers. An *inapparent carrier* is an infected individual whose infection remains subclinical; the carrier never develops observable symptoms but is shedding the organism and exposing others. A *convalescent carrier* is an infected individual who no longer has acute disease but who remains infectious to others because of continued shedding of the organism. The infectious state may remain for weeks to months after symptoms are gone. Cholera and *Salmonella* gastroenteritis are diseases that have a convalescent carrier state. Typhoid Mary is an infamous example of the chronic-carrier type. *Chronic carriers* continue to harbor the viable organism indefinitely and remain infectious to others although they have no symptoms themselves. Hospital workers who are chronic staphylococcal carriers, for example, can be a hazard to the patient whose immune state is compromised.

Some agents are free-living in the environment, where, for example, soil and water serve as the reservoirs. The soil serves as reservoir for tetanus spores and for the rickettsia responsible for Legionnaire's disease. The cholera vibrio lives in organic matter found in water.

Animals are the reservoirs for other diseases of humans. Dogs, bats, and small wild animals are the reservoir for rabies; cows, pigs, and goats for brucellosis; and sheep and cattle for anthrax. Five cases of the plague in Colorado and Arizona in the summer of 1996 were traced to its reservoir in fleas, which live on small wild animals in the mountains. In this case, either the humans or their pets had been exposed while walking through a prairie dog colony. One of the two fatal cases contracted the disease from her cat. In such instances the transmission cycle is complex, involving an intermediate host, the wild animal in this case, the prairie dog, as well as the cat (Centers for Disease Control, 1997a). A useful source of information about reservoirs and transmission cycles of specific infectious conditions is *Control of Communicable Disease in Man,* a handbook published by the American Public Health Association (Benenson, 1990).

Transmission.   The life cycle (transmission cycle) of an infectious agent is dependent on the reservoir where the agent resides and multiplies and on how it is transported from the reservoir to a susceptible human host. Such transport or transmission may be made by direct or indirect means. *Indirect transmission* is generally provided by a *vector,* which is some form of a living organism, or by a *vehicle,* which is an inanimate substance such as dust, water, or food. The malaria parasite, *Plasmodium,* for example, lives and breeds in swamps from where it is transported by the mosquito to the human host. Airborne transmission by droplet nuclei also occurs between one infected person and another host. These particles remain suspended in air. This is also a mode of transmission for influenza. *Direct transmission* is the immediate transfer of an infectious agent from the reservoir, including another infected host, to an appropriate portal of entry in a susceptible host. This may involve direct contact between persons, such as kissing or sexual intercourse, or spread by droplets, as in sneezing and coughing. Direct exposure of susceptible tissues to such agents as bacterial spores lying on soil is another method of direct transmission.

Portals of entry include the conjunctiva of the eye, the portal of entry for conjunctivitis; skin breaks as with hepatitis B, transmitted via needles to the blood; the gastrointestinal tract as with food poisoning, hepatitis A, or cholera; the respiratory tract as with influenza; the genitals as with venereal disease and toxic shock syndrome; and the urinary tract opening as with cystitis. These portals of entry also serve as portals of exit.

The cycle of disease transmission can be broken by eliminating the reservoir, by eliminating the means of transmission, or by eliminating both. In the case of malaria, control efforts have focused both on the elimination of the reservoir by draining swamps and other wet areas and on destroying the mosquito vector by aerial spraying with appropriate insecticides. The cycle of transmission by direct contact can be broken by eliminating direct contact, as with use of condoms during sexual intercourse to prevent sexually transmitted diseases. These examples represent primary prevention.

The Host

Disease can only occur in a susceptible host. Basic to the understanding of host resistance to disease is the concept of immunity. *Immunity* refers to the increased resistance on the part of a host to a specific infectious agent. Immunity can be humoral (antibodies in the blood) or cellular (specific to each type of cell). The role of each varies with the infectious agent and with the immune response of the host. Immunity can be passive or active. Passive immunity is attained either naturally (maternal transfer of antibodies to the fetus) or artificially by inoculation of specific protective antibodies (eg, diphtheria antitoxin for diphtheria prevention). Passive immunity is temporary; in the newborn it usually lasts 6 months, during which time the infant is protected only against infections experienced by the mother and for which she has produced antibodies. Breast feeding extends infant immunity for the duration of the breast feeding. By contrast, active immunity is long-lasting and may protect an individual for life. It is attained naturally by infection, with or without clinical manifestations, or artificially by inoculation with vaccine obtained from fractions of products of the infectious agent, or from the agent itself in killed, modified, or variant form. The principle of active immunity is used in many major vaccination programs, such as those for diphtheria and polio. It was also the basis for the successful program to eradicate smallpox through an international case finding, vaccination, and surveillance program. The last reported case of smallpox was in 1977 and the global erradication was announced in 1980 (WHO, 1996). The dramatic change in incidence of paralytic poliomyelitis cases after introduction of the vaccine can be seen in Figure 6–2.

In contrast to immunity, the term *inherent resistance* refers to the ability to resist disease independently of antibodies or specifically developed tissue response. It usually rests in anatomical or physiological characteristics of the host; it may be genetic or acquired, permanent or temporary. Factors such as general health status or nutrition may affect resistance to disease.

In the natural history cycle, an organism may or may not cause illness once it comes in contact with the human host. Assuming that a host is susceptible, infection

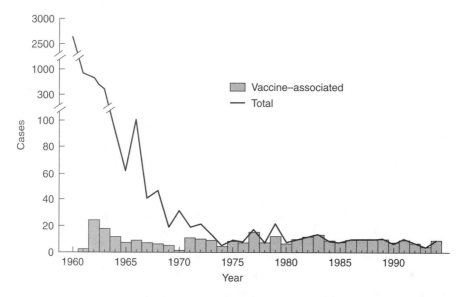

Figure 6–2. Total number of reported paralytic poliomyelitis cases excluding import cases and number of vaccine-associated cases—United States, 1960–1994. (*Adapted from Centers for Disease Control. Paralytic poliomyelitis—United States, 1960–1994.* Morbidity and Mortality Weekly Report, *1997;* 46[4], *Fig. 1.*)

will occur. Infection is defined as the entry and establishment of an infectious agent in a host. The minimum level of physiological reaction occurs when the agent propagates sufficiently to maintain its numbers without producing any identifiable sign of host reaction. This is termed *colonization.* If there is only subclinical infection measurable through antibody tests but the infection is not clinically detectable, the host may never be identified as being infected. When clinical signs and symptoms are observed, infectious disease is present. Hosts at all three levels of infection may be capable of infecting others. As previously mentioned, the term *carrier* refers to infected persons without apparent clinical disease who represent a potential source of infection to others.

METHODS OF CONTROL

Because infectious diseases result from interactions among factors related to the host, the etiological agent, and the environment, methods of control are aimed at modification of these factors and their interactions. The particular factors involved vary from one disease to another. Therefore, specific interventions vary according to the epidemiology of the disease. A review of major approaches to control, however, provides a basis for planning control programs. Approaches to control of infectious disease involve the three levels of prevention discussed in Chapter 2: (1) primary prevention, (2) secondary prevention, and (3) tertiary prevention. In general, measures for control of communicable disease are aimed at preventing the spread of the infectious agent from those environments that harbor it to individuals who are susceptible and who may be exposed. This can be achieved by modifying or eliminating the environment in which the infectious agent lives, thus inactivating the agents by interfering with the means of transmission to the human host or by increasing host immunity—all measures aimed at primary prevention. Control is facilitated by the maintenance of surveillance programs that quickly identify new cases and initiate isolation methods to prevent exposure of susceptibles or institute specific treatments to limit the period of communicability and progression of pathology (secondary prevention). Tertiary prevention plays a smaller role in infectious disease programs than in noninfectious programs because infectious diseases less often result in permanent disability. This is not to say that infectious agents never produce disability. Infectious conditions such as tertiary syphilis or advanced stages of infectious endocarditis are associated with disability and require rehabilitative measures to optimize daily function.

Control approaches within each level of prevention will be discussed here and specific diseases will be used to illustrate an approach to control across the three prevention levels. The presentation of a few specific examples, based on the epidemiology of a particular disease, will be used to illustrate how general approaches are applied to a particular case.

Primary Prevention

Table 6–3 lists three approaches to primary prevention of infectious diseases and the specific methods used in each of the three approaches, along with specific relevant activities. Primary prevention is aimed at intervening before the agent can become lodged in a host and begin to cause pathological changes. As shown in Table 6–3, this level of prevention seeks to keep the agent away from contact with the host by breaking the chain of transmission, inactivating the agent, or increasing host resistance.

Breaking the Chain of Transmission.   The first three methods listed in Table 6–3 for breaking the chain of transmission are aimed at changing the environment. Environmental control programs such as chlorination of water supplies and sewage treatment plants that are targeted at the *reservoir* have had a major impact on the control of infectious diseases. In Italy, Mussolini achieved the eradication of malaria in the vicinity of Rome by drying the "Marais Pontin" swamps which were breeding the malaria parasite, *Plasmodium.* Unfortunately, this was done at the cost of an incredible number of lives, as many of those who worked on this project soon died of malaria. Similarly, under more favorable circumstances, control of dust at construction sites can reduce the spread of organisms whose reservoir is dirt and whose *vehicle* is dust, for example, the organism that causes Legionnaire's disease.

Environmental measures to control infectious diseases may also be aimed at destroying the *vector* that transports the agent (insect or living carrier that transports an infectious agent from its source—infected person or wastes—to a susceptible person or that person's food, water, or surroundings). This is the case for many viral encephalitides that have mosquitoes as vectors. Here attempts have been made to abort urban epidemics by aerial spraying with suitable insecticide. This method, however,

TABLE 6–3. APPROACHES TO PRIMARY PREVENTION OF INFECTIOUS DISEASES

A. Breaking the chain of transmission of infection
  1. Control of animals and other biological vectors of disease (eg, arthropods, snails)
  2. Environmental control of air, dust, or dirt that may harbor infectious agents
  3. Control of general sanitation—food, water, sewage
  4. Personal measures for avoiding exposure or limiting spread of infectious diseases
    a. Good personal hygiene
    b. Proper food-handling procedures
    c. Use of protective clothing or repellents to prevent insect bites
    d. Avoiding water, foods, animals, and insects likely to transmit disease
  5. Use of aseptic technique in management of patients, their excretions and secretions (primary prevention for others)
  6. Chemoprophylaxis before or after exposure to an infectious disease
  7. Rapid case detection and specific chemotherapy to limit infectivity (secondary prevention for the patient, but primary prevention in terms of susceptibles in the environment)
  8. Isolation of infectious cases and quarantine of their contacts
B. Inactivating the infectious agent
  1. Use of physical methods
    a. Heat—pasteurization, adequate cooking of food, heat sterilization of infectious materials
    b. Cold—maintaining foods at low temperatures to inactivate organisms (eg, parasites in meats, contaminants in other foods)
    c. Radiation—ultraviolet light to inactivate infectious agents in air and on surfaces
  2. Use of chemical methods
    a. Chlorinate water supplies and sewage affluents
    b. Disinfect infectious or potentially infectious material
C. Increasing host resistance
  1. Use of immunobiologics—vaccines and toxoids for active immunization and immunoglobulins for passive immunization
  2. Improvement in general health—proper nutrition, exercise, etc.

(Adapted from Chin J. Communicable disease control. In J. Last [Ed.]. Maxcy-Rosenau public health and preventive medicine. Norwalk, Conn.: Appleton & Lange, 1986, p. 184)

may disrupt the ecological balance for other living organisms; the effects of the insecticide should be specific, whenever possible, to the vector being eradicated.

The fourth method listed in Table 6–3 is a form of health promotion aimed at the human host. Encouraging "healthful behavior" to avoid potential harmful agents through good hygiene and use of protective clothing in certain situations can break the chain of transmission.

Measures 5 through 8 in Table 6–3, although involving cases of the disease, still constitute primary prevention because they are aimed at restricting the infection to the human reservoir and preventing the spread to other susceptible human hosts. Although rapid case detection and early treatment may represent secondary prevention for the patient, they contribute to primary prevention for other susceptible hosts. Such control measures require surveillance programs to identify new cases quickly and to subsequently implement methods to keep infectious individuals away from susceptibles. The four methods most frequently used are isolation, quarantine, segregation, and personal surveillance.

Isolation usually refers to the separation of infected persons during the period of communicability from others presumed to be uninfected. Patients with infectious diseases may be confined in isolation wards of a hospital or in the home. Table 6–4 shows the diseases for which isolation precautions are necessary. Different types of isolation are required for different diseases, for example, strict isolation involving a room with special ventilation may be needed for pneumonic plague or viral hemorrhagic fevers, while only drainage/secretion precautions are needed for conjunctivitis. Persons who have been exposed to these patients before their isolation may be

TABLE 6–4. DISEASES REQUIRING ISOLATION PRECAUTIONS

TYPE OF ISOLATION	DISEASES
Strict Isolation (may require room with special ventilation)—private room with door closed; mask, gown, gloves; special handling of waste and contaminated articles required	Pharyngeal diphtheria; viral hemorrhagic fevers; pneumonic plague; smallpox; varicella (chickenpox); zoster in immune-compromised patients
Contact Isolation—private room; mask for close contact or if patient coughing and does not reliably cover mouth; gown and gloves if hand soiling likely; special handling of waste and contaminated articles	Group A *Streptococcus* endometritis; impetigo; pediculosis; major skin, wound, or burn infection; vaccinia; primary disseminated herpes simplex; viral pneumonia; influenza; acute upper respiratory infections; infant/child infected with multiple-resistant bacteria; newborns with gonococcal conjuctivitis; staphylococcocal furunculosis or neonatal disseminated herpes simplex
Respiratory Isolation—private room with door closed; mask for close contact or if patient is coughing and does not reliably cover mouth; special handling of waste and contaminated articles	*Haemophilus influenzae* epiglottitis; infectious erythema; measles; *H. influenzae* or meningococcal meningitis; meningococcal pneumonia; menigococcemia; mumps; pertussis; *H. influenzae* pneumonia in children
Acid-fast bacillus isolation—requires special private room with ventilation and door closed; mask for close contact or if patient is coughing and does not reliably cover mouth; gown if soiling of clothing is likely; special handling of waste and contaminated articles	Tuberculosis
Enteric precautions—Private room desirable but optional; gowns and gloves if soiling of clothes and hands likely; special handling of waste and contaminated articles	Amoebic dysentery; cholera; Coxsackie viruses; acute diarrheal infection; echovirus; enterovirus encephalitis; *Clostridium difficile* or *Staphylococcus*-associated enterocolitis; enteroviral infection; gastroenteritis associated with *Campylobacter, Cryptosporidium, Dietamoeba fragilis, Escherichia coli, Giardia lamblia, Salmonella, Shigella,* or *Vibrio parahaemolyticus; Yersinia enterocolitica;* hand, foot, and mouth disease; hepatitis A; herpangina; viral meningitis caused by enteroviruses; necrotizing enterocolitis; pleurodynia; poliomyelitis; typhoid fever; viral pericarditis, myocarditis, or enteroviral meningitis
Drainage/secretion precautions—gloves and gown if soiling of hands or clothing likely; special handling of waste or contaminated articles	Conjunctivitis; minor or limited abscess; minor or limited burn, skin, wound or decubitus ulcer infection

(*Adapted from* Professional Guide to Diseases. *Springhouse, Pa.: Springhouse Corporation, 1989.*)

incubating the disease and be infectious to others, although they will be free of any signs or symptoms of illness. In the past it was common practice to quarantine those exposed individuals. *Complete quarantine* is defined as the limitation of freedom of movement of well persons exposed to a communicable disease for a period of time no longer than the longest usual incubation period of the disease to prevent direct contact with others not exposed. Complete quarantine, however, is rarely used today. More common is a *modified quarantine,* which selectively and partially limits movement of persons who may be susceptible to a disease and who are known to have been exposed. Nurses and women of childbearing age without a known history of German measles (rubella) or who do not demonstrate mandatory antibody levels would presumably be susceptible to German measles. If they have not been vaccinated and are planning a pregnancy or not using birth control, they should not work on pediatric hospital wards with cases of this disease because maternal infection with rubella may cause severe damage to the fetus, particularly during the first trimester of pregnancy. In another example, individuals who have come in contact with typhoid fever should be excluded from food handling until repeated cultures of the urine and feces have been negative for the typhoid bacterium. In some instances, immune persons have been exempted from provisions required of susceptible persons. For example, after a case of whooping cough in a classroom, only the nonimmune children may be excluded from school for 14 days after the exposure.

Segregation methods have been occasionally applied to facilitate the control of a communicable disease by the separation and observation of a group of individuals. An example would be the establishment of a sanitary boundary to protect uninfected from infected portions of a population. At times, certain areas of a city have been declared "off limits" to military personnel. In certain cases, *personal surveillance* methods may be used. This is the practice of close medical or other supervision of contacts to promote recognition of infection or illness but without restricting their movements. This is extremely useful in the field of sexually transmitted diseases. Sexual contacts of AIDS patients, for example, are closely monitored for HIV status or symptoms of the disease. These individuals are also discouraged from donating blood and unprotected sexual activity.

For susceptible persons such as hospital personnel and family members who must be exposed to infectious individuals in order to care for them, proper use of aseptic techniques in the management of the patient, secretions, and excretions can provide appropriate protection. Proper management also includes appropriate disposal of contaminated materials to protect others who may come in contact with these materials.

Inactivating the Agent.   Inactivation of the agent is a second method of primary prevention. Such inactivation, whether by chemical or physical means, can be generally effective as in the use of fungicides to destroy potentially infectious agents at their sources. In other instances of intervention aimed at inactivating organisms, available methods must focus on inactivating the organism in a particular vehicle (eg, pasteurization of milk aimed at the agent for brucellosis). Although pasteurization is effective at controlling the spread of brucellosis by consumption of milk, it is not an effective general control measure. Brucellosis can also be spread to handlers of infected animals such as farmers or butchers.

Increasing Host Resistance.   Primary prevention can influence inherent resistance of the host through health education programs and infant feeding programs aimed at maximizing health status. Another approach to primary prevention aimed at the host is the immunization of susceptibles in the population. Immunization is performed with vaccines obtained from fractions or products of the agent or from the agent itself in killed, modified, or variant form. *Vaccine* is a general term that applies to specific and actively immunizing agents, regardless of their origin, used against viral, rickettsial, or bacterial diseases. *Toxoids* are vaccines derived from denatured proteins that have lost their toxicity but retain much of their original antigenicity. The killed poliomyelitis virus vaccine (Salk) confers protection against the paralytic disease but not against infection; the live-attenuated poliomyelitis vaccine (Sabin) is thought to confer lifelong protection against subsequent infection by wild polio virus strains. Diphtheria toxoid used in combination with tetanus toxoid and pertussis vaccine (the DPT vaccine) in a series of three intramuscular injections given 4 to 6 weeks apart beginning at 2 or 3 months of age and boosters at 15 months, 4 years, and 6 years, is a routine procedure. Vaccines are available for prevention of many of the common infectious diseases, including cholera, anthrax, hepatitis A and B, influenza, measles, mumps, plague, pneumococcal disease, rabies, tetanus, and tuberculosis; however, it is important that vaccines be appropriately used. A number of recent epidemics of vaccine-preventable diseases have occurred because children did not receive the recommended number of vaccine doses. Figure 6–3 shows cases of measles in a 1996 outbreak in Utah by age and number of doses of measles-

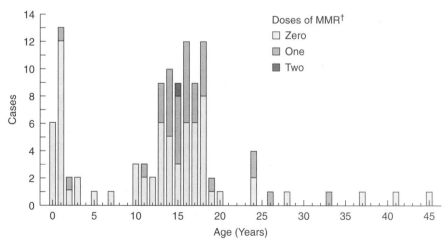

* n = 107.
†Measles-mumps-rubella vaccine.

Figure 6–3. Age distribution of persons with measles and vaccination history, southwestern Utah, 1996. (*Adapted from Centers for Disease Control. Measles outbreak—Southwestern Utah, 1996.* Morbidity and Mortality Weekly Report, *1997; 46[33], 768, Fig. 2; Massachusetts Medical Society, Waltham, Mass.*)

mumps-rubella vaccine previously received. The majority of cases did not have any vaccinations. Nearly all of the remainder had only one dose, rather than the two recommended. The measles attack rate was calculated among students at the high school where the outbreak originated, since vaccination records were available. Among those students who were unvaccinated, the attack rate was 33%. Among recipients of one dose of the vaccine it was 1%. There were no cases at the school among those vaccinated with two doses of vaccine (Centers for Disease Control, 1997b).

It is not necessary to achieve 100% immunity in the population to achieve control. A high degree of resistance by a group to invasion and spread of an infectious agent may be reached if a high proportion of individuals in the group are immune. This concept is termed *herd immunity.*

Secondary Prevention

Case Finding.   As a form of secondary prevention, case finding detects the disease early so that treatment can be instituted and progression of the illness stopped. As a result of detecting and treating the disease early, spread to others in the community is limited; thus, case finding as a form of secondary prevention of an infectious disease also contributes to primary prevention by restricting the infection to the human reservoir and preventing spread to other susceptible human hosts. Case finding can be done by following up on known contacts, as with sexual partners of those with venereal diseases or persons who may have eaten food prepared by someone with hepatitis. Once located, these contacts are tested for the disease and treated if disease is present. Case finding can also occur through screening programs. Blood tests required for marriage licenses are one way of screening for venereal disease. Tuberculin testing in inner city schools or among homeless populations is designed to detect cases of tuberculosis in potentially high-risk populations.

Public Education.   Health education also plays a role in secondary prevention. Awareness of early signs and symptoms can enable an individual to seek care early. Knowledge of what behaviors contribute to spreading a disease may influence individuals with the disease to modify their behavior. Behavioral change may accomplish two things: (1) interrupt spread to other persons (primary prevention), for example, if a person with AIDS avoids unprotected sexual contact with well individuals; and (2) improve the prognosis for the sick person, again using AIDS as an example, since those individuals with a weakened immune system are more susceptible to other infections. A person with AIDS therefore, may prolong survival by avoiding situations, such as crowds, that are likely to expose him or her to infections.

Tertiary Prevention

As mentioned previously, residual disability is less common for diseases of infectious etiology than for those with noninfectious causal agents. Examples of infectious diseases resulting in disability, however, can be found. Leprosy, stage 3 syphilis, impaired vision resulting from severe conjunctivitis, hearing impairment caused by repeated or severe ear infections, paralytic polio, and AIDS are illustrative of the variety of forms of disability possible. Tertiary prevention is aimed at minimizing the degree of disability and enabling the patient to live the fullest life possible within the limitations imposed by his or her illness. Medical technology, vocational rehabilitation, and physical rehabilitation are all aspects of tertiary prevention. Rehabilitation planning will be specific to the disease entity.

INVESTIGATION OF AN EPIDEMIC

The investigation of an epidemic, whether of an infectious communicable nature or not, follows basically the same process. The word *epidemic* refers to any marked upward fluctuation in disease incidence, whereas the term *endemic* implies the habitual presence of a disease or agent of disease within a given area. A third term, *pandemic*, is used to describe epidemics that include large areas of the world, ie, a worldwide epidemic.

Figures 6–4 and 6–5 illustrate the epidemic fluctuation of rates. Many diseases such as pneumonia and influenza fluctuate on a seasonal basis, cyclical cycle, or both, every several years. Such fluctuations usually occur within a range, where the usual peaks and lows represent the range of expected rates. A peak that substantially exceeds the upper range of usual rates represents an epidemic. Other rates such as the malaria rates in Figure 6–4 and the foodborne botulism rates in

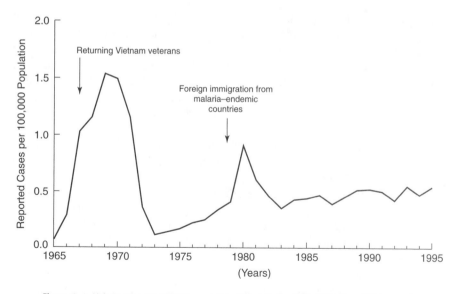

Figure 6–4. Malaria cases per 100,000 population, United States, 1965–1995. Since 1985, approximately 1,000 cases of imported malaria have been reported annually in the United States. Recent immigrants and visitors accounted for 50% of these cases. (*Adapted from Centers for Disease Control. Summary of notifiable diseases, United States, 1995.* Morbidity and Mortality Weekly Report, *1995; 44[53], 42.*)

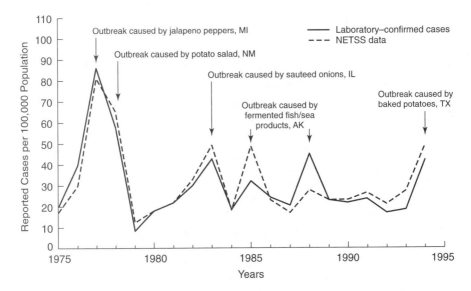

Figure 6–5. Rates of foodborne botulism, 1975–1995. Although they occur infrequently, outbreaks of foodborne botulism can rapidly kill many persons. Such outbreaks require prompt and effective communications between clinicians and public health officials. (*Adapted from Centers for Disease Control. MMWR summary of notifiable diseases, United States, 1995.* Morbidity and Mortality Weekly Report, *1995; 44[53], 24.*)

Figure 6–5 show long-term trends. For malaria, there were sudden increases in rates, for example, around 1950 and again in the mid-1960s, which represent epidemics and are related to specific events, in these cases veterans returning to the United States, first from Korea, then from Vietnam. Figure 6–4 shows one peak from the returning Vietnam veterans in the late 1960s and early 1970s and another peak in 1980 attributed to foreign immigration. The epidemic peaks for botulism in Figure 6–5 are related to specific contaminated foods eaten by large numbers of individuals.

The investigative process for an outbreak of infectious disease should proceed in an orderly fashion, encompassing the five basic steps discussed below, although the steps may not occur in this order depending on the particular circumstances of the outbreak. Sometimes, for example, it may be possible and desirable to institute measures to manage the epidemic and reduce the spread before results of hypothesis testing are obtained. These measures would be based on general principles of disease control and the best information available as to the probable source of infection.

Verification of the Diagnosis and Confirmation of an Epidemic. The first indication that an epidemic may be occurring is based on review of reported cases. United States federal regulations require that diseases identified as notifiable should be reported to the local health department, which subsequently reports these cases to the Centers for Disease Control. Since 1995, there are 52 infectious diseases that are notifiable under these standards. These are shown in Table 6–5.

Both for purposes of notification and investigation, a standard definition of a case is needed. The criteria used to define a case can strongly affect rates. Further, inclusion of noncases in a set of cases for study of an epidemic increases the difficulties in delineating a cause. Thus, although clinical knowledge and experience are necessary to make a diagnosis of an infectious disease, requiring laboratory evidence to confirm it is more precise. Rates based only on clinical diagnosis and those based on laboratory confirmation can be quite discrepant.

To establish the true epidemic nature of a disease, it is essential to have some estimates of previous incidence rates (preferably based on the same case criteria) in order to identify an apparent epidemic that is, in fact, due to better reporting of an endemic situation. The availability of a new treatment, for instance, may attract a large number of patients whose disease had not previously been reported.

An *epidemic* or *attack curve* is essentially an incidence curve on which the number of diseased persons in the population is plotted by time of onset of disease. The existence of an epidemic depends on the presence of a communicable agent and on the availability of susceptible individuals to be infected by the agent. Figure 6–6 illustrates the situation of a *common source epidemic*, also called a *point source epidemic*. This type of epidemic is characterized by the simultaneous exposure of a large number of susceptibles to a common infectious agent. Because

TABLE 6–5. INFECTIOUS DISEASES DESIGNATED AS NOTIFIABLE, UNITED STATES, 1995

Acquired immunodeficiency syndrome (AIDS)	*Haemophilus influenzae,* invasive diseases	Poliomyelitis, paralytic
Anthrax	Hansen's disease (leprosy)	Psittacosis
Botulism	Hantavirus pulmonary syndrome	Rabies, animal
Brucellosis	Hemolytic-uremic syndrome, postdiarrheal	Rabies, human
Chancroid		Rocky Mountain spotted fever
Chlamydia trachomatous, genital infection	Hepatitis A	Rubella
	Hepatitis B	Salmonellosis
Cholera	Hepatitis, C/non-A, non-B	Shigellosis
Coccidioidomycosis	Human immunodeficiency virus (HIV) infection, pediatric (age 13 years or younger)	Streptococcal disease, invasive, group A
Congenital rubella syndrome		*Streptococcus pneumoniae,* drug-resistant
Congenital syphilis		
Cryptosporidiosis	Legionnaire's disease	Streptococcal toxic-shock syndrome
Diptheria	Lyme disease	Syphilis
Encephalitis, California	Malaria	Tetanus
Encephalitis, Eastern equine	Measles	Toxic-shock syndrome
Encephalitis, St. Louis	Meningococcal disease	Trichinosis
Encephalitis, Western equine	Mumps	Tuberculosis
Escherichia coli 0157:H7	Pertussis	Typhoid fever
Gonorrhea	Plague	Yellow fever

(*From Centers for Disease Control. MMWR summary of notifiable diseases, United States, 1995.* Morbidity and Mortality Weekly Report, 1995; 44[53].)

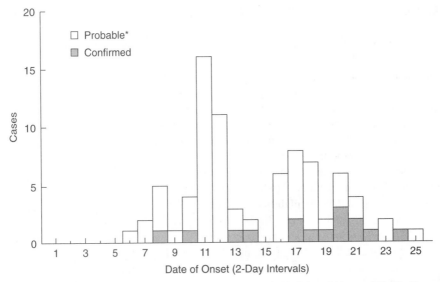

*A probable case was defined as onset of diarrhea (two or more loose stools during a 24-hour period) with either fever or bloody stools while at the resort or within 11 days of leaving the resort. A confirmed case additionally required *Shigella sonnei* isolated from stool. A total of 82 cases were identified, including 67 probable and 15 confirmed.

Figure 6–6. Example of an epidemic curve based on a point source epidemic. Number of confirmed and probable cases of *Shigella sonnei* by date of onset—Idaho, August 6–24, 1995. (*Adapted from Centers for Disease Control.* Shigella sonnei *outbreak associated with contaminated drinking water—Island Park, Idaho, August 1995.* Morbidity and Mortality Weekly Report, *1996; 45[11], 230.*)

nearly all the susceptibles have been infected at the same time, the epidemic terminates when the supply of susceptible persons is exhausted. The explosive increase in the number of cases of a disease over a short period of time, often only hours, is characteristic of an epidemic of food poisoning originating from a single event, such as a church supper. Some epidemics related to a common source show a more scattered pattern of new cases, as shown in Figure 6–6. This occurs when the common source is a contaminated product that is widely distributed and consumed at different times by individuals or small groups. In this epidemic of *Shigella sonnei*—the most common source of bacillary dysentery in the United States—the average duration from arrival at a resort in Idaho to onset of diarrhea was 4 days (range 1–11 days). Relative risk for illness among those who drank tap water or used ice from machines was 17.6 (confidence interval 2.5–123.0) compared with those who did not drink the water or use ice. Onset of illness was restricted to the dates between August 6 and 24, 1995. No cases occurred before that date and within one incubation period after control measures were instituted—restricting use of tap water and ice from the machines and providing bottled water to drink—no further cases occurred. The source of contamination was a sewer line from a nearby housing construction site that was draining improperly (Centers for Disease Control, 1996).

Figure 6–7 illustrates a situation in which only a few susceptible individuals are initially infected. After an incubation period, however, these infected individuals are the source for secondary cases. A stepwise progression in the number of diseased persons is to be expected as those exposed to each new group of infected individuals develop symptoms after an incubation period. The epidemic would continue as long as any susceptibles remained, especially if additional susceptible individuals were brought into the epidemic area. The drop-off in rates also is stepwise. The duration of the epidemic is relatively long, usually months. This type of epidemic is called a *propagated epidemic*. In the measles epidemic shown in Figure 6–7, the drop-off in rates was influenced by the mass vaccination campaign.

Identification of Affected Persons and Their Characteristics. Each case of a disease has to be identified to obtain a complete picture of the epidemic. In addition to the usual information about name, age, sex, occupation, place of residence, recent movements, symptoms of the disease, and time of onset, the epidemiological history taking is concerned with the circumstances related to the illness and is guided by what is suspected as the cause (eg, what has been eaten, in the case of suspected food poisoning). Also important is the individual's history of infectious diseases, immunization, recent travel, and associations with people or animals who are ill.

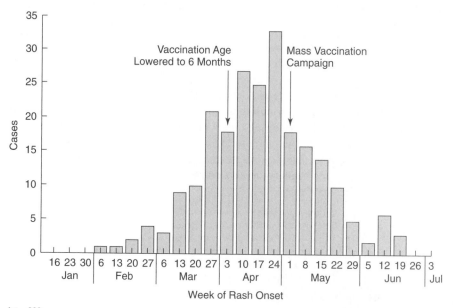

* n = 228.

Figure 6–7. Example of an epidemic curve in a propagated epidemic. Number of measles cases by week of rash onset—Guam, 1994. (*Adapted from Centers for Disease Control, measles outbreak—Guam, 1994. Morbidity and Mortality Weekly Report. 1995, 44(36):657*).

The search for additional cases of the disease helps complete the disease picture. Large-scale serological surveys have been carried out on populations that have subsequently experienced epidemics of infectious diseases. A similar postepidemic serological survey would indicate the percentage of the population infected by the epidemic agent and who developed serum antibodies. If careful record of clinical illness was taken during the epidemic, results of such surveys provide useful data on the frequency of inapparent or asymptomatic disease. In addition to serological testing, which may be useful for the identification of asymptomatic cases, the epidemiologist attempts to identify environmental changes that set the stage for the epidemic.

Formulation and Testing of a Hypothesis.   The descriptive characteristics of the population should make it possible to pinpoint a common experience shared only by the patients and also to obtain age- and sex-specific incidence rates by identifying the total population at risk. Disease incidence is compared for persons exposed to the hypothesized cause and those not exposed. It might be instructive to study those individuals seemingly exposed but unaffected and compare their characteristics with those of the exposed and affected group. Statistical tests are helpful in evaluating the postulated source. All links in the infectious process should be included in the hypothesis: the agent, the reservoir, the mode of transmission to the human host, the mode of entry in the host, and host susceptibility to infection. In instances in which the total population (or a representative sample) of exposed and unexposed individuals cannot be obtained, a case control approach must be used, comparing the ill population with well persons (controls) in regard to exposure to the hypothesized source.

Management of an Epidemic.   In addition to the treatment of patients, control measures to reduce the spread of the epidemic (isolation measures) or to prevent its recurrence (improvement in the environment and vaccination of the population) are important. The success or failure of control measures may be helpful in confirming or refuting the hypothesis on which these measures were based. Health education leading to appropriate behavior change is a long-range measure of great importance.

Continued surveillance and monitoring of infection, which can now be carried out, have been useful in defining thresholds, predicting outbreaks, and providing strategic information for health programs and economic deployment of resources. Surveillance requires data on:

- Infective persons or sources
- Susceptible persons at risk
- Effective contact rate between susceptible persons and infective persons or sources
- Time period of effective contact
- Persons removed by isolation, immunity, or death
- Removal rate

Surveillance systems have been useful in monitoring hospital infections as well as community-wide infections. Existing surveillance systems are discussed in Chapter 12.

Even when a disease has been virtually eradicated in one country, measures must be taken to prevent its entry from another region where it may be endemic. All links of the chain of transmission of a disease must be kept under scrutiny to maintain surveillance of a disease. The World Health Organization provides guidelines for surveillance of diseases that are likely to spread through international travel. Individual countries set up requirements for immunization and inspection of goods coming from endemic or epidemic areas of the world. In addition to the reporting of cases, which was discussed earlier, surveillance of diseases can use additional sources of information such as death certificates and data from public health laboratories, entomological and veterinary services, and estimates of the immune status of a young population based on the amount of DPT vaccine used in relation to number of births. Infectious disease surveillance systems should also be designed for early identification of new problems. The emergence during the past 30 years of Legionnaire's disease, toxic shock syndrome, hantavirus pneumonia, and AIDS serves as a reminder of the importance of surveillance systems.

INTERNATIONAL INFECTIOUS DISEASE CONTROL

The World Health Organization has stated that the infectious disease burden today comprises a global crisis (WHO, 1996). Not only does infection cause disease directly, but infectious agents such as the hepatitis virus play a role in the development of many types of cancer. Infectious diseases have been classified by the WHO into three categories: "old diseases-old problems"; "old diseases-new problems"; and "new diseases-new pathogens" (WHO, 1996). The first category, "old diseases-old problems," includes diseases that, given the commitment and resources available, can be eradicated (measles, poliomyelitis, dracontiasis) and those that could be eliminated as public health problems (leprosy, neonatal tetanus, measles, intestinal worms, hepatitis, and typhoid). Immunization of children against six vaccine-preventable diseases—diphtheria, pertussis, tetanus, poliomyelitis, measles, and tuberculosis—would be required to accomplish this. The estimated cost of such an immunization program would be $0.50 per capita. Additional factors for this eradication process would involve using an integrated approach to the management of sick children ($1.60 per capita); providing adequate clean drinking water and basic sanitation, as well as collecting household garbage and instituting basic hygienic measures such as hand washing after defecation and before food preparation; establishing school health programs to treat parasite infections and micronutrient deficiencies and provide health education ($0.50 per capita); and case managing sexually transmitted diseases ($11 per capita). Intensive two-dose vaccination campaigns have already begun to have some impact on measles incidence (Fig. 6–8).

The category of "old diseases-new problems" includes tuberculosis, malaria, dengue, and other vectorborne diseases. Drug and pesticide resistance have become a problem, requiring use of more expensive or toxic drugs. These diseases are becoming more prevalent in areas of the world where they were relatively well controlled in the past. Early diagnosis and prompt treatment, vector control measures to prevent

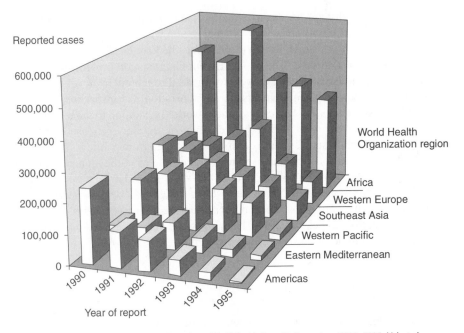

Figure 6–8. Reported incidence of measles—World Health Organization regions, 1990–1995. (*Adapted from Centers for Disease Control.* Morbidity and Mortality Weekly Report, *1997; 46[RR-11], 5, Fig. 1.*)

epidemics, research on new treatment regimens, improved diagnostics, drugs, and vaccines, and surveillance mechanisms and procedures with laboratory support for early detection, confirmation, and communication are suggested strategies.

Finally, the third category, "new diseases-new pathogens" includes Ebola and other viral hemorrhagic fevers, hantavirus pulmonary syndrome, HIV/AIDS, foodborne and waterborne infections due to new organisms such as *Cryptosporidium* or new strains of bacteria such as *Escherichia coli* O157:H7 and cholera, O139. Some 29 new diseases have emerged in the last 20 years (WHO, 1996). A need remains for speedy responses to outbreaks of important new infections wherever they occur, intensive research on the natural history of new diseases and on methods of prevention, treatment, and control. A global surveillance program is crucial (WHO, 1996).

COMMON INFECTIOUS DISEASES IN THE UNITED STATES

During the period from 1992 to 1994, the ten most frequently reported nationally notifiable infectious diseases for all ages and both sexes in the United States were (in descending order) gonorrhea, AIDS, salmonellosis, shigellosis, primary and secondary syphilis, tuberculosis, hepatitis A, hepatitis B, Lyme disease, and hepatitis C/non-A, non-B. The incidence by age group and gender are shown in Table 6–6. Although women use health services more often than men, for seven of these

TABLE 6–6. TEN MOST COMMONLY REPORTED NATIONALLY NOTIFIABLE INFECTIOUS DISEASES AMONG CHILDREN, ADOLESCENTS, AND ADULTS,[a] BY SEX—UNITED STATES, 1992–1994[b]

AGE GROUP/ RANK	DISEASE	FEMALES No. of Cases	Rate per 100,000 Population	DISEASE	MALES No. of Cases	Rate per 100,000 Population
Children						
1	Gonorrhea	24,291	29.8	Salmonellosis	25,457	29.2
2	Salmonellosis	22,062	26.6	Shigellosis	22,272	25.6
3	Shigellosis	21,520	26.0	Hepatitis A	11,688	13.4
4	Hepatitis A	11,247	13.6	Gonorrhea	7,477	8.8
5	Pertussis	5,919	7.1	Pertussis	5,812	6.7
6	Congenital syphilis	4,367	5.3	Congenital syphilis	4,552	5.2
7	Lyme disease	2,633	3.2	Lyme disease	3,262	3.7
8	Tuberculosis	2,539	3.1	Tuberculosis	2,580	3.0
9	Meningoccocal disease	1,774	2.1	Meningoccocal disease	2,209	2.5
10	Mumps	1,412	1.7	Mumps	1,963	2.3
Adolescents						
1	Gonorrhea	218,018	878.0	Gonorrhea	164,079	627.4
2	1°/2° Syphilis	5,936	23.4	1°/2° Syphilis	3,067	11.4
3	Hepatitis A	2,639	10.4	Hepatitis A	3,019	11.3
4	Salmonellosis	2,280	9.0	Salmonellosis	2,531	9.5
5	Hepatitis B	1,812	7.2	Hepatitis B	1,011	3.8
6	Shigellosis	1,523	6.0	Tuberculosis	870	3.3
7	Tuberculosis	840	3.3	Shigellosis	865	3.2
8	Lyme disease	631	2.5	Lyme disease	717	2.7
9	Pertussis	476	1.9	AIDS	683	1.8
10	AIDS	425	1.2	Meningococcal disease	475	1.8
Adults						
1	Gonorrhea	344,433	122.0	Gonorrhea	531,384	205.2
2	AIDS	34,872	12.1	AIDS	187,211	71.0
3	1°/2° Syphilis	31,893	11.0	Tuberculosis	46,160	17.5
4	Salmonellosis	30,286	10.5	1°/2° Syphilis	39,504	15.0
5	Tuberculosis	23,184	8.1	Hepatitis A	25,729	9.8
6	Hepatitis A	18,258	6.3	Salmonellosis	24,943	9.5
7	Shigellosis	14,274	5.0	Hepatitis B	21,640	8.2
8	Hepatitis B	13,987	4.9	Lyme disease	10,152	3.9
9	Lyme disease	11,024	3.8	Hepatitis C/non-A, non-B	9,413	3.6
10	Hepatitis C/non-A, non-B	4,980	1.7	Shigellosis	8,054	3.1

[a]Children were defined as persons aged <15 years; adolescents, aged 15–19 years; and adults, aged ≥ 20 years. For AIDS cases, children were persons aged <13 years and adolescents were persons aged 13–19 years.
[b]Persons for whom age was not reported are excluded.

ten diseases, the reported incidence is lower in women. Gonorrhea, however, is higher for women in all age groups. Rates of AIDS incidence increased faster in recent years for women than for men but rates overall decreased for the first time in 1994 (Fig. 6–9). Women between 15 and 44 years of age accounted for 84% of cases. As of October 31, 1995, 501,310 cases of AIDS had been reported to the Centers for Disease Control (CDC). Of these, 10% were reported during 1981 to 1987, 41% during 1988 to 1992, and 49% during 1993 to October 1995. The proportion of AIDS cases among women increased from 8% of cases in 1981 to 1987 to 18% during 1993 to October 1995. The proportion attributed to intravenous drug use increased from 17% in 1981 through 1987 to 27% during 1993 through October 1995, and the proportion attributed to sexual transmission between heterosexuals from 3% to 10% (Centers for Disease Control, 1995). Sexually transmitted diseases such as gonorrhea, syphilis, and AIDS can be prevented through public education programs about safe sex together with prompt identification and follow up of sexual contacts of individuals with these diseases and proper treatment of infected persons.

Cases of salmonellosis, shigellosis, and hepatitis A were highest among children. Most of these cases of disease are preventable. For example, appropriate use of vaccines could prevent pertussis, mumps, and hepatitis A. Foodborne diseases have been increasing in incidence during the 1990s. These can be prevented by targeting education programs to food handlers about proper hand washing, safe storage and preparation of food, and the potential for serious disease outbreaks if food is mishandled. Better monitoring of imported foods is also needed.

The United States, like the rest of the world, is experiencing a resurgence of old diseases like tuberculosis and cholera and an emergence of new pathogens, such as hantavirus. Many cases of old diseases are introduced from other countries. Because of this, the CDC has generated new efforts to strengthen prevention and control. These include expanding and coordinating surveillance systems for early detection, tracking and evaluation of emerging infections; developing more effective international surveillance networks for the anticipation, recognition, control, and

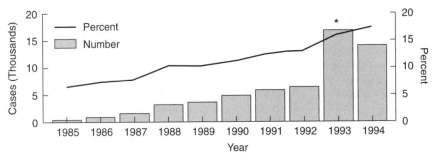

* The AIDS surveillance case definition was expanded in 1993.

Figure 6–9. Number and percentage of AIDS cases among women aged ≥ 13 years—United States, 1985–1994. (*Adapted from Centers for Disease Control. Update: AIDS among women—United States, 1994.* Morbidity and Mortality Weekly Report, *1995; 44[5], 81, Fig. 1.*)

prevention of emerging infectious diseases; improving surveillance and rapid laboratory identification to ensure early detection of antimicrobial resistance; strengthening and integrating programs to monitor and prevent emerging infections associated with food/water, new technology, and environmental sources; expanding epidemiologic and prevention effectiveness research; improving laboratory and epidemiological techniques for rapid identification of new pathogens and syndromes; ensuring timely development, appropriate use, and availablility of diagnostic tests and reagents; augmenting rapid response capabilities for vaccine delivery and expansion of evaluation of vaccine efficacy; and developing methods and enhancing infrastructures for improved communication of public health information to ensure prompt implementation of prevention strategies (Centers for Disease Control, 1997d).

CLINICAL CONTRIBUTIONS TO CONTROL OF INFECTIOUS DISEASES

While most of what was discussed earlier relates to public health strategies for control of infectious diseases, we should not ignore the contribution of clinical services. Particularly in a climate where managed care is becoming an increasingly common way of delivering health care services, strategies for prevention and early detection of infectious diseases make important contributions to assuring the health of the population. In the 1989 Report of the U.S. Preventive Services Task Force "Guide to Clinical Preventive Services" (Fisher, 1989) preventive interventions for clinical practice were evaluated and synthesized. These recommendations are based on extensive review of the literature and debate and synthesis of critical comments from expert reviewers to identify which interventions have proven efficacy and effectiveness. The recommendations for infectious disease prevention include screening, immunizations, and counseling. These recommendations are listed in Table 6–7. Unless clinicians adopt these recommendations as a routine part of practice, however, infectious diseases will continue to regularly occur. In 1993, the CDC recommended routine screening for chlamydia in all sexually active females under 20 years of age. In 1996, chlamydia was the most commonly reported infectious disease in the United States and had a prevalence rate of 5 to 15%. Despite this, screening by primary care providers serving adolescents was generally low. While 100% of health care providers in community health clinics surveyed in North Carolina in 1996 reported routinely screening for chlamydia, only 15% of those in private for-profit settings did so. In health departments, 78% screened for this disease. Rates for private non-profit settings and university health centers were 89% and 50%, respectively. Providers in general medical or emergency specialties were more likely to screen (56%) than those in internal medicine or family practice (10%) or those in obstetrics/gynecology (22%) (Centers for Disease Control, 1997e,f).

    Specific counseling recommendations for prevention of HIV infection and other sexually transmitted diseases include advice that abstaining from sex or maintaining a mutually faithful monogamous sexual relationship with a partner known

TABLE 6–7. RECOMMENDATIONS FOR CLINICAL PREVENTIVE SERVICES FOR INFECTIOUS DISEASES

Screening Tests	Target Population
Hepatitis B surface antigen	Pregnant women at first prenatal visit; repeat in third trimester for high-risk women
Tuberculin skin testing	High-risk individuals (household members of persons with TB; staff members at risk of contact with TB patients; recent immigrants or refugees from countries where TB is common; persons with underlying medical disorders [eg, HIV infection])
Syphilis serologic testing	High-risk individuals (prostitutes, those with multiple sexual partners in areas with high syphilis rates, sexual contacts of patients with active syphilis); pregnant women at first prenatal visit and at delivery (also at 28 weeks if at high risk)
Gonorrhea screening	High-risk individuals (as per syphilis); pregnant women at first prenatal visit and repeated in late pregnancy if at high risk
Human immunodeficiency virus (HIV)	Individuals seeking treatment for sexually transmitted diseases; intravenous drug users; homosexual and bisexual men; other high-risk individuals
Chlamydial screening	High-risk individuals (at sexual disease clinics/other high-risk health care facilities; age less than 20; multiple sexual partners or partner has multiple contacts); pregnant women at high risk
Genital herpes simplex	Pregnant women with active lesions
Asymptomatic bacteriuria	Persons with diabetes mellitus; pregnant women; preschool children; persons over age 60

Immunizations	Target Population
Childhood	All children without established contraindications
Diptheria-pertussis-tetanus (DPT)	Ages 2, 4, 6, and 15 months; repeat between age 4 and 6 years
Oral poliovirus	Ages 2, 4, 6, and 15 months; repeat between age 4 and 6 years
Measles-mumps-rubella (MMR)	Age 15 months
Haemophilus influenzae type B	Age 18 months
Monovalent measles	Age 9 months in areas with more than five cases among preschool-aged children during each of previous 5 years (in addition to MMR as above)
Adulthood	
Pneumococcal vaccine	Once for persons 65 and older and for selected high-risk groups (medical conditions that increase risk of infection, patients living in special environments or social settings with identified increased risk)
Influenza vaccine	Annually for persons 65 and older; selected high-risk groups (as per pneumococcal vaccine)
Hepatitis B vaccine	Sexually active homosexual men; intravenous drug users; others at high risk
Tetanus-diptheria toxoid booster	Every 10 years for adults
Measles and mumps	All adults who lack evidence of immunity

Counseling	Target Population
HIV infection prevention	Sexually active adolescent and adult patients
Prevention of other sexually transmitted diseases	Sexually active adolescent and adult patients

(*Compiled from Fisher M. [Ed.]* Guide to clinical preventive services: An assessment of the effectiveness of 169 interventions. *Report of the U.S. Preventive Services Task Force. Baltimore: Williams & Wilkins, 1989.*)

not to be infected are the most effective ways to prevent these conditions. Counseling should also include information about the indications and proper methods for use of condoms and spermicides in sexual intercourse and health risks associated with anal intercourse. Intravenous drug users should be warned not to share drug paraphernalia or use unsterilized needles and syringes and advised to enroll in a drug treatment program. Of course, this also implies routinely taking a sexual history from these individuals.

Preventive efforts have been associated with dramatic reductions in morbidity and mortality from infectious diseases. When these efforts become lax, rates of morbidity and mortality increase. The benefits of preventing infectious disease or detecting it early, as opposed to the difficult and often unsuccesful treatment of advanced disease argue for ongoing collaborative efforts between the public health and clinical communities—both to ensure the health of the public and to contain costs of health care.

REFERENCES

Benenson A. (Ed.). (1990) *Control of communicable diseases in man.* Washington, D.C.: American Public Health Association.

Centers for Disease Control. (1995) MMWR summary of notifiable diseases, United States, 1995. *Morbidity and Mortality Weekly Report, 44*(53).

Centers for Disease Control. (1997a) Fatal human plague—Arizona and Colorado, 1996. *Morbidity and Mortality Weekly Report, 46*(27), 617–620.

Centers for Disease Control. (1997b) Measles outbreak—Southwestern Utah, 1996. *Morbidity and Mortality Weekly Report, 46*(33), 768 (Fig. 2).

Centers for Disease Control. (1997c) *Shigella sonnei* outbreak associated with contaminated drinking water—Island Park, Idaho, August 1995. *Morbidity and Mortality Weekly Report, 45*(11), 230.

Centers for Disease Control. (1997d) The CDC Prevention Strategy. CDC home page.

Centers for Disease Control and Prevention. (1997e) Chlamydia screening practices of primary-care providers—Wake County, North Carolina, 1996. *Morbidity and Mortality Weekly Report, 46*(35), 819–822.

Centers for Disease Control. (1997f) Chlamydia trachomatous genital infections—United States, 1995. *Morbidity and Mortality Weekly Report, 46*(9), 193–198.

Fox J., Hall C., Elveback L. (1970) *Epidemiology: Man and disease.* Toronto, Ont.: Collier-MacMillan Canada Ltd.

Fisher M. (Ed). (1989) *Guide to clinical preventive services: An assessment of the effectiveness of 169 interventions.* Report of the U.S. Preventive Services Task Force. Baltimore: Williams & Wilkins.

Koenig R. (1996a) A shared European concern. *Science, 272,* 1412.

Koenig R. (1996b) Koch keeps new watch on infections. *Science, 272,* 1412–1414.

Pennisi E. (1996) U.S. beefs up CDC's capabilities. *Science, 272,* 1413.

World Health Organization. (1996) *Executive Summary; The World Health Report 1996.* World Health Organization home page. Available at www.who.org.

7

Epidemiology and Control of Diseases of Noninfectious Etiology

ost major causes of death, serious illness, and disability in the United States today are related to violence and chronic diseases of noninfectious etiology. Chronic diseases of the heart, cancer, and stroke alone accounted for 62.1% of deaths in 1995 (U.S. Bureau of the Census, 1997). Accidents, suicide, and homicide accounted for another 6.1%. These major health problems are not caused by infectious agents. Although the natural history differs for each, these diseases as a group share certain commonalities of natural history not shared by diseases of infectious origin. Because we are using the natural history of disease as the basis for our discussion of disease control, we have chosen to classify all diseases as infectious or noninfectious. Although this approach is simplistic, it facilitates conceptualization of natural history and control issues, as well as approaches to research. It is necessary to recognize, however, that diseases classified here as noninfectious include acute and chronic conditions, physical and mental diseases, and conditions caused by numerous types of agents including physical, chemical, nutrient, psychological, and behavioral, or a combination of these. To minimize the complexity of discussion, this chapter has been organized as follows: (1) morbidity and mortality impact of chronic diseases; (2) major contrasts in the natural history of these diseases compared with those caused by infectious agents; (3) methodological issues in the study of noninfectious etiology; (4) major categories of etiological agents; and (5) public health and clinical approaches to control of these diseases.

MORBIDITY AND MORTALITY IMPACT OF DISEASES OF NONINFECTIOUS ETIOLOGY

Table 7–1 shows age-adjusted rates for the 15 major causes of death in the United States in 1995. Overall, heart disease, cancer, stroke, chronic obstructive pulmonary disease, and chronic liver disease account for about three quarters of all U.S. deaths (Centers for Disease Control, 1997). Although rates of these major killers are the highest among older age groups, these diseases represent a major proportion of

TABLE 7–1. NUMBER OF DEATHS AND AGE-ADJUSTED DEATH RATES[a] FOR THE 15 LEADING CAUSES OF DEATH[b] —UNITED STATES, 1995

RANK[b]	CAUSE OF DEATH (ICD-9)	NUMBER OF DEATHS (IN THOUSANDS)	AGE-ADJUSTED DEATH RATE FOR 1995
1	Diseases of the heart	738.8	138.2
2	Malignant neoplasms, including neoplasms of lymphatic and hematopoietic tissues	538.0	129.8
3	Cerebrovascular disease	158.1	26.7
4	Chronic obstructive pulmonary disease and allied conditions	104.8	21.2
5	Accidents and adverse effects	89.7	29.2
6	Pneumonia and influenza	83.5	13.0
7	Diabetes mellitus	59.1	13.2
8	Other infectious and parasitic diseases	49.6	17.4
9	HIV Infection	31.3	unavailable
10	Suicide	30.9	11.0
11	Homicide and legal intervention	21.6	8.8
12	Chronic liver disease and cirrhosis	24.8	7.5
13	Nephritis, nephrotic syndrome, and renal failure	23.8	4.0
14	Septicemia	21.1	4.1
15	Atherosclerosis	16.8	2.3
	All Causes	2,312.2	502.9

[a]Per 100,000 population, age-adjusted to 1940 U.S. population.
[b]Based on number of deaths.
(From U.S. Bureau of the Census. Statistical abstract of the United States; 1997 [117th ed.]. Washington, D.C.: U.S. Government Printing Office, 1997.)

deaths at younger ages as well. Male mortality is higher for all these causes of death than is female mortality. Except for accidents and adverse effects, chronic obstructive pulmonary disease, and suicide, rates for blacks are higher than for whites (Table 7–2). Calculation of "potential years of life lost" is one method of measuring the loss to society resulting from death at young or early ages. It has been estimated that three categories of death represent 52% of potential years of life lost in the United States—diseases of the circulatory system, cancer, and cerebrovascular disease. Injuries contribute another 10%. Accidents, suicide/homicide, and cancer, however, contribute a larger percentage of years of life lost than of deaths because these are often killers of young persons (Centers for Disease Control, 1990a).

Diseases of the circulatory system and musculoskeletal system are major contributors to causing limitation of activity. Chronic diseases are major causes of disability and decreased quality of life. They represent a major source of medical care expenditures in the United States, $425 billion in 1990, or 61% of total U.S.

TABLE 7–2. RATIO OF AGE-ADJUSTED DEATH RATES[a] FOR THE 15 LEADING CAUSES OF DEATH, BY SEX AND RACE—UNITED STATES, 1992

		RATIO	
RANK[b]	CAUSES OF DEATH (ICD-9)[c]	Male:Female	Black:White[d]
1	Diseases of the heart (390-398, 402, 404-429)	1.7	1.6
2	Malignant neoplasms, including neoplasms of lymphatic and hematopoietic tissues (140-208)	1.9	1.5
3	Cerebrovascular diseases (430-438)	1.5	1.4
4	Chronic obstructive pulmonary diseases and allied conditions (490-496)	1.7	0.8
5	Accidents and adverse effects (E800-E949)	2.6	1.3
	Motor vehicle accidents (E810-E825)	(2.4)	(1.0)
	All other accidents and adverse effects (E800-E807, E826-E949)	(3.0)	(1.6)
6	Pneumonia and influenza (480-487)	1.7	1.4
7	Diabetes mellitus (250)	1.1	2.4
8	HIV infection (042-044)	7.0	3.7
9	Suicide (E950-E959)	4.3	0.6
10	Homicide and legal intervention (E950-E959)	4.0	6.5
11	Chronic liver disease and cirrhosis (571)	2.4	1.5
12	Nephritis, nephrotic syndrome, and nephrosis (580-589)	1.5	2.8
13	Septicemia (038)	1.3	2.7
14	Atherosclerosis (440)	1.3	1.1
15	Certain conditions originating in the prenatal period[e]	1.2	3.2
	All Causes	1.7	1.5

[a] Age-adjusted rates per 100,000 based on 1940 population.
[b] Rank based on number of deaths.
[c] International Classification of Disease Codes, ninth revision (ICD-9) are shown in parentheses.
[d] Both groups include Hispanics.
[e] Based on infant mortality rates.
(From Centers for Disease Control. Mortality patterns—United States, 1992. Morbidity and Mortality Weekly Report, 1995; 43[6S], 8,Table D.)

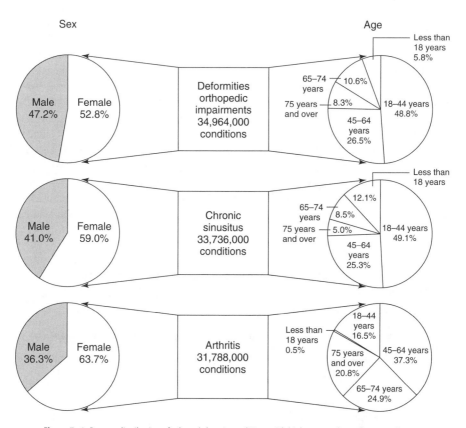

Figure 7–1. Percent distribution of selected chronic conditions with highest prevalence, by sex and age: United States, 1990–1992. (*Adapted from Collins J. G. Prevalence of selected chronic conditions: United States, 1990–1992. National Center for Health Statistics.* Vital Health Statistics, *1997;* [10]*194.*)

medical care expenditures (Centers for Disease Control, 1997). For many individuals, effects on quality of life from these conditions may begin in childhood or early adulthood. Figure 7–1 shows the percent distribution of three chronic conditions: orthopedic impairments and deformities, chronic sinusitis, and arthritis by gender and by age. Nearly 6% of orthopedic deformities and impairment and 12% of chronic sinusitus occur among children under age 18. Prevalence of these conditions, particularly arthritis, is higher for females than for males. Because of the impact of these diseases, understanding their natural history is crucial so prevention and control programs can be developed.

NATURAL HISTORY

As with infectious diseases, the natural history of chronic diseases involves interaction of host, agent, and environment. One can also view the progression of these diseases using the stages presented under our discussion of infectious disease in

Chapter 6: susceptibility, presymptomatic disease, and clinical disease. Although the framework for understanding the natural history applies to both infectious and noninfectious etiological agents, there are important differences. These are listed in Table 7–3 and discussed below.

Characteristics of the Agent

One important difference between infectious diseases and noninfectious diseases is the absence of a single necessary agent. Infectious diseases cannot occur without exposure to the single infectious agent necessary to cause the disease. Although there may be additional agents or circumstances whose presence or absence increases or decreases the likelihood of acute infection, they are not necessary for the disease to occur. When diseases are caused by noninfectious agents there is rarely, if ever, a single necessary agent. This is a function, in part, of the system used for disease classification. Although many infectious diseases are classified in terms of the causal agent (eg, tuberculosis after the tubercle bacillus), most diseases caused by noninfectious agents are classified on the basis of manifestations rather than on the basis of etiology. Cardiovascular disease, renal disease, and neoplasms are all manifestation-based classifications. Numerous agents may lead to similar manifestations. Fire, chemicals, and the sun can all produce burns. Different chemical agents may produce cancer at the same site. Any of several combinations of lifestyle factors seem to produce the manifestations we call cardiovascular disease. In diseases of infectious etiology, however, even those classified by manifestation have a single necessary agent (eg, rheumatic heart disease is caused by the *Staphylococcus* agent).

A related difference between infectious and noninfectious diseases is that the known "causes" of noninfectious diseases are often risk factors representing physiological states known to increase an individual's risk for developing a disease. As such, these risk factors represent physiological changes that have already begun. For example, obesity, elevated cholesterol levels, and hypertension are risk factors for coronary heart disease. These physiological states often involve cellular changes that are steps in the development of disease. Although some reversal of damage may occur with treatment, some residual is likely to remain. Genetic makeup may also relate to risk for developing a disease. Having the BRCA1 gene, for example,

TABLE 7–3. DIFFERENCES IN NATURAL HISTORY FOR INFECTIOUS AND NONINFECTIOUS DISEASES

INFECTIOUS DISEASE	NONINFECTIOUS DISEASE
Single necessary agent	No single necessary agent
Agent-disease specificity	Seldom agent-disease specificity
Causes are known	Causes unknown, intervention often based on risk factors
Short incubation period	Long latency period
Single exposure usually sufficient	May require multiple exposure to same or multiple agents
Usually produces acute disease	Most often produces chronic disease
Acquired immunity possible	Acquired immunity unlikely
Diagnosis based on tests specific to disease agent	Diagnosis often dependent on nonspecific symptoms or tests

may be associated with a breast cancer that is faster growing than tumors in women without the BRCA1 gene (Breast Cancer Consortium, 1997).

Time Frame

Another difference between infectious and noninfectious diseases is the length of time required between initial exposure to causal agents and onset of detectable physiological signs and symptoms (latency period for noninfectious diseases; incubation period for infectious diseases). With many infectious agents, signs and symptoms of the related disease become evident in hours, days, or weeks, or at most a few months. In the case of most noninfectious agents, it is often years or decades before illness is apparent. The reason for the short time required by infectious agents is that if the human host is not immune, the agents are able to multiply rapidly until their number is sufficient to produce disease. Because the agents in conditions of noninfectious etiology are not living organisms, there is no multiplication. Therefore, multiple low-dose exposures may be required to cause illness; this is the case with certain chemicals. In other instances, such as asbestosis, only a single exposure is thought to be necessary, but the mechanism of physiological response can take as many as 30 years before damage to the lung is sufficient to produce signs and symptoms. In still other instances, such as cancers, it is suspected that the causal mechanism may require exposure to at least two agents that produce damage to the genetic material of cells. A final situation is exhibited by conditions such as cardiovascular or cerebrovascular diseases; these seem to evolve subsequent to chronic conditions or states of high risk such as hypertension, smoking, diabetes, and high blood cholesterol.

Exceptions to the long latency periods of diseases of noninfectious etiology do occur, for example, in chemical agents that cause acute episodes of poisoning. Awareness of the probable latency period for a particular condition is important both in planning etiological investigations and in planning control measures, as will be discussed later in this chapter.

Nature of the Disease

Another difference between diseases of infectious and noninfectious etiology is that, more often than not, diseases of noninfectious or unknown etiology are chronic in nature. The term *chronic disease* is used in the sense defined by the 1957 Commission on Chronic Diseases—all impairments or deviations from normal that have one or more of the following characteristics: is permanent; leaves residual disability; is caused by nonreversible pathological alterations; requires special training of the patient for rehabilitation; or may be expected to require long periods of supervision, observation, or care (Commission on Chronic Disease, 1957).

The high frequency with which chronicity is observed in diseases of noninfectious etiology is probably a function of the long latency period characteristic of these conditions. When a disease process is proceeding slowly over time, the body is likely to make adaptive responses that will, in turn, contribute to the overall ability of the physiology to respond to stresses. These adaptive responses, although facilitating short-term function, may be detrimental over the long term. The residual disability of these diseases requires ongoing medical treatment and rehabilitation programs. For example, patients with diabetes are likely to require indefinite ongoing supervision of prescribed medications such as insulin, control of diet, modification of lifestyle, and frequent screening for eye changes, cardiovascular status, and so forth.

In contrast, the short incubation period required for multiplication and establishment of an infectious agent leaves little time for adaptive response and an acute illness, often of rather abrupt onset, ensues. Physiological response to the infection is agent-specific; antibodies against the particular agent are produced, and this immune response, when combined with drug treatment to aid in killing the organism, usually results in recovery. The patient may be ill for a period ranging from a few days to several months and recover without residual disability; however, if the illness is severe or the patient is debilitated, they may die from the illness. Death is most frequently seen with debilitated or immune-compromised patients such as those found in hospital settings. Patients who recover rarely require long-term followup, except for diseases such as hepatitis that may have residual disability or AIDS, which is progressive. As previously pointed out, there are infectious illnesses with chronic stages. These result either from residual damage, as with rheumatic heart disease, or from inactive stages of an organism that has survived the immune response of the host, as with the herpes simplex virus that produces shingles and the syphilis organism that, if unrecognized and untreated with antibiotics goes on to attack the neurological system.

Some noninfectious agents can produce both acute and chronic disease. Beryllium serves as an example. Beryllium may cause chronic disease characterized by granulomatosis lesions of the lung and enlarged lymph nodes in conjunction with the lesions. The chronic disease develops, in most cases, without being preceded by an acute phase. Beryllium can also produce acute episodes characterized by a pneumonia-like process that includes fever, chills, cough, sputum production, and shortness of breath with transient inflammation of the upper air passages and upper bronchi. The acute episodes can last up to 3 months and may cause death. It has been estimated that about 6% of acute cases will develop into a chronic condition. The chronic condition caused by beryllium exposure is symptomatically characterized by a progressive shortness of breath, cough, slight sputum production, weight loss, occasional nausea, and low-grade fever. Shortness of breath may be the sole symptom. Other cases are characterized by a rapidly progressive disease causing emaciation and death within months. Some individuals with massive prolonged exposure show no clinical or radiographical evidence of any disease. The relationship between exposure and the natural history of beryllium lung disease is not well understood (Meyer, 1994; Rossman, 1996; Newman et al, 1996).

Synergism in Disease Causation

Synergistic effects of two or more agents are frequently seen in causation models of noninfectious agents. As one example, workers in a grocery store in Ohio experienced an outbreak of phytophotodermatitis (Centers for Disease Control, 1985). All cases occurred among cashiers, baggers, and produce clerks. None occurred among shelf stockers, delicatessen clerks, meat clerks, or managers. Development of the rash was traced to contact with fresh vegetables and flowers, which contain psoralens. Risk of developing phytophotodermatitis, however, increased substantially among workers who used tanning salons. Risk of developing the rash was 4.3 times greater for exposure both to psoralen and ultraviolet light (tanning salons) than psoralen alone (Fig. 7–2).

In another example of synergism, nonsmoking workers exposed to asbestos have been reported to have a risk of developing lung cancer eight times that of nonsmoking, nonexposed individuals. However, smokers who are exposed to asbestos have 90 times the risk of the nonsmoking, nonexposed individuals (Selikoff et al, 1968). This is of concern because control efforts often must settle for minimizing rather than eliminating workplace exposures. It was hoped that if exposures to harmful environmental agents, such as asbestos, could be kept low, then the latency period before onset of symptoms would be so long that the average individual would not have health problems related to the exposure until old age. This expectation was based on accumulating evidence that higher doses contribute both to increased disease risk and to length of the latency period (Seidman et al, 1979). The presence of synergism, however, may shorten latency periods and produce illness in the prime of life even with low level exposure. The concepts of initiation and promotion are relevant. While one agent may initiate the process of cancer development, numerous other agents, called *promoters,* can play the role of speeding up the process. Additional research is needed to clarify these issues. In the meantime, law-

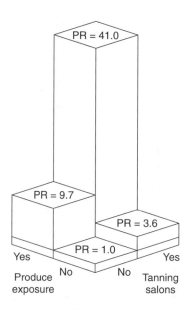

Figure 7–2. Risk of rash among grocery workers, by exposure to fresh produce and use of tanning salons: Ohio, April–August 1984. (*Adapted from Centers for Disease Control.* Phytophotodermatitis *in Ohio.* Morbidity and Mortality Weekly Report, *1985;* 34[1], 13.)

makers, planners of control programs, economists who consider the cost–benefit effects of control efforts, and many others concerned with the health of the public are forced to make decisions based on present levels of knowledge.

METHODOLOGICAL ISSUES IN THE STUDY OF DISEASES OF NONINFECTIOUS ETIOLOGY

Natural History

The natural history characteristics of diseases must be considered in the design of studies investigating etiology. The lack of a single necessary agent causing a disease makes it more difficult to isolate the effect of any individual factor. Synergistic effects of other agents and effects of known causes of a disease must be controlled. The long latency period between exposure and onset of disease increases the difficulties associated with obtaining information on exposure in retrospective study designs or in tracking exposed populations to assess disease incidence in prospective study designs. The chronic nature of many of these diseases, together with their relatively lower frequency of occurrence, often means that prevalence cases are studied rather than incidence cases. This produces a wide spectrum of stages in the natural history among the cases. Because factors may have independent effects and converse effects on the processes of disease development, disease progression, and survival, interpretations of causality for prevalence cases may be difficult.

Rates Used to Study Chronic Disease Causation

Incidence and prevalence rates (discussed in Chapter 3) are used to measure the frequency of chronic diseases in populations. While both are used to study etiology, prevalence is particularly relevant for health planning, since it provides a measure of the ongoing caseload that is likely to need services. This is because prevalence is a function of both disease incidence and duration. When a disease has a relatively short latency or there is good historical data on exposure and a population can be tracked over time to determine whether the disease of interest has developed, as with many occupational-related diseases, prospective or historical cohort studies can be conducted to study etiology. These studies yield incidence rates that can be compared for a group exposed to a putative causal agent and a comparison group. Relative risk ratios based on comparing the incidence in the exposed versus the nonexposed comparison group can then be computed to determine the excess risk associated with the exposure. When a disease has a long latency and historical cohorts with the required data are unavailable for study or when a disease of interest occurs infrequently, cross-sectional case-control studies are likely to be used to explore causal associations. These studies rely on use of prevalence cases of the disease and a comparison group that does not have the disease. An odds ratio is used as the measure of association between the exposure and the disease. These measures were discussed in more detail in Chapter 4.

Case Identification: Defining Numerators of Morbidity Rates

Identifying a case of a disease of noninfectious etiology is more difficult than is defining a case of an infectious disease. In infectious diseases, definitive identification of a case is possible by obtaining a sample of the appropriate body fluid or secretion and growing the organism in a laboratory culture. If the criteria for case status demand a positive culture or a transformation to a positive antibody status, then separation of cases from noncases is possible with a high degree of validity. For most diseases of noninfectious etiology, definition of case status may depend on presence or absence of a cluster of symptoms with or without positive values on specified laboratory tests. Differentiation of specific diagnoses within a broad disease classification may be difficult (eg, differentiating specific diagnosis, such as emphysema and asthma, within the broader category of chronic obstructive lung diseases). Particularly for research using medical records, the need to rely on stated diagnoses may be problematic because criteria for arriving at the recorded diagnosis may vary by institution or physician. Changes in medical practice take time to diffuse, so physicians at one institution may use new diagnostic measures earlier than physicians elsewhere. For example, diagnosis of cardiovascular events such as myocardial infarction (MI) has until recently required hospitalization for a series of tests. Now new blood tests called cardiac treponin I can be done on an outpatient basis to determine whether a patient has had a mild MI (Galvani et al, 1997). But while major medical centers may be using these tests, many physicians practicing in other settings have yet to adopt them.

For conditions where some subjectivity of judgment is needed for diagnosis, consistency is hard to achieve. Studies have demonstrated a lack of agreement among multiple psychiatrists making psychiatric diagnoses based on the same information for patients with similar symptoms who differ by race, sex, or socioeconomic status (Warner & Peabody, 1995; Basco et al, 1994). Studies using psychiatric diagnoses, therefore, may need to build into the design blind review procedures of all cases to establish diagnosis using standardized criteria for all cases. Similar, although probably less severe problems, could be expected for different subcategories of other noninfectious diseases, for example neuromuscular conditions. Cutoffs for labeling blood pressure levels as hypertension or abnormal blood sugar values as diabetes vary from clinician to clinician and may vary over time as better data on the predictive validity of various test levels indicating progression of clinical disease become available. These issues are discussed further in Chapters 12, 15, and 16. The importance of setting clear criteria for valid classification of cases versus noncases in studies of noninfectious diseases cannot be overemphasized.

Identifying the Appropriate Population for Rate Denominators

In order to derive incidence or prevalence rates, it is necessary to determine the appropriate population from which the cases arose, ie, the *population at risk*. This may be employees of a particular plant, residents of a geographic area, patients receiving a specific treatment, or a population susceptible to developing the disease of interest. One would need to be careful to exclude from the denominator individuals who could not possibly develop the disease—for example, women who have had hysterectomy if studying the relationship between hormone replacement therapy and endometrial cancer. Similar exclusions would need to be made for both the study group and the comparison group. Since it is generally not possible to study all individuals who might have and not have an exposure for a cohort study or all cases who have a disease and all individuals who might be available for a comparison group for a case-control study, one must usually select a sample of those available to study. If the sampling strategy gives each individual an equal probability of being selected for the sample, the sampling method is called *random sampling* or *probability sampling*. This approach has the best chance of assuring that characteristics of people in probability samples are similar to those of the population from which they were selected. Other methods are more likely to be biased, for example selecting patients only from a medical center practice, studying only individuals willing to participate, or studying only cases that meet certain criteria. However, there may be good reason for using these other approaches. One must be aware of the potential effect of such bias on the results when reading results of the study.

Measuring Exposure

The ability to measure exposure accurately is an important methodological consideration in the study of diseases of noninfectious etiology. Although investigations of infectious diseases require demonstration of exposure to a source of the infectious agent, quantity of the infectious agent is less of an issue than agent qualities such as virulence or pathogenicity. In the case of noninfectious agents, whether lifestyle related agents such as cigarette smoke or fat content of the diet, or occupational/environmental agents such as benzene, lead, or pesticides, the amount or level of exposure is important. A single agent can produce acute illness with high dose exposures or can produce chronic illness with continuing low dose exposure. One does not necessarily lead to the other. The acute illness associated with lead intoxication is not an early stage of the disease associated with long-term, low level chronic lead exposure.

Determination of dose of exposure is problematic. It must be decided whether dose is a function of the nature of the metabolite of the agent, enzymatic alteration, or level of the original xenobiotic agent. Should environmental levels be used as a measure of exposure or should levels in the body be used? If the latter, what is the appropriate place to measure the dose—plasma levels, brain concentration, kidney, some other organ? For agents with long tissue residence, biological measures reflecting cumulative burdens may be more appropriate. Studies must often settle for indirect, crude measures, such as the number of cigarettes smoked daily. Information on whether the cigarettes are filtered, their levels of tar, nicotene, and other chemicals, what percent of each cigarette is actually smoked, and so on, is often unavailable.

An undifferentiated, broad range of exposures among an exposed population may make it more difficult to study effects because the exposed group may be diluted by the presence of substantial numbers of individuals with relatively low levels of exposure to the agent. Furthermore, precise identification of exposure levels enables the investigator to evaluate at what level of exposure hazard to health begins, an important piece of information in planning control measures. Demonstration of a dose effect (ie, increases in disease frequency associated with increasing levels of exposure) helps to establish a causal role for the agent.

Another important aspect of measuring exposure is the constancy of the exposure. Likelihood of effects may differ in constant exposure and intermittent exposure. For example, in our own work investigating health effects associated with the occupational exposure of nurses to antineoplastic drugs, this becomes a crucial factor. Although some antineoplastic drugs reach peak rates of excretion within 6 hours, others peak closer to 24 hours. A nurse who handles large amounts of these drugs only twice a week, on Monday and Thursday, has ample time between handling sessions to eliminate the drugs from their body. A nurse who handles a moderate amount of the drugs daily may never achieve total clearance of the drugs, thus experiencing a constant exposure. The constant exposure is more likely to be associated with effects than is the intermittent exposure even if the total dosage of exposure were the same.

It is not the intent of this text to discuss in depth such methodological issues related to epidemiological research. For those interested in designing epidemiological studies these issues are covered extensively in methodological texts. However, it has been the author's intent to raise issues that should be kept in mind when reading the epidemiological literature so that the reader can evaluate whether a study has addressed the important issues relevant to the particular study. The specific natural history characteristics discussed in this chapter for diseases of noninfectious etiology should be addressed.

The Issues of Conflicting Findings and Causality

Clinicians are often put on the spot by patients who have read a report of a medical study in the newspaper or in another lay publication. The questions usually relate to some agent that has been shown to "cause" a particular disease. The proliferation of such reports in the lay press puts considerable pressure on health professionals to keep up with their reading of the literature so that they can respond appropriately to requests for advice regarding the personal implications of such study reports. A dilemma arises, however, for many clinicians attempting to read the epidemiological literature because contradictory findings are often reported. It is probably useful to keep in mind, first of all, that there is a bias in favor of publication of studies with positive findings. Particularly if it is the first study to test a particular hypothesis, editors are likely to find positive findings more interesting and are more likely to publish such findings. Once positive findings have been published, negative findings from subsequent studies stand a greater chance of being published. As the literature develops with regard to a particular hypothesis, a variety of findings may therefore result. This is particularly true for studies of noninfectious causal agents. In reviewing a body of literature, one can discount findings from severely biased studies, particularly if those are the ones that consistently produce findings that contradict those from less biased studies. However, some criteria for making inferences about causality are required. These are discussed below.

Infectious Disease Causality

Determining cause for infectious agents has been possible for many years, since Robert Koch (1843–1910) introduced his five postulates for demonstrating a causal relationship. These postulates require that the organism: (1) be found in *all* cases of disease (possible because it is a single *necessary* agent); (2) be isolated from patients and grown in pure culture; (3) reproduce the disease when the pure culture is inoculated into a susceptible animal; (4) be recoverable from the diseased animal; and (5) not be present as a nonpathogenic organism when the disease is not present. In general, these postulates have stood the test of time; carrier states are now known to exist, invalidating postulate number 5. Viruses cannot be grown on lifeless culture media but require living cells. In addition, more recent technology has led to the identification of disease-specific antibodies that can provide immunological proof of presence of an infection and case status.

Noninfectious Disease Causality

Causality in disease of noninfectious etiology must rely more heavily on strictly epidemiological evidence. Epidemiological evidence requires well-designed studies to demonstrate that the incidence of a disease is higher among those exposed than those not exposed (prospective studies) or that exposure to the putative causes should be present more commonly among those with the disease than among those without (case-control studies). Elimination or reduction of the putative cause should decrease the incidence of disease. The cumulative body of studies available must be reviewed as an entirety. After eliminating from consideration those studies in which the findings could be predicted *a priori* by the presence of biases in the design, the remaining study findings can be evaluated using the criteria discussed in Chapter 2—temporal correctness, consistency of findings, specificity of the relationship, strength of the relationships demonstrated (including dose effect), and biological plausibility—to determine the level of evidence supporting an etiological role for the factor.

MAJOR CATEGORIES OF ETIOLOGICAL AGENTS

Noninfectious disease agents include physical, chemical, nutrient, genetic, and psychological agents. For purposes of the discussion to follow, these agents are considered as they relate to three specific areas of focus: (1) occupational health, (2) general environmental health, and (3) lifestyle factors, such as smoking which has a major impact on health status. Further discussion of lifestyle factors as disease agents is integrated in Chapters 7 through 10.

Occupational Health

Many human diseases can be traced to exposures associated with the work environment, including substances or working conditions that pose risks to health or accidents and injuries on the job. In addition, substances to which workers are exposed may interact with lifestyle behaviors such as alcohol consumption and smoking to increase risks of occupational illness or injury. The role of employers in recent years in creating a safer environment, providing health information to employees, and offering health promotion activities has increased during the 1970s and 1980s, due in part to activities of the Occupational Safety and Health Administration and National Institute of Occupational Safety and Health. The number of disabling occupational injuries decreased from 2.2 million in 1970 to 1.7 million in 1989. The current rate is 3.6, but because of changes in methodology cannot be compared with previous years (U.S. Bureau of the Census, 1997). Rates of work-related deaths decreased from 1.04 per 100,000 female workers in 1980 to 0.66 in 1993. Comparable figures for male workers were 12.46 and 7.21 respectively (Wagener et al, 1997). Decreases surpassed goals set in the 1979 report *Healthy People: The Surgeon General's Report on Health Promotion and Disease Prevention for 1990* (U.S. Department of Health, Education, and Welfare, 1979). The historically high risk groups, including workers in mining, construction, transportation, and farming industries have also experienced lower rates in fatal injuries over time. Data for 1994 and 1995 shows decreasing rates of nonfatal work-related injuries as well (U.S. Bureau of the Census, 1997).

Causal Agents in the Workplace.   Control of work-related exposures that pose hazards to worker health is a major potential target for primary prevention. Epidemiological investigations play an important role in identifying chemicals, metals, or other substances associated with adverse health outcomes and in confirming as hazards to human health any substances initially implicated by animal studies. The cumulative body of evidence from laboratory and epidemiological studies provides a basis for control and regulatory decisions.

A list of the leading work-related diseases and injuries in the United States is shown in Table 7–4. Additional concerns are the effects of occupational exposures on reproductive function, including sexual dysfunction, abnormal sperm or decreased sperm count, chromosome abnormalities, fetal loss, low birth weight, birth defects, increased infant mortality, and childhood morbidity, including cancer.

Chemicals are prime agents affecting the health of the working population. Each year thousands of new chemicals are developed. Many of these are potential mutagens, teratogens, or carcinogens. More than 6 million chemicals have been registered with the Chemical Abstracts Service. Of these, more than 50,000 are thought to be regularly used in commerce, but fewer than 1,000 have been studied for their potential for cancer causation (U.S. Public Health Service, 1993). The World Health Organization's International Agency for Research on Cancer, which routinely evaluates evidence for carcinogenicity of chemicals, has evaluated 782 compounds and, based on available evidence, declared 66 as carcinogenic to humans, 51 as probably

TABLE 7–4. THE TEN LEADING WORK-RELATED DISEASES AND INJURIES—UNITED STATES, 1990[a]

1. Occupational lung diseases: asbestosis, byssinosis, silicosis, coal workers' pneumoconiosis, lung cancer, occupational asthma
2. Musculoskeletal injuries: disorders of the back, trunk, upper extremity, neck, lower extremity; traumatically induced Raynaud's phenomenon
3. Occupational cancers (other than lung): leukemia; mesothelioma; cancers of the bladder, nose, and liver
4. Severe occupational traumatic injuries: amputations, fractures, eye loss, lacerations, and traumatic deaths
5. Occupational cardiovascular diseases: hypertension, coronary artery disease, acute myocardial infarction
6. Disorders of reproduction: infertility, spontaneous abortion, teratogenesis
7. Neurotoxic disorders: peripheral neuropathy, toxic encephalitis, psychoses, extreme personality changes (exposure-related)
8. Noise-induced: loss of hearing
9. Dermatological conditions: dermatoses, burns (scaldings), chemical burns, contusions (abrasions)
10. Psychological disorders: neuroses, personality disorders, alcoholism, drug dependency

[a]The conditions listed under each category are to be viewed as *selected* examples, not comprehensive definitions of the category. (*From U.S. Public Health Service.* Healthy people 2000: National health promotion and disease prevention objectives. *Washington, D.C.: 1990, p. 65.*)

carcinogenic to humans, 210 as possibly carcinogenic to humans, 454 with data insufficient to determine carcinogenicity, and 1 as probably not carcinogenic to humans. Evidence from human studies is evaluated for evidence of causal relationships of the chemical with occurrence of human cancers. This evidence is supplemented with data from carcinogenesis bioassays and other experimental studies of animals, toxicity data, and other biological data (Stellman & Stellman, 1996). The National Institute of Occupational Safety and Health estimates that more than 7 million American workers are potentially exposed on a regular basis to chemical carcinogens in the workplace, and that approximately 12 to 20% of cancer deaths are due to occupational exposures (Landrigan, 1996). Chemicals can also cause respiratory inflammation, dermatitis, asthma, neurotoxicity, liver toxicity, and a variety of other adverse effects on human health.

Metals and naturally occurring minerals are a group of occupational agents. Mineral dusts and fibers, such as silica and asbestos, are physical agents that produce occupational disease. Silicosis and asbestosis are both respiratory conditions, each common to particular groups of exposed workers. Groups such as miners, quarry workers, tunnel drillers, excavators, and stonemasons experience a high incidence of silicosis. Asbestosis has been associated with workers in asbestos mines or processing plants, shipyard workers, construction workers, and auto repair workers. Lead, nickel, mercury, arsenic, beryllium, and tin are among the many metals associated with occupational diseases. Risks from these occupational exposures may extend beyond the work force at the particular exposure site. Asbestos dust carried home on the clothing of workers, for example, has been associated with asbestosis and mesothelioma among family members in the household of those working with asbestos.

Four occupational exposures have potential impact on cardiovascular health: (1) metals, dusts, and trace elements; (2) occupational inhalants and other chemical exposures; (3) noise; and (4) psychosocial stress. Congestive heart failure resulting from restrictive lung disease (cor pulmonale) has been observed in occupational respiratory diseases such as silicosis and chronic beryllium disease. Other metals such as antimony, cobalt, and lead have also been implicated. Carbon monoxide may precipitate acute cardiovascular events (eg, changes in cardiac rhythm) in persons with preexisting coronary artery disease. Carbon disulfide, a common solvent, increases the risk of cardiovascular disorders, including coronary artery disease and hypertension. Other solvents, halogenated hydrocarbons, have precipitated sudden death, likely caused by cardiac arrhythmias, in workers exposed to high levels. Some of these solvents have been associated with arrhythmias at or below concentrations permitted by occupational standards. Workers exposed to nitroglycerine and nitrates during manufacture of explosives experienced a "rebound vasospasm" effect with an increased risk of cardiac chest pain, MI, and sudden death after withdrawal from exposure (Centers for Disease Control, 1985).

Single exposures to noise lead to transient increases in blood pressure. Chronic occupational exposure to noise has been associated with sustained increases in blood pressure. Increases in serum cholesterol and changes in circulating hormones have also been observed in association with exposure of humans to noise. Evidence suggests that psychological stress in the work setting is related to cardiovascular disease, particularly hypertension. Work overload, role conflicts, limited autonomy, nonsupportive supervisors, and lack of job mobility have predicted cardiovascular disease risk in several studies (Centers for Disease Control, 1985).

Investigating Occupational Exposures.   *Agent factors* to be considered in investigating occupational exposures include size and shape of particles (eg, asbestos dust), route of exposure (eg, lead by oral ingestion versus respiratory inhalation), and whether the substance is in free or compound, organic or inorganic, or liquid or vapor form.

Environmental factors pertinent to investigations of occupational disease include the conditions present in the work environment that influence the likelihood that workers will come in contact with an agent (eg, engineering containment measures), general cleanliness and ventilation of the work area, lighting of the work area, and temperature of the work area, which may affect volatility of certain chemicals and thus influence respiratory dose. Excessive temperature may, in itself, be an agent. Male workers exposed to high temperatures on the job, for example, may experience infertility as a result of sperm mortality. The social and psychological aspects of the work environment may also play a role. Scheduled breaks, positioning of workstations for physical comfort of the worker, and the opportunity for conversation with coworkers may be related to morale and fatigue levels that are factors in occupational accidents.

Host factors to be considered in occupational studies include lifestyle behaviors that may increase risk of disease from occupational exposure to an agent. Smoking is one such major factor that seems to have a synergistic effect on many exposures, leading, for example, to an enormous increase in risk for a variety of respiratory conditions when compounded by exposure to other agents that cause respiratory diseases. The increase in lung cancer for workers exposed to both asbestos and tobacco smoke was previously discussed. Smoking has also been linked to increased risk of mortality from cancers of the head and neck, urinary tract, pancreas, and bladder, leukemia, and myeloma; many of these cancers are also associated with particular occupational exposures making interaction between the two an ongoing concern. Alcohol use, quality of personal relationships, sleeping patterns, eating patterns (eg, eating on the job while handling hazardous chemicals), and diet can all affect risk for various occupational diseases or injuries. Genetic constitution may also affect susceptibility to a given occupational exposure.

Assessing Exposure.   Exposure assessment, although essential to epidemiological studies of occupational exposure and disease often cannot be measured directly, particularly in case-control studies of diseases with long latency periods and historical cohort studies. Thus, exposure assessment must rely on company records, which under ideal circumstances include industrial hygiene measurements of ambient levels of the hazardous agent, but often must be inferred indirectly through job titles or site of employment. Records may include information on use of protection against exposure. In cross-sectional studies and prospective cohort studies, it may be possible to obtain direct measures of exposure, using industrial hygiene measures or measures of biological dose using serum or other body fluid samples. Clearly, the more complete and accurate the information available regarding exposures incurred by individuals, the easier it will be to more precisely relate cancer risks to such exposures.

A second issue is assessing exposure to other host and environmental factors that can confound the relationship between the occupational exposure and the disease outcome of interest when their effect is not controlled—for example, smoking. Studies where exposure and outcome data are assessed from employment records and death certificates are often unable to obtain this crucial information. Information available on these other factors in records is often not valid and reliable.

Assessing Outcomes.   Assessment of outcome is done differently, depending on the study design. Acute illnesses caused by occupational exposures can be asssessed by physical examination, laboratory tests, and so on. But diseases such as cancer, because of their long latency periods often require use of historical cohort or other designs where outcome is assessed long after an exposure has occurred. Many occupational mortality studies thus rely on death certificate data to assess outcome. Accuracy of these data varies by disease condition.

Prevention of Occupational Exposures.   Since the two major routes of exposure to occupational chemicals are through respiratory and skin exposure, protective engineering controls and personal protective systems are an important means of prevention. Occupational risk reduction targets under the "Healthy People 2000 Objectives" are focused on increasing the proportion of worksites with over 50 employees that mandate use of occupational protection systems to 75%; reducing the number of workers exposed to noise levels >85 dB to 15% or less; eliminating exposures leading to blood lead concentrations >25 mg/dl of whole blood; and increasing hepatis B immunization among occupationally exposed workers to 90% (U.S. Public Health Service, 1993).

Environmental Health

The field of environmental health encompasses exposures in the community or residential environment. Many of the same substances encountered in occupational settings may be present in the general community environment.

Sources of Exposure.   Presence of industrial chemicals and other substances in the general community environment may result from contamination of air, water, and soil by industrial activities or inadequate methods of waste disposal. Exposure to these substances is, in general, at a lower dose than exposure to similar substances in occupational environments. Exceptions may occur near a particular landfill or dump site in which large quantities of waste substances have been disposed.

Other industrial products are distributed widely throughout the community as a function of their use. Pesticides, herbicides, and chemical fertilizers, for example, become airborne during spraying, drain off fields into streams, or soak into the ground after rain. Some of those chemicals are subsequently ingested by fish, stored in fatty tissue, and later consumed by humans. They may also seep into underground aquifers or rivers used for drinking water by humans and many animals. Eventually the entire ecosystem can be exposed. Even the food we eat can be contaminated with these chemical products. A study of organochlorine pesticide in the U.S. diet for the years 1965 through 1970 found DDT, Addrin, Dieldrin, and heptachlor epoxide in doses ranging from 1 to 87 μg of daily intake. These data are based on Food and Drug Administration market basket survey of diets that simulate the daily intake for young men, 16 to 19 years of age, in five major cities. The DDT total (DDT-T) consisting of DDT, DDE, and DDD is fat-soluble and likely to be stored in body tissues and released slowly in the body over a period of time. Fortunately, use of DDT reached a peak in 1966 and began declining until 1973, when its use was banned for all but essential public health needs (Krus, 1980). More recently, presence of Alar on apples produced a major health scare in 1989 and resulted in growers stopping use of the chemical. Increasingly, there are reports of chemicals in drinking water supplies, including arsenic, asbestos, radon, agricultural chemicals, and hazardous waste. Drinking water may be contaminated at the source, as a consequence of treatment processes, or can enter as the water is conveyed to the user, as with seepage of lead from old pipes (Morris, 1995).

Other potentially hazardous products are widely used in housing. Wood paneling and other products embedded with formaldehyde, for example, are commonly used in residential dwellings. Such products have been associated with adverse health effects, particularly respiratory problems, in mobile homes or newer housing where better insulation decreases the exchange of indoor and outdoor air. As a result, formaldehyde vapors inside these dwellings can reach toxic levels during the winter months.

By-products of heating homes, factories, and public buildings contribute to general environmental exposures. Burning coal, for example, produces emissions that pollute the air with particulates and sulfer dioxide. Automobile exhausts also contribute to the air pollution problem. Such by-products also have contributed to acid rain and its widespread effects on tree growth and the death of fish and other life forms.

Radiation is another ubiquitous agent. In addition to the naturally occurring radioactive atoms within living plants and animals that come from natural radioactive substances found in rocks, soil, and cosmic rays, there are numerous forms of human-produced radiation, such as that from medical and dental x-rays, fallout from atomic explosions and weapons testing, and accidental radioactive leaks and wastes from nuclear power reactors like that from Chernobyl some years ago. Although there has been a decrease in nuclear fallout from weapons testing since the 1963 Nuclear Test Ban Treaty, any such environmental radiation contaminates the food supply. Fallout on the land is absorbed and concentrated by plants that are eaten by humans and animals subsequently consumed by humans. Similarly, fallout on the sea, lakes, and rivers is available to marine plants and animals that concentrate the substances. Radioactive concentration can cumulatively increase at every step of the food chain. The most important food contaminant is strontium 90, a long-life radioactive element that is deposited in bone (Krus, 1980).

Many products used in the home for cleaning, redecorating or remodeling, or hobbies and crafts are potentially toxic agents if found by unsupervised children or if precautions are not followed during use, such as appropriate ventilation of the work area. Some of these products may require use of protective garments, such as gloves, masks, or goggles, to prevent skin burns, eye irritation or damage, and other effects. Fumes from gas cooking stoves have been associated with respiratory diseases such as asthma. Household dust can be a disease agent for susceptible individuals. Prescription and nonprescription drugs are other potential environmental agents in the home setting. Throw rugs, structural features such as stairs, the temperature of the water, and numerous other factors common to most home environments are potential agents for illness or injury.

Investigating Environmental Exposures.   The study of environmental agents uses methods similar to those discussed under occupational health. The major differences are in emphasis. Dose levels of many environmental exposures are considerably lower than those in occupational settings where workers are directly handling materials. Thus larger populations must be studied to detect the lower incidence of health effects likely to result. Also, routine availability of data on levels of contamination is less likely. Classification of persons as exposed or unexposed must often be based on residence in a contaminated or uncontaminated area, so ecological studies are more commonly used. Mobility of individuals may complicate definition of an exposed population, particularly in ecological-type studies; large numbers of individuals moving in or out of an area may lead to dilution of the population exposed and a major problem with misclassification of exposure. There may be more confounding variables to consider because individuals in a study may be scattered over a wide geographic area in which a variety of other exposures must be considered. Collection of data on health status and relevant behaviors may also be difficult and expensive.

Additional considerations in environmental studies include:

1. Wider ranges of ages exist among the exposed population than is true in occupational studies. Children and older people may be especially susceptible to a particular exposure.

2. Although workers are likely to be exposed for about 8 hours per day, residents of an area may be exposed 16 to 24 hours per day.
3. Meteorological conditions may play a much more important role in estimates of exposure. Air pollution levels may be much higher on the downwind side of a plant than on the upwind side.
4. Seasonal effects must be considered. A spring thaw may dilute pollutant levels in water. People are more likely to be outdoors and in contact with soil in warmer weather.

Although this list is far from exhaustive, it does point out the kind of thinking that must go into the design of environmental studies. Environmental epidemiology has become an increasingly important field following the publicity focused in recent years on the Environmental Protection Agency's toxic waste Superfund sites such as the Hanford nuclear facility. The need to apply epidemiological methods to the identification of health effects in communities that may result from hazardous substances is becoming increasingly urgent.

Lifestyle and Illness

Poverty, stress, insufficient exercise, being overweight, drug use, heavy alcohol consumption, risky sports activities, and poor nutrition are among the lifestyle factors that are associated with health status (Centers for Disease Control, 1997). However, none of these have been demonstrated to have the impact of cigarette smoking on health. For more than a decade, the U.S. Public Health Service has identified cigarette smoking as the most important preventable cause of death in our society. In 1964, the U.S. Surgeon General's Advisory Committee on Smoking and Health concluded, after reviewing more than 7,000 research articles relating to smoking and disease, that cigarette smoking is a cause of lung cancer and laryngeal cancer in men, a probable cause of lung cancer in women, and the most important cause of chronic bronchitis (U.S. Public Health Service, 1964). Additional diseases, including emphysema, cancer of the cervix, cerebrovascular disease, and cardiovascular disease were also found, on the basis of epidemiological evidence, to be associated with smoking. Each of the last five surgeon generals has identified cigarette smoking as one of the most significant causes of death and disease in the United States. For the first time, in 1986, lung cancer mortality equaled breast cancer as a cause of cancer deaths in women. Smoking is responsible for more than one of every six deaths in the United States. About 400,000 Americans die each year from diseases caused by smoking, including heart disease, lung cancer, other cancers, chronic obstructive pulmonary disease, and stroke (Centers for Disease Control, 1990b).

All the surgeon generals' reports since 1964 have documented the benefits of smoking cessation. The executive summary of the most recent report (Centers for Disease Control, 1990b) presents the following conclusions about the benefits of quitting:

1. Smoking cessation has major and immediate health benefits for men and women of all ages. Benefits apply to persons with and without smoking-related disease.

2. Former smokers live longer than continuing smokers. For example, persons who quit smoking before age 50 have one half the risk of dying in the next 15 years compared with continuing smokers.
3. Smoking cessation decreases the risk of lung cancer, other cancers, heart attack, stroke, and chronic lung disease.
4. Women who stop smoking before pregnancy or during the first 3 to 4 months of pregnancy reduce their risk of having a low birth weight baby to the same rate as that of women who never smoked.
5. The health benefits of smoking cessation far exceed any risks from the average 5-lb (2.3-kg) weight gain or any adverse psychological effects that may follow quitting.

The role of the other lifestyle factors associated with illness are discussed in Chapters 8 through 12.

CONTROL OF DISEASES OF NONINFECTIOUS ETIOLOGY

Treatment of chronic disease is a huge burden on the health care system and in 1990, consumed 61% of total U.S. health care expenditures. However, disease control expenditures (in 1989) accounted for only 3% of state health department expenditures, equivalent to $0.99 per capita. The per capita public health expenditure for chronic disease prevention and control amounted to $1.21 in 1994 (Centers for Disease Control, 1997). The share of prevention spending by states relative to federal spending has declined; in 1989, 77% of prevention and control spending was from state funds, but by 1994 only 39% was by states and 45% was by the federal government. Priorities for spending on prevention and control are aimed at cancer, tobacco, and youth (Centers for Disease Control, 1997).

Primary Prevention

Primary prevention of diseases of noninfectious origin is complex, difficult, and sometimes not possible because of the lack of a simple necessary agent, inadequate evidence for causes other than risk factors indicative of existing physiological change, the ubiquitous distribution of many agents in the occupational and general environment, and the probable synergistic effects among agents. Basic approaches, similar to those for control of infectious agents, emphasize two methods:

1. Removal of agent(s) from the environment or minimizing the amount of the agent present.
2. Protection of the susceptible host from exposure.

These measures can be effective when a causal agent is known, although because of the multiple cause problem, each and every agent must be eliminated to assure control of disease incidence. As mentioned before, however, often no specific agent(s) has been identified; the state of knowledge is such that only risk factors are known. In these instances, primary prevention may not be possible—for example, risk factors for breast cancer include early age at menarche, late age at first full-term pregnancy, family history of breast cancer, and possessing the BRCA1 gene. It is difficult to intervene and change any of these risk factors, except perhaps age at first full-term pregnancy. But if age at first full-term pregnancy is a risk factor because high-risk women have difficulty conceiving or carrying an infant to term, then intervention here is also difficult.

In other instances, such as with some of the risk factors for heart disease shown in Table 7–5 (eg, obesity, elevated blood cholesterol, and high blood pressure), causal precedents might be diet, lack of exercise, and stress. Under these assumptions, efforts aimed at primary prevention of heart disease must focus on such factors as maternal diet during pregnancy, the diet of the child during early life, regular exercise, and health education programs regarding the hazards of smoking, a known agent. Essentially, individuals must be persuaded to change their lifestyle.

Specific protection as an approach to primary prevention can be used when specific agents can be identified. In occupational settings, exposure to harmful substances may be eliminated or minimized by engineering equipment to enclose harmful substances or by designing safety equipment that can be worn by the worker. Right-to-know laws may influence worker awareness of potential hazards and motivate workers to seek means for self-protection. Injuries resulting from automobile accidents can be prevented by building and maintaining safe roads, engineering safer cars, wearing seat belts, training drivers, and regulating speed. Much lung cancer can be prevented through health education programs aimed at convincing people not to begin smoking in the first place and, if they already smoke, to quit. Smoking has been identified as a specific agent for a number of noninfectious diseases and has been identified as the leading preventable cause of death in the United States (Centers for Disease Control, 1995b). This is one instance where primary prevention efforts aimed at preventing smoking initiation and promoting cessation have been extensive. National health objectives for the year 2000 for reduction in tobacco use include, preventing initiation of use, particularly among young persons,

TABLE 7–5. RISK FACTORS FOR THE TEN LEADING CAUSES OF DEATH—UNITED STATES, 1993

CAUSE OF DEATH	RISK FACTOR
Heart disease	Smoking, hypertension, elevated serum cholesterol (diet), lack of exercise, diabetes, stress, family history, obesity, high blood pressure
Malignant neoplasms	Smoking, work site carcinogens, environmental carcinogens, alcohol, diet
Cebrovascular disease (stroke)	Hypertension, smoking, elevated serum cholestrol, stress
Chronic obstructive pulmonary disease	Smoking, air pollution
Accidents and adverse effects	Alcohol, drug abuse, fires, product design, handgun availability, failure to wear seat belts, speed, roadway design, vehicle engineering
Influenza and pneumonia	Smoking, vaccination status
Diabetes	Obesity
HIV infection	Unsafe sex, contact with blood of exposed individuals
Suicide	Stress, alcohol and drug abuse, gun availability
Homicide	Poverty, stress, alcohol and drug abuse, gun availability, urban environment
Cirrhosis of the liver	Alcohol abuse

and addressing public policies focusing on smoke-free air by limiting smoking in public places and tobacco advertising as well as increasing excise taxes on tobacco products. Efforts to reduce tobacco use historically focused on smoking cessation. Because the impact of this approach has been limited, more recent tobacco prevention and reduction efforts have relied on a public health approach directed at changing public policies regarding tobacco use. Sale and use of tobacco have been regulated and taxes on tobacco products increased. By June 30, 1995, there were 1,238 state laws addressing tobacco use (Centers for Disease Control, 1995a). In 1997, President Clinton asked Congress to pass legislation limiting access to cigarette advertising and cigarettes for youth.

Evidence shows that public health efforts promoting smoking cessation are having some effect. Smoking prevalence among adults decreased from 40% in 1965 to 29% in 1987 and has continued to drop slowly since then, although there is variation by geographic area of the United States. Nearly one half of all living adults who ever smoked have quit. About three quarters of a million smoking deaths were avoided or postponed as a result of smokers quitting or decisions not to start. The smoking decline has been slower among women than men and smoking prevalence remains higher among blacks, blue-collar workers, and less educated persons than in the overall population. Of concern is the high rate of children beginning to smoke, especially girls. Future control efforts need to target these groups. Among U.S. adults who have ever smoked daily, 91% tried their first cigarette and 77% became daily smokers before the age of 20 years (Centers for Disease Control, 1995b). Thus, an important prevention strategy is preventing young persons from trying cigarettes, beginning with children in the primary grades. Because the age of beginning to smoke has gotten earlier over time, smoking cessation programs need to be implemented among younger age groups as well.

Primary Prevention Activities in Clinical Settings.   The Report of the U.S. Preventive Services Task Force (Fisher, 1989) identified several primary prevention/health promotion activities for diseases of noninfectious etiology that are particularly appropriate for primary care settings. These include, in addition to smoking prevention and cessation programs, counseling on excercise and nutrition, as well as on how to prevent motor vehicle, household, and environmental injuries, unintended pregnancies, and dental diseases. Other recommended primary prevention targets for clinical settings included estrogen prophylaxis for asymptomatic women who are at increased risk for osteoporosis, who lack known contraindications, and who have received adequate counseling about potential benefits and risks and aspirin prophylaxis for men aged 40 and over who are at significantly increased risk for MI and who do not have any contraindications to the drug.

Secondary Prevention

As previously mentioned, because knowledge is limited regarding the etiology of many diseases caused by noninfectious agents, the best information regarding the natural history of these diseases often does not specify a particular agent, but rather physiological factors associated with higher risk of developing the disease. Because of this, secondary prevention assumes major importance. If tests or other means are available to identify persons at high risk, specific treatment can be instituted to halt the disease progression and perhaps to reverse some damage. In the case of occupational or environmental exposures to known agents, secondary prevention is based on the screening or monitoring of exposed groups for early signs of disease. Worker notification programs may be required to alert former employees to their increased risk and to educate them regarding the appropriate action for them to take. Detection must be followed by prompt treatment.

Recommended Secondary Prevention Activities in Clinical Settings.   For diseases like breast cancer, where the current level of knowledge does not permit primary prevention, secondary prevention is crucial. Teaching self-breast examination to women, particularly those at high risk because of age, family history, prior benign breast disease, or other factors, may improve chances of detecting a lump before metastasis. Mammography screening, physician palpation, and breast self-examination also facilitate early detection and make treatment more likely to be successful. The validity of the various screening procedures varies, both inherently and by personal characteristics such as age of the woman and build of the woman. Decisions need to be made with regard to the cost-effectiveness and ethical concerns relative to each procedure when planning a program. These issues are discussed in Chapters 14 and 16. For diseases such as cardiovascular disease, early detection programs necessarily focus either on identification of early physiological risk factors, including the high-density lipoprotein to low-density lipoprotein ratio, obesity, high blood pressure, or diabetes, or on identification of behavioral risk factors such as smoking, high fat diet, inactivity, or stressful lifestyles. Changes in diet and activity, smoking cessation programs, stress reduction programs, and treatment of diabetes and high blood pressure are all interventions aimed at halting or slowing the rate of cardiovascular disease progression.

Tertiary Prevention

Many of the diseases of noninfectious origin first present to the medical care system as advanced disease (eg, the patient with atherosclerosis who first presents as an acute heart attack or the patient with chronic obstructive lung disease who seeks help only when he or she has an acute lung infection that overtaxes the limited function of their severely damaged respiratory system). Because of this, tertiary prevention plays a crucial role in management of these diseases. Objectives of tertiary intervention are: (1) to prevent further damage from occurring; (2) to minimize the symptoms that interfere with daily life; and (3) to help the patient function maximally within the restrictions imposed by the disease.

Prevention of further damage is often accomplished through modifying harmful habits or states that contribute to a decline in function and to progression of the disease process (eg, smoking cessation, weight reduction, regular physical activity, diet modification, and control of blood sugar levels in diabetics). These can all assist in preventing further damage for a patient with atherosclerotic heart disease. This same patient may require medications to minimize symptoms, such as angina, that interfere with normal daily activities. Vocational retraining may be required to enable the individual to secure a job that he or she is physically capable of performing.

Because of the chronic nature of many of the diseases caused by noninfectious agents, because the disease is often quite advanced before illness is diagnosed and treated, and because of the irreversible nature of many of these diseases, tertiary prevention must be the focus for a major portion of persons with these diseases. Improvements in medical technology during the past several decades have contributed greatly to the length and quality of life for many patients with these conditions.

REFERENCES

Basco M. R., Bostic J. Q., Daview D., Witte B., Barnett V., Kasner M., Walker D., Hendrickse W., Rush A. J. (1994) Psychiatric diagnoses in community mental health: Accuracy and cost. *AHSR FHSR Annual Meeting Abstract Book, 11*, 8–9.

Breast Cancer Consortium. (1997) Pathology of familial breast cancer: Differences between breast cancers in carriers of BRCA1 or BRCA2 mutations and sporadic cases. *Lancet, 349*, 1505–1510.

Centers for Disease Control. (1995b) Health-care provider advice on tobacco use to persons aged 10–22 years—United States, 1993. *Morbidity and Mortality Weekly Report, 44*(44).

Centers for Disease Control. (1990c) *Health United States, 1989.* Hyattsville, Md.: Public Health Service.

Centers for Disease Control. (1990a) Mortality patterns—United States, 1987. *Morbidity and Mortality Weekly Report, 39*(12).

Centers for Disease Control. (1985) Phytophotodermatitis in Ohio. *Morbidity and Mortality Weekly Report, 34*(1), 11–13.

Centers for Disease Control. (1997) Resources and priorities for chronic disease prevention. *Morbidity and Mortality Weekly Report, 46*(13), 286–287.

Centers for Disease Control. (1995a) State laws on tobacco control—United States, 1995. *Morbidity and Mortality Weekly Report, 44*(SS-6).

Centers for Disease Control. (1990b) The Surgeon General's 1990 report on the health benefits of smoking cessation (executive summary). *Morbidity and Mortality Weekly Report, 39*(RR-12).

Commission on Chronic Diseases. (1957) *Chronic illness in the United States.* Vol. 1. Cambridge, Mass.: Harvard University Press.

Fisher M. [Ed.] (1989) Guide to clinical preventive services: An assessment of the effectiveness of 169 interventions. *U.S. Preventive Services Taskforce,* Baltimore: Williams and Wilkins.

Galvani M., Ottani F., Ferrini D., Ladenson J. H., Destro A., Baccos D., Rusticali F., Jaffe A. S. (1997) Prognostic influence of elevated values of cardiac troponin I in patients with unstable angina. *Circulation, 95*(8), 2053–2059.

Krus C. Sanitary control of food. In J. Last (Ed.). (1980) *Maxcy-Rosenau public health and preventive medicine.* New York: Appleton-Century-Crofts, pp. 875–919.

Landrigan P. J. (1996) The prevention of occupational cancer. *CA—A Cancer Journal for Clinicians, 46*(2), 67–69.

Meyer K. C. (1994) Beryllium and lung disease. *Chest, 106*(3), 942–946.

Morris R. D. (1995) Drinking water and cancer. *Environmental Health Perspectives, 103*(suppl. 8), 225–231.

Newman L. S., Lloyd J., Daniloff E. (1996) The natural history of beryllium sensitization and chronic beryllium disease. *Environmental Health Perspectives, 104*(suppl. 5), 937–943.

Rossman M. D. (1996) Chronic beryllium disease: Diagnosis and management. *Environmental Health Perspectives, 104*(suppl 5), 945–947.

Seidman H., Selikoff I. J., Hammond, E. C. (1979) Short-term asbestos work exposure and long-term observation. *Annals of the New York Academy of Sciences, 330,* 61–89.

Selikoff I. J., Hammond E. C., Chung J. (1968) Asbestos exposure, smoking and neoplasia. *Journal of the American Medical Association, 204*(27), 106–112.

Stellman J. M., Stellman S. D. (1996) Cancer and the workplace. *CA—A Cancer Journal for Clinicians, 46*(2), 70–92.

U.S. Bureau of the Census. (1997) *Statistical Abstract of the United States, 1997* (117th Ed.). Washington, D.C.: U.S. Government Printing Office.

U.S. Bureau of the Census. (1996) *Statistical Abstract of the United States, 1996* (116th ed.). Washington, D.C.: U.S. Government Printing Office.

U.S. Department of Health and Human Services. (1979). Smoking and health. *A report of the Surgeon General* (DHHS Publication No. PH579-50066). Washington D.C.: U.S. Government Printing Office.

U.S. Public Health Service. (1993) Agency for Toxic Substances and Disease Registry: *Annual Report.* Atlanta.

U.S. Public Health Service. (1993) *A public health service progress report on healthy people 2000.* Occupational Safety and Health Administration, Washington D.C.

U.S. Public Health Service. (1964) *Smoking and health. Report of the Advisory Committee to the Surgeon General of the Public Health Service.* PHS Publication No. 1103. Washington, D.C.: U.S. Department of Health, Education, and Welfare. Public Health Service, Center for Disease Control.

Warner M. D., Peabody C. A. (1995) Reliability of diagnoses made by psychiatric residents in a general emergency department. *Psychiatric Services, 46*(12), 1284–1286.

Wegener D. K., Walstedt J., Jenkins L., et al. (1997) Women: Work and health. *Vital Health Statistics, 3*(31), DHHS Publication No. (PHS) 97-1415. National Center for Health Statistics, Hyattsville, Md.

Epidemiology and the Life Cycle

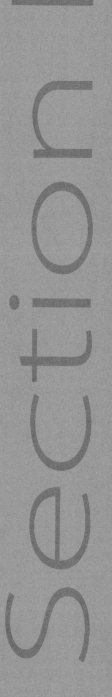

Patterns of Morbidity and Mortality During Pregnancy and Infancy

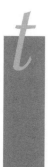

*t*he health of an infant cannot be separated from the health of the parents, particularly the mother. Health from infancy to adulthood is profoundly affected by conception, gestation, birth, and by the nurturing received early in life. This chapter describes the trends in reproductive health and childbearing in the United States and discusses risk factors that affect reproductive health. National goals for pregnancy and infant health and the important health services that support healthy reproduction and healthy infants are also discussed.

REPRODUCTIVE PATTERNS

Two rates are commonly used in reporting rates of births and as measures of fertility. The crude birth rate (CBR) is readily available and thus is often used to compare rates across countries or over long periods of time. It is calculated as the number of births occurring in a given year divided by the total population at midyear and multiplied by 1,000. The second rate used is the birth rate, computed as the number of registered live births in a year divided by the number of women between 15 and 44 years of age multiplied by 1,000. This rate better reflects fertility among women of reproductive age.

The CBR in the colonial United States was 43 births per 1,000 population, reflecting the large families characteristic during that time. Comparably high rates are seen today in some developing countries. By the 1930s, the CBR in the United States had dropped to 18 births per 1,000 population and a high proportion of women of childbearing age remained childless. This low birth rate was interpreted as intrinsic to an industrial society, and many sociologists predicted continued low fertility. Immediately after World War II there was an anticipated postwar "baby boom" as people compensated for delayed marriage and childbearing. What was unpredicted was the sustained period of increase in birth rate, peaking at a crude rate of 25 births per 1,000 population in 1957. This rate reflects an increase in the pace of childbearing at that particular time; women married earlier and had their first births earlier after marriage. It does not reflect a return to large families, but rather a shift back to a two-child family from an earlier time when many women remained childless or bore only one child. After 1957, the CBR began to drop again. The crude birth rate in 1996 in the United States was 14.8 per 1,000 population (U.S. Bureau of the Census, 1996).

The fertility of women in the United States decreased substantially between 1957 and the mid-1970s (Fig. 8–1). In 1957, the fertility rate was 122 births per 1,000 women aged 15 to 44 years. By 1976, the fertility rate was 65 per 1,000 women aged 15 to 44 years. Since 1976, the fertility rate has varied little, ranging from 65.0 to 68.4. The decline in fertility after 1957 through 1976 was due to

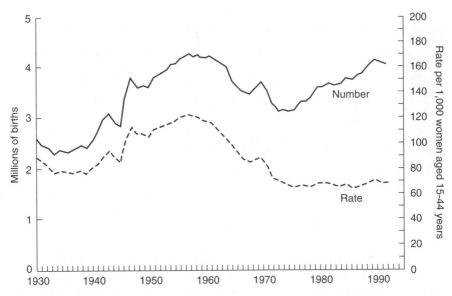

NOTE: Beginning with 1959, trend lines are based on registered live births: trend lines for 1930–59 are based on live births adjusted for underregistration.

Figure 8–1. Live births and fertility rates: United States, 1930–1992. (*Adapted from Ventura S. J., Martin J. A., Taffel S. M., et al. Advance report of final natality statistics, 1992.* Monthly Vital Statistics Report, *1994; 43, 5 [suppl.]. Hyattsville, Md. National Center for Health Statistics.*)

women desiring fewer babies on the average and postponing conception of the first child. In 1967, the average woman in the United States wanted to have three children; by 1976, most American women wanted and expected to have only two children (U.S. Bureau of the Census, 1978). The decline also reflects the increasing ability of women to prevent unwanted pregnancies and births by better accessibility to abortion services and more effective contraceptive methods.

Differences by Age and Race

For women in the age group 20 to 29, birth rates have not changed substantially since 1975, although they are slightly higher since 1990 than in the preceeding 15 years (Fig. 8–2; Table 8–1). The birth rate for women aged 30 to 34 years, however, was 80.8 per 1,000 in 1993, higher than it had been for more than 20 years. The rate

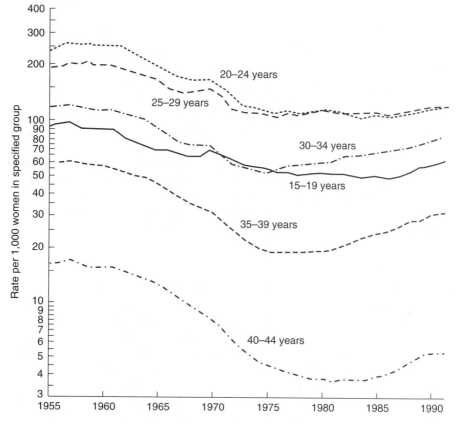

NOTE: Beginning with 1959, trend lines are based on registered live births: trend lines for 1955–59 are based on live births adjusted for underregistration.

Figure 8–2. Birth rates by age of mother: United States, 1955–1991. (*Adapted from National Center for Health Statistics. Monthly Vital Statistics Report, 1993; 42, 3, [suppl.], Fig. 2.*)

TABLE 8–1. BIRTH RATES[a] BY AGE OF MOTHER—UNITED STATES, 1970–1993

	AGE OF MOTHER						
YEAR	10–14 Years	15–19 Years	20–24 Years	25–29 Years	30–34 Years	35–39 Years	40–44 Years
1993	1.4	59.6	112.6	115.5	80.8	32.9	6.1
1990	1.4	59.9	116.5	120.2	80.8	31.7	5.5
1985	1.2	51.3	108.9	110.5	68.5	23.9	4.0
1980	1.1	53.0	115.1	112.9	61.9	19.8	3.9
1975	1.3	55.6	113.0	108.2	52.3	19.5	4.6
1970	1.2	68.3	167.8	145.1	73.3	31.7	8.1

[a]Birth rates are live births per 1,000 women in a specified age group.
(*Compiled from National Center for Health Statistics. Advance report of final natality statistics, 1988.* Monthly Vital Statistics Report, *1990;*
39,4 [suppl.]. Washington, D.C.: Public Health Service; and U.S. Department of Commerce. Statistical abstract of the United States, 1996
[116th ed.]. *Washington, D.C.: U.S. Government Printing Office, 1996.*)

for women aged 35 to 39 years has also been increasing since 1975, and since 1984, so has the rate for women aged 40 to 44. The result of this trend has been an upward shift in the age of childbearing to later years. This is most often attributed to more women entering the work force and delaying pregnancies until their careers or financial stability has been established.

Levels of childbearing among women aged 10 to 19 years declined somewhat in the early 1970s, and remained reasonably stable until they began increasing again after the mid-1980s (see Table 8–1). Although teenage fertility rates again appear to be stabilizing, the impact of teenage mothers and infants is still a major public health problem. Approximately 23% of black infants born in 1993 were born to teenage mothers compared to 11% of white infants (Fig. 8–3). Other U.S. population groups with high teenage birth rates include Native Americans, Eskimos, Aleutian Islanders, and Hawaiians.

Adolescent Pregnancy: An Urgent Problem

Adolescent pregnancies are associated with higher rates of maternal and infant complications. Maternal morbidity and mortality is higher among adolescents, and their infants are more likely to be born prematurely or with a low birth weight. Adolescent motherhood is also associated with lower educational and occupational attainment. The younger the adolescent, the greater the risk for untoward complications.

Promoting the health of adolescents is a particularly difficult task because of the special physiological and psychological characteristics of this age group. Teenage pregnancy has emerged repeatedly as an area of health needs unmet in our society; yet schools have traditionally been reluctant to allow health education programs on sex and contraception. This reluctance stems frequently from small but vocal parent groups who believe that sex education programs do not restrict themselves to just the transmitting of information but also affect the development of personal values. Clearly parents should help plan health education programs in schools

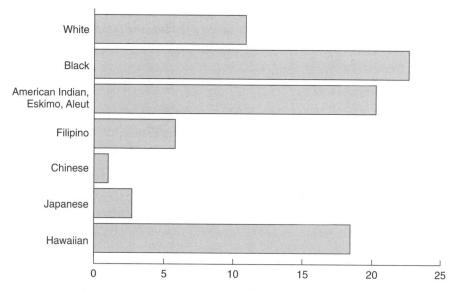

Figure 8–3. Births to teenage mothers as a percent of total births, by race—United States, 1993. (*Adapted from U.S. Bureau of the Census.* Statistical abstracts of the United States, 1996 [116th ed.]. Washington, D.C.: U.S. Government Printing Office, 1996, Fig. 2.2, p. 73.)

and should be aware of the content that is presented. Effective school programs providing information on sex and contraception and content on risk taking and decision making are needed to counteract the vast "pro-sex" influence of television, movies, music, and advertising.

Health services are also needed to provide sexual counseling to adolescents. Data from the 1988 National Survey of Family Growth show that the proportion of young teenagers aged 15–17 years who were sexually experienced had been increasing during the 1980s, from 33% in 1982 to 38% in 1988 (Centers for Disease Control, 1991); since 1990, however, this proportion has remained stable (Abma et al, 1997). For that percentage of adolescents who choose to become sexually active, knowledge of and easy access to contraceptive methods is urgent. Family planning programs should be especially adapted to the needs of adolescents and to encourage their use by this population.

Services for pregnant adolescents are crucial. Of the nearly 200,000 births to girls aged 12 to 17 years each year, 12,220 are to girls 14 years of age or younger (U.S. Bureau of the Census, 1996). An almost equal number of these individuals have miscarriages or induced abortions. Early pregnancy detection is an important health service component because teenage pregnancies are at high risk of adverse outcomes for both the mother and the infant. Early diagnosis can lead to initiation of prenatal care at a time when it can be most effective. Once a pregnancy is diagnosed, the teenager needs assistance in making decisions as to continuing the pregnancy, keeping the infant, releasing the infant for adoption, or abortion. She should have counseling on the advantages or disadvantages of each of these alternatives. In the event that abortion is chosen, early identification of pregnancy is more likely to permit abortion during the first trimester when a suction procedure or saline injection can be used. These procedures are safer for the mother than the alternative, dilatation and curettage (D & C).

Factors Influencing Fertility

Closely related to the trend of postponing first pregnancies to an older age is concern about the potential for increased risk of infertility. Epidemiologists use two measures to assess the ability of a population to conceive and maintain pregnancies. *Subfecundity* is *the perceived difficulty in conceiving or carrying a baby to term*, and *infertility* is *the state of being surgically sterile or having had at least 12 months of unprotected intercourse without conceiving a pregnancy*. The major difference in these two terms is that infertility refers to the inability to conceive a pregnancy whereas subfecundity includes both the inability to conceive and maintain a pregnancy. In 1995, 24% of women of reproductive age were surgically sterile for contraceptive reasons, 3% were surgically sterile for noncontraceptive reasons, another 10% had impaired fecundity, and 63% were fecund (able to bear children) (Abma et al, 1997).

Age and Race.   Both impaired fecundity and infertility increase with age. Pregnancy loss is a common occurrence in the United States. Overall, one in six women experiences at least one pregnancy loss; by age 40 to 44 years, the figure is one in four. About 16% of pregnancies end in miscarriage or stillbirth. Most of the increase observed over time in women with subfecundity is among the 35 to 44 year age group. From 1988 to 1995 there was a 1.8% increase in subfecundity (from 8.4% to 10.2%), likely reflecting the postponement of first pregnancy until later years. Among women 15 to 24, 4.4% have received services for infertility. Parallel figures for women aged 25 to 34 and 35 to 44 are 17.1 and 22.9%, respectively (Abma et al, 1997).

Contraception.   In 1995, contraception was used by 76.4% of currently married women, 69.1% of those formerly married, and 46.6% of women who have never been married. Use is more common among whites (66%) than blacks (62.2%) and Hispanics (58.9%). Use is also more common among older than younger women. Surgical sterilization is the leading method of birth control in the United States. In 1995, 18% of women reported having had a tubal ligation, 5% a hysterectomy, and 8% had partners with a vasectomy. Among women with three or more births, nearly 67% had undergone surgical sterilization and 13.2% of married women reported that their partner had undergone a vasectomy (Abma et al, 1997). The birth control pill was the second most common form of contraception, used by 20.4% of never married women, 25.6% of married women, and 34% of formerly married women. Condoms were the third most common form of contraception.

Births to Unmarried Women

Marital status of the parent can affect the outcome of a pregnancy and the health of the infant. The younger a woman is at the time of her first marriage, the more likely it is that she is already pregnant. Marriage subsequent to a pregnancy often predisposes couples to an economic disadvantage, because the traditional time in which a couple usually establishes an income and home before having children is lost. Economic disadvantage is associated with poor housing, malnutrition, and lack of health care and may, therefore, be threatening to the health of the mother and the infant.

Women today are more likely than women in the past to bear children out of wedlock (Fig. 8–4). This is true across age, race, and socioeconomic groups and relates to changing patterns of marriage and cohabitation. In 1995, about 38% of women of childbearing age (15 to 44) had never been married. Nearly half of all women aged 25 to 39 have had an unmarried cohabitation with a man at some time in their lives and about 10% of women in their 20s are currently cohabiting. Compared with 1982, the percent of women cohabiting in 1995 was higher in every age group (Abma et al, 1997).

In 1970, 5.6% of births to white women and 37.6% of births to black women were to unmarried women. By 1993, the corresponding figures were 23.6 and 68.7%, respectively (Table 8–2). More than 1.24 million babies were born to unmarried mothers in 1993, a rate nearly twice that of 1980 and more than three times that of 1970. These increases occurred while births to married women did not increase and marital fertility rates declined. The reasons for this increase are not totally clear. It is due in part to the increased number of baby boomers in the 15 to 44–year age range, the postponement of marriage, and increasing divorce rates (National Center for Health Statistics, 1990a). Another contributing factor to the increasing rates of births to unmarried women may be the trend of decreasing rates of induced abortions. In a report on induced abortions in 14 states providing this information to the National Center for Health Statistics, the abortion ratio (number of abortions per 1,000 live births) declined 9% from 1982 to 1987 (National Center for

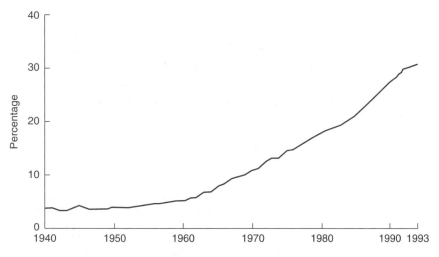

Figure 8–4. Percentage of births out-of-wedlock—United States, 1940–1993. (*Adapted from Ventura S. J. Births to Unmarried Mothers—United States, 1980–1993. National Center for Health Statistics. Vital and Health Statistics, 1995, Hyattsville, Md. 21, 53.*)

TABLE 8–2. CHARACTERISTICS OF LIVE BIRTHS BY RACE—UNITED STATES, 1993

RACE	NO. OF BIRTHS (1,000)	BORN TO TEENS (%)	BORN TO UNWED MOTHERS (%)	BEGINNING PRENATAL CARE (%)		LOW BIRTH WEIGHT (%)
				First Trimester	Third Trimester	
White	3,150	11.0	23.6	81.8	3.9	6.0
Black	659	22.7	68.7	66.0	9.0	13.3
Native American, Eskimo	39	20.3	55.8	63.4	10.3	6.4
Aleutian Islander, Asian, and Pacific Islander	15.3	5.7	15.7	77.6	4.6	6.6
Hispanic origin	654	17.4	40.0	66.6	8.8	6.2
Total:	4,000	12.8	31.0	78.9	4.8	7.2

(Compiled from Lewis C. T., Matthews T. J., Heuser R. I. Prenatal care in the United States, 1980–1994. National Center for Health Statistics. Vital Health Statistics; 1996, 21,54.)

Health Statistics, 1990a; Kochanek & Hudson, 1989). Approximately 83% of the abortions reported in 1991 occurred in unmarried women (U.S. Department of Commerce, 1996). As more unmarried women decide to maintain pregnancies rather than obtain induced abortions, the birth rate for unmarried women will continue to increase. Unfortunately, births of unmarried women are associated with an increased rate of mortality, fetal death, and low birth weight. Unmarried women giving birth need social support, such as adequate housing and nutrition, and often times, special medical care.

Timing and Spacing of Pregnancies

Other factors affecting pregnancy outcomes are the timing of pregnancy and spacing between children. Pregnancies at either end of the childbearing age range are at increased risk of complications. The spacing between pregnancies influences both the likelihood of complication and the ability of parents to meet the infant's needs. An interval between pregnancies of less than 24 months and longer than 48 months is associated with a higher incidence of low birth weight (National Center for Health Statistics, 1990a). For example, in 1988, babies born within 18 months of a previous birth were almost twice as likely to be of low birth weight as compared with babies born 1½ to 5 years after a previous birth.

When pregnancies occur at less than 24-month intervals, the mother has less time to restore her health, predisposing her to an increased rate of complications, and the family has less time to adjust to the stress introduced by new family members. When the interval between pregnancies is greater than 48 months, however, the incidence of complications also increases. This increased incidence may be related to having unplanned pregnancies or perhaps to problems associated with infertility.

Black infants are more likely than white infants to be born at very short intervals, and intervals between successive births tend to be shorter for young mothers than for older mothers. For example, the proportion of white infants born within 18 months of a previous birth was 12% in 1992 compared with a rate of 20% of black births (Ventura et al, 1994). The percentage of short interval births has remained relatively stable since 1980. These infants are more likely to be of low birth weight (9.1% of short interval births versus 4.6% of those born at 2 to 3 years after a previous live birth).

Health Practices During Pregnancy

The impact of tobacco and alcohol use during pregnancy continues to be a public health concern. In 1979, the Surgeon General (Office of the Assistant Secretary for Health and the Surgeon General, 1979) issued the following warning about smoking and drinking during pregnancy:

> Smoking slows fetal growth, doubles the chance of low birth weight, and increases the risk of stillbirth. Recent studies suggest that smoking may be a significant factor in 20 to 40 percent of low weight infants born in the United States and Canada. Studies also indicate that infants of mothers consuming large amounts of alcohol may suffer from low birth weight, birth defects, and/or mental retardation.

Since the above statement was issued, warnings regarding the impact of tobacco use have become highly visible on tobacco products and advertisements. Likewise, warnings on the risk of alcohol use during pregnancy are becoming increasingly visible in establishments serving alcohol. Alcohol use during pregnancy is associated with a variety of adverse effects, including low birth weight and fetal alcohol syndrome. Despite these public warnings, substantial proportions of women continue to use these substances during pregnancy, although use has decreased. In 1993, 15.8% of women smoked during pregnancy (Ventura et al, 1994).

Adequate nutrition and weight gain during pregnancy have a major impact on pregnancy outcome, including effects on birth weight, length of gestation, and fetal growth (Ventura et al, 1994). Women who gain less than 14 lbs during pregnancy produce infants of low birth weight four times more frequently than women who gain 30 to 35 lbs. Black mothers are two times more likely than white mothers to gain less than 16 lbs during pregnancy.

Substance abuse has reached epidemic proportions across the United States and has affected every socioeconomic group. The National Institute of Alcohol Abuse and Alcoholism indicated that in the early 1980s, 2.25 million women in the United States were problem drinkers (Ouellette, 1983). A 1986 National Institute of Drug Abuse survey revealed that one in ten women of childbearing age had used cocaine in the previous year (Clayton, 1986). Approximately 375,000 infants are exposed each year to addictive substances, and the overall incidence rate of illicit substance abuse during pregnancy has been reported to be 11% (Chasnoff et al, 1989). Cocaine use, particularly the "crack" form, has become increasingly widespread in urban and inner-city populations. Complications that have been associated with co-caine use during pregnancy include placental abruptio, intrauterine growth retarda-tion, preterm labor, and spontaneous abortions. The neonatal effects of cocaine use are associated with the poor intrauterine growth patterns, the possibility of teratoge-nesis, and distinct neurobehavioral effects.

Substance use may be abating, particularly during pregnancy. In 1994, only 12% of 18 to 25 year olds reported having used marijuana in the previous month, al-though 25% reported having used it at least once during their lifetime. Similarly, 1% reported using cocaine in the previous month, while 3% reported having used it at least once in the past. The same patterns were also seen for other drugs, such as in-halants, hallucinogens, heroin, and stimulants. Alcohol was the most commonly used drug. Nearly 64% of the 18 to 25 year olds and 56% of those 26 and older reported having used alcohol in the past month. Corresponding figures for use at any time in the past were 87 and 91%, respectively. Current cigarette use was also lower than previous use at any time by about two thirds for both 18 to 25 year olds (27% versus 68%) and those 26 years old and older (U.S. Department of Commerce, 1996).

Birth certificate data on use of alcohol during pregnancy in 1991 indicate that reported alcohol use declined for mothers of all racial groups from 1990 to 1991. In 1991, 2.9% of births were to mothers who reported alcohol use, with black mothers slightly more likely than white mothers (3.4% versus 2.7%) to use alcohol during pregnancy. Asian and Hispanic mothers were even less likely than either blacks or whites to use alcohol during pregnancy. The highest reported rate of alcohol use was among American Indian women (7.3%) (Ventura et al, 1994). It is thought that alcohol use during pregnancy is substantially underreported on the birth certificate. Studies that used personal interviews and written questionnaires found levels closer to 20% (Serdula et al, 1991).

Birth certificate data for 1991 for the United States showed that 17.8% of women who gave birth that year smoked during pregnancy, a decline from 18.4% in 1990 and 19.5% in 1989. White mothers were more likely to smoke than black mothers (18.8% versus 14.6%). Smoking was uncommon among Asian and His-panic women (2% and 8%, respectively) although among Hawaiian women the fig-ure was 19.4%. Smoking is highest among American Indian mothers (22.6%).

The public health goals regarding substance abuse and use during pregnancy include identification of high-risk populations, education regarding the effects on pregnancy and infant health, referral systems for women with substance abuse prob-lems, increased treatment programs targeted to pregnant women, prevention or identification of obstetrical and neonatal complications associated with substance abuse, and social support services to promote appropriate parenting of the drug-exposed newborn.

Prenatal Care

The importance of prenatal care in reducing maternal–infant morbidity and mortal-ity is well recognized. Babies born to women who receive no prenatal care are three times more likely to die in infancy (Hughs et al, 1986). The risk of having a low birth weight infant is three times as high for women with no prenatal care as it is for women who begin prenatal care during the first trimester (Institute of Medicine, 1985). In 1993, 79% of births were to women whose prenatal care commenced in the first trimester. Nearly 5% of the mothers in the United States did not begin prenatal care until the third trimester or received no care at all (see Table 8–2). These rates have improved only slightly since the early 1980s. Much of the lack of improvement in early receipt of prenatal care is associated with the increasing proportion of births to unmarried mothers (Lewis et al, 1996). The crucial importance of improving rates of early prenatal care is emphasized by its inclusion in the "Year 2000 Health Objectives for the Nation" (U.S. Department of Health and Human Services, 1991).

A substantial racial differential can be found in the use of prenatal care. In 1993, 82% of white mothers began care in the first trimester whereas only 66% of black mothers began care this early. Four percent of white mothers received delayed or no prenatal care, compared with 9% of black mothers. Black women, however, showed greater improvement in obtaining earlier prenatal care in recent years than white women.

A considerable proportion of teenage mothers is at high risk for receiving delayed or no prenatal care. In 1994, only 50% of white mothers and 42% of black mothers 15 years and younger began prenatal care in the first trimester (Lewis et al, 1996). A major biological problem for pregnant teenagers is that the demands of the growing fetus are superimposed on the nutritional needs of the teenager. This competition for nutrients may result in a low birth weight baby. In addition, toxemia is more common in young mothers. Depending on the age of the mother, the reproductive system may not be mature, predisposing her to fetopelvic disproportion. All these factors make it even more desirable that pregnant teenagers receive appropriate counseling about sex education and contraception and be strongly urged to seek help at the earliest sign of pregnancy.

Timing of the first prenatal visit correlates highly with educational attainment (Fig. 8–5). In 1988, 92% of mothers with college degrees began care in the first trimester compared with only 56% of mothers having less than a high school education. The more children a woman has had, the more likely she is to obtain insufficient prenatal care, and unmarried women are three times as likely to obtain late or no prenatal care. Poverty is one of the most important correlates of insufficient prenatal care, and women residing in inner cities and isolated rural areas are more likely not to receive adequate prenatal care (Centers for Disease Control, 1995a).

AIDS in Women—Impact on Childbearing

The number of new acquired immunodeficiency syndrome (AIDS) cases in women increased through the 1980s, peaking in 1994 at 6,615 new cases, then decreasing to 4,881 new cases in 1995. The proportion of AIDS cases that were among women increased from 8% in the period 1981 to 1987 to 18% during the period 1993 to October 1995 (Centers for Disease Control, 1995b). Among all cases of AIDS in

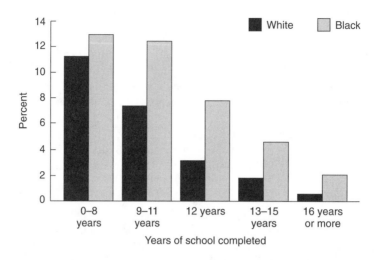

Figure 8–5. Percent of live births where mothers received late or no prenatal care, by educational attainment and race of mother—United States, 1994. (*Adapted from Lewis C. T., Matthews T. J., Heuser R. L. Prenatal care in the United States, 1980–1994. National Center for Health Statistics. Vital Health Statistics, 1996; 21, 54.*)

women in 1995, 61.4% occurred among women of childbearing age (15–40 years) and another 27.3% among women between 40 and 49 years of age. An estimated 7,000 women infected with the human immunodeficiency virus (HIV) delivered infants in the United States during 1993. With the perinatal transmission rate generally estimated to be between 15 to 30%, approximately 1,000 to 2,000 infants were perinatally infected with AIDS (Centers for Disease Control, 1995c). However, the rate of perinatal transmission from infected mothers is unknown and the rate has been reported as high as 65% (Scott et al, 1985). It is believed that the HIV virus is transmitted from infected women to their fetuses during pregnancy or labor and delivery. The virus also has been isolated from breast milk (Thiry et al, 1985). Testing for the HIV virus at prenatal visits is an important part of care. In 1995, approximately 48% of women aged 15 to 44 years had an HIV test at some time in their lives, 23% in connection with prenatal care (Abma et al, 1997).

Work and Reproduction

Reproductive hazards associated with the workplace are currently the focus of a great deal of political, economic, and scientific controversy. Between 1947 and 1984, the number of American women in the work force nearly tripled, from 16.7 million to 46.5 million. Seventy-five percent of these women are of reproductive age (La Dou, 1990). In 1994, more than 65% of all live births were to women who had worked at some time in the year before delivery (U.S. Department of Commerce, 1996). Almost 80% of all employed women work in just 20 occupations, including health care, textiles, cosmetology, electronics, and other jobs with potential exposure to reproductive toxins.

Much of the controversy regarding reproductive hazards is related to how to restrict exposure to these hazards. A major concern is how to protect the reproductive health of a man or woman and the health of the fetus without practicing selective job discrimination. The relative dearth of epidemiological data on the effects of workplace hazards on reproduction complicates these problems. Animal studies and case reports lend evidence that exposure to numerous occupational hazards can have negative effects on reproduction. Reported and demonstrated health effects include menstrual disorders, decreased sperm count and mobility, abnormal sperm morphology, impotence, decreased fertility, spontaneous abortions, low birth weight, fetal brain damage, and birth defects (Rothstein, 1990). Table 8–3 lists some of the numerous substances under review for possible effects on male or female reproductivity.

Maternal Mortality

In 1900, deaths of pregnant women or those who died from complications of childbirth were major contributors to overall population mortality figures. Large decreases in maternal mortality during the past 50 years have greatly contributed to declines in the overall mortality rate.

TABLE 8–3. OCCUPATIONAL EXPOSURES UNDER REVIEW FOR REPRODUCTIVE EFFECTS

Chemical and Pharmaceutical Agents	Job Stress and Biological Agents
Antineoplastic drugs	Cytomegalovirus
Hormones	Rubella virus
Anesthetic gases	Toxoplasmosis
Vinyl chloride	Lyme disease
Organic solvents	Hepatitis B virus
Methyl mercury	Human immunodeficiency virus (HIV)
Ethylene oxide	**Metals**
Pesticides/herbicides	Lead
Polycyclic aromatic hydrocarbons	Cadmium
Styrene	Mercury
Trichlorethylene	Boron
Benzene	Manganese
Formaldehyde	
Physical Agents	
Radiation	
X-rays	
Heat	

(Compiled from Office of Technology Assessment, U.S. Congress. Reproductive health hazards in the workplace, 1985, p. 7; and Shortridge L. A. Advances in the assessment of the effect of environmental and occupational toxins on reproduction. Journal of Perinatal and Neonatal Nursing, 1990; 3, 1–11.)

Maternal death is defined by the Committee on Maternal Mortality of the International Federation of Gynecologists and Obstetricians to be "death of any woman dying of any cause while pregnant or within 42 days of termination of pregnancy, irrespective of the duration or site of pregnancy" (Roehat, 1981). However, vital statistics do not reflect all deaths occurring to pregnant women but only those deaths assigned to complications of pregnancy, childbirth, and the puerperium.

The maternal mortality ratio (often used as a rate), calculated as number of maternal deaths divided by the number of live births, has gradually decreased over the years as shown in Table 8–4. In 1940, maternal mortality was 320 per 100,000 live births to white women and 782 per 100,000 live births to black women. By 1992, there were 7.8 maternal deaths for each 100,000 births in the United States. This decrease has resulted in large part from the greater use of hospitals for delivery, the recognition and special care of pregnant women at high risk, the availability of antibiotics, improvements in anesthesia, and intensive research on the preventable causes of maternal deaths.

Although substantial improvements have been made in the overall maternal mortality rates, improvements still need to be made in the rates for disadvantaged ethnic groups and mothers of low socioeconomic status. This is best reflected in the differences in maternal mortality ratios for whites and blacks, as shown in Table 8–4. In 1992, black women were four times as likely as white women to die of maternal causes. Black women are more likely to be of a lower socioeconomic class and have less likelihood of receiving early and periodic prenatal care. They may also have poorer nutrition and more frequent exposure to infectious agents or hazardous agents in their place of employment. Even though maternal mortality ratios in the United States have decreased dramatically during the 20th century, the racial differentiation reflects significant inequality in the attainment of preventive health care services and socioeconomic status.

Maternal age may also affect the risk for maternal mortality. The lowest mortality is associated with women in the 20- to 29-year age group. Extremes of childbearing years, particularly those younger than 15 or older than 35, represent a higher risk for maternal mortality.

TABLE 8–4. MATERNAL MORTALITY RATES[a] BY RACE—UNITED STATES, 1940–1992

RACE	1940	1950	1960	1970	1975	1980	1985	1990	1991	1992
All	376.0	83.3	37.1	21.5	12.8	9.2	7.8	8.2	7.9	7.8
White	319.8	61.1	26.0	14.4	9.1	6.7	5.2	5.4	5.8	5.0
Black	781.7	223.0	105.6	59.8	31.3	21.5	20.4	22.4	18.3	20.8

[a]Maternal deaths per 100,000 live births.

(From National Center for Health Statistics. Health, United States, 1989. (DHHS Pub. No. [PHS] 90–1232). Public Health Service, Washington, D.C.: U.S. Government Printing Office, March, 1990; and U.S. Bureau of the Census. Statistical abstract of the United States, 1996 [116th ed.]. Washington, D.C.: U.S. Government Printing Office, 1996.)

A total of 318 deaths in the United States were reported as pregnancy-related during 1992. These deaths, shown in Table 8–5, were primarily of three categories:

1. Pregnancies with abortive outcomes
2. Direct obstetrical causes
3. Indirect obstetrical causes

Direct maternal deaths result from obstetrical complications of the pregnancy, labor, or puerperium and from interventions or any sequelae of these. Indirect maternal deaths are not directly due to obstetrical causes but result from previously existing diseases or a disease that developed during pregnancy, labor, or the puerperium and that was aggravated by pregnancy.

During the 1970s the likelihood of deaths from illegally induced abortions was virtually eliminated. Spontanaeous abortions, however, still contribute to maternal mortality. During this same time period, the rate of death from ectopic pregnancies has increased. Since 1970, there has been an epidemic in the number of ectopic pregnancies in the United States. In 1992, there were 28 deaths due to ectopic pregnancies and many more such pregnancies that did not result in death. The most commonly cited reason for this increase is the increase in gonorrhea with its resultant pelvic inflammation now easily detected through improved diagnostic technology.

As shown in Table 8–5, in 1992, blacks were five times more likely than whites to die from all abortive outcomes. Blacks have both a higher incidence of ectopic pregnancies and a reduced likelihood that diagnosis and treatment would be sought early on for the symptoms of an ectopic pregnancy. Until risk factors that

TABLE 8–5. NUMBER OF MATERNAL DEATHS AND MATERNAL MORTALITY RATES[a] BY RACE FOR SELECTED CAUSES— UNITED STATES, 1992.

CAUSE OF DEATH	NUMBER	ALL RACES	WHITE	BLACK
Pregnancy with abortive outcome	52	1.3	0.8	3.9
Ectopic pregnancy	28	0.7	*	*
Spontaneous abortion	9	*	*	*
Legal abortion	5	*	*	*
Other	10	*	*	*
Direct obstetrical causes	249	6.1	3.9	15.9
Hemorrhage	39	1.0	*	*
Toxemia	53	1.3	0.7	4.2
Puerperium complications	95	2.3	1.5	5.9
Other	62	1.5	1.2	3.1
Indirect obstetrical causes	17	0.4	0.2	1.3
All deaths	318	7.8	5.0	20.8

[a]Rates per 100,000 live births in a specified group.
* Number of deaths too small to calculate rates.
(Compiled from Kochanek K. D., Hudson B. L. National Center for Health Statistics. Advance report of final mortality statistics, 1992. Monthly Vital Statistics Report, 1995; 43, 6 [suppl.]. Hyattsville, Md.: National Center for Health Statistics.)

lead to ectopic pregnancies are established and controlled, early detection remains the most effective means of reducing the morbidity and mortality associated with this condition.

The leading causes of maternal mortality in 1992 resulted directly from obstetrical complications of the pregnancy, labor, or puerperium. Toxemia was the leading single cause of death in this category. This disease has often been associated with young maternal age, poor nutritional patterns, and lack of prenatal care. The maternal mortality rate could be further decreased by preventive health measures to lower the incidence of these known risk factors.

Infant Morbidity and Mortality

The chances of live birth and survival through the first year of life have steadily improved in the United States. Table 8–6 shows fetal, neonatal, and postneonatal mortality ratios by race for 1970 to 1992. Each of these ratios provides information useful for investigating causes of mortality for the fetus and newborn infant. Fetal mortality is generally related to maternal health status or to toxic exposures that may have affected the viability of the germ cell. Neonatal mortality reflects mortality during the first 4 weeks of life and is often related to low birth weight, congenital malformations, respiratory problems, or other conditions present at birth. Postneonatal mortality, in contrast, is more frequently due to adverse environmental or social circumstances, delay in seeking care for treatable conditions, or nutritional deficit or other social conditions amenable to public health intervention. Another measure often reported is the infant mortality ratio, which reflects the sum of the neonatal and postneonatal deaths, representing total mortality during the first year of life.

All of these measures reflect decreasing fetal and infant mortality. Fetal and neonatal mortality in 1992 for both whites and nonwhites were at levels 50% lower than comparable rates in 1970. Postneonatal mortality dropped approximately 30% for whites and 40% for nonwhites. However, all three types of mortality remain 80 to 100% higher for nonwhites than for whites.

TABLE 8–6. FETAL, NEONATAL, AND POSTNEONATAL MORTALITY RATIOS[a] BY RACE—UNITED STATES, 1970–1992

YEAR	FETAL MORTALITY		NEONATAL MORTALITY		POSTNEONATAL MORTALITY	
	White	Nonwhite	White	Nonwhite	White	Nonwhite
1970	12.4	22.6	13.8	21.4	4.0	9.5
1980	8.2	13.4	7.4	13.2	3.5	7.0
1985	7.0	11.3	6.0	11.0	3.2	5.8
1990	6.4	11.9	4.8	9.9	2.8	5.6
1992	6.3	11.7	4.3	9.2	2.6	5.2

[a]Deaths per 1,000 live births.

(1970–1985 data From National Center for Health Statistics. Advance report of final mortality statistics, 1988. Monthly Vital Statistics Report, 1990; 39,7 [suppl.]. Washington, D.C.: Public Health Service. 1990 and 1992 data from Kochanek K. D., Hudson B. L. Advance report of final mortality statistics, 1992. Monthly Vital Statistics Report, 1995; 43, 6 [suppl.] Hyattsville, Md.: National Center for Health Statistics.)

If one assumes that neonatal deaths reflect prenatal and perinatal circumstances and that postneonatal deaths result from environmental factors, different preventive health strategies are needed to decrease the number of deaths in each of these categories. It is important to note that much, if not all, of the racially related difference in mortality are socioeconomically associated. Infant mortality declines as socioeconomic class rises. The racial difference observed in infant mortality rates could be considerably offset by improving the quality of living conditions, parenting skills, and access to health care for impoverished families.

Compared with other nations of the world, the U.S. infant mortality rate in 1996 was ranked 12th among countries with populations of 5 million or more (Table 8–7) (U.S. Department of Commerce, 1996). This placement is due in part to better success in this country at bringing to term infants with defects and delivering live infants of very low birth weight. In 1992, nearly 300,000 infants were born weighing less than 5.5 lbs. In that same year, 34,648 babies died before reaching their first birthday (U.S. Department of Commerce, 1996). Clearly, despite progress, the fate of a child born in the United States today is by all means not assured.

Low Birth Weight Infants

The low birth weight of an infant has been associated with an elevated risk of infant mortality, congenital malformations, and other physical and neurological impairments. Although only an approximate 7% of all newborns are of low birth weight, this group of infants accounts for more than half of all infant deaths and nearly three fourths of all neonatal deaths (McCormick, 1985). Either low birth weight or gestational age can be used to estimate the physical maturity of a newborn infant. Weight

TABLE 8–7. COUNTRIES WITH THE LOWEST INFANT
MORTALITY RATES, 1996

COUNTRY	RATE
Japan	4.4
Denmark	4.8
Finland	4.9
Netherlands	4.9
Hong Kong	5.1
Australia	5.5
Germany	6.0
Canada	6.1
France	6.2
Austria	6.2
Belgium	6.4
United States	6.7

(*Compiled from U.S. Bureau of the Census.* Statistsical abstract of the United States, 1996 [116th ed.]. *Washington, D.C.: U.S. Government Printing Office, 1996.*)

at birth is more commonly used in epidemiology because it is accurately and completely recorded. Although accurate physical assessment of gestational age may be done in some birth settings, often the accuracy of gestational age depends on the mother's correct recollection of the date of her last menstrual period. Infants weighing 2,500 g (5.5 lbs) or less at birth are considered to be of low birth weight. Low birth weight infants may be preterm (ie, born before 37 weeks' gestation) or full term but small for their gestational age.

Rates of low birth weight have fluctuated over the past 30 years. From 1975 through 1985, a 9% decrease in the incidence of low birth weight occurred, from 73.9 per 1,000 live births in 1975 to 67.5 per 1,000 in 1985 (Table 8–8). However, the rate of infants born with low birth weight increased again in subsequent years. Although the initial decline was observed for both white and black infants, the decline was nearly twice as great for white infants (9%) as for black infants (5%) the subsequent increases were also greater for blacks. These substantial and persistent differences between black and white infants for the risk of low birth weight can be attributed in part to relatively more black women being represented in the risk groups of unmarried, adolescent, less than high school education, and with late or no prenatal care. Other factors related to the higher rates of low birth weight among black infants include poorer nutritional status and higher rates of unwanted pregnancies. Anemia and poor pregnancy weight gain are also more prevalent in black pregnant women (Taffel et al, 1989).

Other characteristics such as previous stillbirths and miscarriages, short intervals between pregnancies, and mothers younger than 18 years of age or older than 35 years of age are also associated with low birth weight. Clearly, the problem of low birth weight is one that merits particular emphasis in health promotion programs in the United States.

Infant mortality rates declined even more sharply than did rates of low birth weight. This disproportionate decline in rates can be explained by the fact that low birth weight contributes greatly to the infant mortality rates and that any small

TABLE 8–8. RATES[a] OF LOW AND VERY LOW BIRTH WEIGHT, BY RACE—UNITED STATES, 1975–1994

BIRTH WEIGHT	1975	1980	1985	1990	1994
2,500 g or less					
All races	73.9	68.4	67.5	70.0	73.0
White	62.6	57.0	56.4	57.0	61.0
Black	130.9	124.9	124.2	133.0	132.0
1,500 g or less					
All races	11.6	11.5	12.1	NA	NA
White	9.2	9.0	9.4	NA	NA
Black	23.7	24.4	26.5	NA	NA

[a]Rates per 1,000 live births.
(From Centers for Disease Control. Low birth weight—United States, 1975–1987. [DHHS (PHS) Publication No. (CDC) 90–8017]. 1990 and 1994 data from U.S. Bureau of the Census. Statistical abstract of the United States, 1997 [117th ed.]. Washington, D.C.: U.S. Government Printing Office, 1997.)

changes in the incidence of low birth weight will result in a large improvement in infant survival. Also, advances in perinatal and neonatal medicine have increased the survival of many infants of low birth weight.

Changes in the incidence of low birth weight among newborns have been attributed to federally funded programs implemented in the 1960s and early 1970s that targeted intervention toward socioeconomic factors associated with low birth weight, including prenatal care and nutrition programs, such as the Maternal and Infant Care (MIC) projects, community health centers, Medicaid, food stamps, and Women, Infant, and Children (WIC) supplemental feeding. These programs improved the health status and nutrition of pregnant women. The late 1960s also brought about efforts to regionalize prenatal and neonatal services to ensure that all pregnant women and their newborn infants would have rapid access to an appropriate level of care. Increased availability of effective contraceptive methods, as well as increased access to family planning and abortion services also occurred during this time period and resulted in a decrease in the proportion of births to high-risk women. Some of the increase in rates of low birth weight in the 1990s may be attributable to cuts in these programs.

Over the years, there has been improvement in the outcome of infants of all birth weights but particularly of those infants weighing 1,000 to 2,500 g. These improvements have been largely due to better intrapartum and neonatal care, fetal monitoring techniques, and improved neonatal care. Use of electronic fetal monitoring, for example, has been increasing over time. In 1991, it was the most frequently used medical procedure in pregnant women. Labor induction or stimulation of labor were used in 121 of 1,000 live births among whites and 105 of 1,000 live births among blacks. Ultrasound for confirming conditions such as unclear vaginal bleeding and for dating gestational age was used in 54% of pregnant women, but less among blacks than whites. Amniocentesis was used for 76% of live births in 1991 compared with 68% in 1989, and 45% in 1980. Appropriately, use was higher among older women than among younger women. Finally, tocolysis, used to delay premature delivery, was employed in 16 of 1,000 live births (U.S. Department of Health and Human Services, 1996).

During the next decade, primary prevention strategies should be directed toward narrowing the gap between the incidence rates of low birth weight in black versus white infants. This is one of the goals identified in the "National Goals for the Year 2000" (U.S. Department of Health, Education, and Welfare, 1991). The prevention of unintended pregnancies could substantially reduce the difference in the low birth weight between black and white infants (Hogue & Yip, 1989). In addition, ensuring adequate nutritional status of all pregnant women would result in decreased rates of infants of low birth weight. Iron supplementation for pregnant women with borderline or frank anemia should lead to a modest reduction in the relative risk of low birth weight among black infants. Care should begin before conception to include family planning. Increasing the socioeconomic conditions of black women should have a direct impact on the risk of having an infant with a low birth weight. Social support and family planning services should be made more, not less, accessible, particularly for young high-risk black women.

Leading Causes of Death During Infancy

The decline in the infant mortality rate from the 1960s to the 1980s was phenomenal. Neonatal death rates decreased 56% from the 1960s to the 1980s, whereas post-
natal deaths decreased 27%. The neonatal period, the first 28 days after birth, is the
time when the risk of infant death is greatest; 64% of all infants who died in 1988
died during the first 28 days of life (National Center for Health Statistics, 1990b).
Between 1980 and 1992, infant mortality rates dropped another 25% from 12.6 of
1,000 live births to 8.5 of 1,000 life births and neonatal mortality dropped from 8.5
to 5.4. Postneonatal mortality dropped from 4.1 to 3.1. The infant mortality rate for
births to white women was 6.9 compared to 16.8 for black women (Kochanek &
Hudson, 1995).

Congenital anomalies are the leading cause of infant mortality in the United
States. The rate of deaths from these anomalies in 1995 was 183.2 per 100,000 live
births, accounting for more than 25% of infant deaths. Such anomalies also contribute to childhood morbidity, disability, and years of life lost (Table 8–9). The
leading congenital anomalies resulting in death of children younger than 1 year and
their related number of deaths in 1995 are congenital anomaly of the heart (2,337),
digestive system (988), musculoskeletal system (507), genitourinary system (473),
and circulatory system (439). Clearly, complications of pregnancy and birth, such
as respiratory distress syndrome, low birth weight, and hypoxia, are major factors
contributing to infant mortality. The other major causes of infant mortality and associated rates for blacks and whites are listed in Table 8–9.

TABLE 8–9. TEN LEADING CAUSES OF DEATH UNDER 1 YEAR OF AGE—UNITED STATES, 1992

		DEATH RATE[a]		
CAUSE OF DEATH	TOTAL NO. OF DEATHS	All Races	Whites	Blacks
All causes	34,628	8.5	6.9	16.8
1. Congenital anomalies	7,449	1.8	1.8	3.0
2. Sudden infant death syndrome (SIDS)	4,891	1.2	1.0	2.2
3. Disorder related to short gestations and unspecified low birth weight	4,035	1.0	0.6	2.2
4. Respiratory distress syndrome	2,063	0.5	0.4	1.0
5. Newborn affected by maternal pregnancy complications	1,461	0.4	0.3	0.7
6. Newborn affected by complications of umbilical cord, placenta, and membranes	993	0.2	0.2	0.5
7. Infections specific to the neonatal period	901	0.2	0.2	0.4
8. Accidents/adverse effects	819	0.2	0.2	0.4
9. Hypoxia/asphyxia (intrauterine)	613	0.2	0.1	0.3
10. Pneumonia/influenza	600	0.1	0.1	0.3
All other causes	10,803	26.6	20.3	58.6

[a]Per 1,000 live births.
(*From Kochanek K. D., Hudson B. L. Advance report of final mortality statistics, 1992. Monthly Vital Statistics Report, 1995; 43,6 [suppl.].
Hyattsville, Md.: National Center for Health Statistics.*)

Advances have been made in the prenatal diagnosis of congenital defects. Diagnostic ultrasound may be used to detect fetal anomalies such as hydrocephaly, microcephaly, anencephaly, ascitis, myelomeningocele, and polycystic kidneys. Amniotic fluid analysis can provide information on chromosomal aberrations and the detection of neural tube defects through α-fetoprotein analyses. Prenatal diagnosis enables one to prevent the birth of an affected infant. Use of birth control can prevent conception of future affected infants, if desired. Screening and abortion of fetuses of high-risk pregnant women could result in a savings of the cost of a lifetime of care for severely mentally or physically handicapped individuals. What cannot be accurately estimated in dollars is the emotional and psychological savings to the family when such births are prevented.

Rapid advances are being made in fetal medicine. Surgical techniques have been performed on fetuses with congenital defects that surely would have led to death *in utero* or at birth if intervention had not taken place. Clearly, the area of fetal medicine and prenatal diagnosis opens new prospects for primary and secondary prevention in the coming years.

Significant improvements have occurred in the diagnosis and treatment of other congenital defects, and many deaths can now be prevented. Significant advances in palliative care and open heart surgery have decreased the mortality of those with congenital heart defects. In recent years, organ transplants for defects such as biliary atresia have increased the survival of infants who otherwise would not survive past the first year of life.

As shown in Table 8–9, the second leading single cause of death in infants is sudden infant death syndrome (SIDS). In the United States it is the number one cause of death in infants after the first week of life. It occurs five times more frequently among infants of low birth weight. The cause of the disease is still unknown although its occurrence was recorded almost 2,000 years ago in the New Testament. Preventive efforts toward SIDS have recently begun. Such efforts became possible with the identification of high-risk groups such as premature infants and siblings of children who have died from SIDS. Apnea monitors have been installed in homes to permit closer surveillance of high-risk infants and possibly to prevent some of the deaths from SIDS.

Health problems developing after the neonatal period are most often related to environmental factors. Parent–child bonding has been shown to be a crucial attachment process during the early days and weeks of life and can affect the subsequent physical and emotional growth of the infant. Infants with inadequate attachment appear to have more growth problems or to be more prone to develop failure to thrive. Failure to thrive is a term applied to infants who fail to grow, but no clear organic etiology can be found to explain this. Instead the problem seems to arise from situations of environmental, sensory, or parental deprivation. Placement of a child in a nurturing environment often brings improvement, but prevention of the problem by thorough prenatal and postpartum assessment and anticipatory guidance is clearly more desirable.

Lastly, respiratory diseases and other conditions, such as diarrhea, result in many infant visits to the physician. In the past, these diseases were major causes of death during infancy. Today there is less mortality from these causes than in the past, but a tremendous amount of time is spent by the health industry in controlling these acute illnesses.

MAJOR FOCI OF PREVENTIVE EFFORTS

Prepregnancy Health Services

The health of our infants is largely dependent on the health of mothers and fathers. Health services are needed throughout the stages of gestation, birth, early life, and parenting. These health services need to target known factors affecting pregnancy and infant health (Table 8–10). The optimal type of health service begins in anticipation of pregnancy. Nurses and health educators should develop and implement

TABLE 8–10. FACTORS INFLUENCING PREGNANCY AND INFANT OUTCOMES

DEMOGRAPHIC RISKS	LIFESTYLE AND ENVIRONMENTAL FACTORS
Age (under 17 years; older than 34 years)	Smoking
Race (black)	Alcohol consumption
Low socioeconomic status	Substance abuse
Unmarried	Poor nutritional status
Low level of education	Toxic or occupational exposures, or both
	Inadequate prenatal care
Current Pregnancy	Lack of social support
Uterine anomalies	Stress
Isoimmunization	
Poor weight gain	**Preexisting Medical Conditions**
Multiple gestation	Heart disease
Incompetent cervix	Diabetes, insulin-dependent
Irritable uterus	Sickle-cell anemia
Anemia	Polyhydramnios
Bleeding	Thyroid disease
Pyelonephritis	Epilepsy
Premature rupture of membranes	Hepatitis
Preeclampsia	Asthma
Placenta previa	Tuberculosis
Deep venous thrombosis	Hypertension
Oligohydramnios	Malignancy
Hyperemesis	
Active herpes	**Obstetrical History**
Selected infections (eg, bacteriuria, rubella,	History of preterm delivery, infant death, or
cytomegalovirus)	congenital anomaly
Positive serology	Parity (more than 5)
	Eclampsia
	Short interval since last pregnancy

(*Compiled from Institute of Medicine.* Preventing low birthweight. *Washington, D.C.: National Academy Press, 1985; and Ohio Department of Health.* Prenatal risk assessment form. *DHS, Columbus, Oh, 3535 [1/88].*)

health education programs in schools and in health care settings. Mass media sources should be used to promote health practices beginning at the preschool level and continuing throughout life. Areas to be emphasized in such programs of primary prevention include needs of the body for maintaining health, activities that promote health and prevent disease, family planning and sex education, knowledge of the menstrual cycle and pregnancy, harmful factors during pregnancy such as smoking, infections, drugs, and radiation, and the need for early prenatal care.

Food supplementation programs to ensure the health of the women and children in our society need to be maintained. Awareness of the political process and active involvement by those in the health professions, including lobbying efforts to maintain these programs must be ongoing. Medical services to detect and treat sexually transmitted and other communicable diseases and chronic problems, such as hypertension, should be accessible to the entire population regardless of socioeconomic class. Accessible mental health services are needed for those with predictable or nonpredictable life stresses. The relationship between accessibility to family planning services and decreased infant and maternal mortality is clear. These sources, including an outreach component, should be available to all persons contemplating or engaging in sexual activity. Pregnancy testing services should be readily available with referral for counseling, genetic screening, family planning, and infertility services as requested or needed.

Prenatal Services and the Recognition of High-risk Pregnancies

Much research has accumulated in the past three decades as to the identification of those pregnancies with the greatest risks for maternal or infant problems. Figure 8–6 illustrates that services to identify and treat any conditions existing before pregnancy should begin with comprehensive health services for all adolescents and young women. It is hoped that women or adolescents carrying the greatest risk for abnormal pregnancy and outcome can be identified at this point, and appropriate counseling and family services provided so that these individuals can make responsible

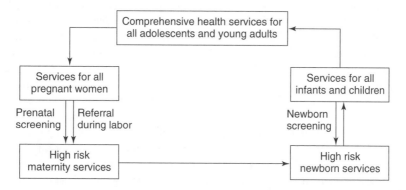

Figure 8–6. Health services network to improve maternal–infant health status.

decisions regarding the timing of childbearing. Table 8–10 outlines those factors associated with a higher likelihood of a high-risk pregnancy. These are danger signals of potential threats to the mother and newborn. Optimally, primary prevention should begin before conception. Nurses and other health care professionals functioning in school and community settings with adolescents can be particularly helpful in recognizing individuals with potential or actual risk factors and in providing or referring these individuals to appropriate resources and services.

More effective strategies to ensure prenatal care for all pregnant women are of the highest priority. Prenatal care not only results in improved pregnancy outcomes but is also cost-effective. Japan and many western European countries provide prenatal care with minimal barriers or preconditions, resulting in high rates of first trimester enrollment (Institute of Medicine, 1988). The most frequently described barriers to prenatal care present in the United States are: (1) financial barriers, (2) inadequate system capacity, (3) organization, practices, and atmosphere of prenatal services, and (4) cultural and personal barriers. A 1988 report by the Institute of Medicine revealed a "fundamentally flawed, fragmented, and overly complex" maternity care system in the United States. It was suggested that the best prospects for improving prenatal care utilization lie in reorganizing the nation's maternity care system. Outreach programs should not be a substitute for more accessible, responsive services. Efforts should not be directed to assisting women through the barriers of the health care system, but instead toward removing the obstacles.

Initial screening would occur at the time of pregnancy diagnosis. Screening tests recommended by the U.S. Preventive Services Task Force for pregnant women at the first prenatal visit include: blood pressure, hemoglobin and hematocrit, ABO/Rh blood typing, Rh(D) and other antibody screens, VDRL/RPR, hepatitis B surface antigen, urinalysis for bacteriuria, gonorrhea culture, and for high-risk groups, hemoglobin electrophoresis, rubella antibodies, and testing for chlamydia and HIV. The task force also recommends a screening history for genetic and obstetric history, dietary intake, tobacco/alcohol/drug use, risk factors for intrauterine growth retardation and low birth weight, and prior genital herpetic lesions (Fisher, 1989). The woman and fetus should have continual assessment to detect potential threatening health conditions such as hypertension, diabetes, or abnormal fetal development. Screening, diagnosis, and counseling for fetal genetic disorders should be available, along with second trimester abortion services if desired by the parents. Education on behaviors promoting healthy pregnancies and also information on the labor and delivery process should be introduced early in pregnancy. Childbirth education classes should remain available to all couples. Education on breastfeeding and parent–child bonding should also be available prenatally. Parents can be taught early infant development, stimulation techniques to promote development, and accident prevention measures that should be taken with all infants. Special prenatal programs can be developed for adolescents, particularly those programs geared to permit the teenager to continue her educational or vocational training. Social and legal services are needed to assist women and families with proper housing and food. Adoption services and counseling should also be available.

Appropriate referrals are important for all women diagnosed as high risk during this prenatal period. Approximately two thirds of high-risk newborns can be anticipated through careful prenatal evaluation. In addition to the services needed by all pregnant women, the high-risk mother requires constant, careful surveillance of herself and her infant. Such monitoring can include periodic amniotic fluid analyses to detect stress in the fetus, sonography or fundal height measures to assess fetal maturity, and careful management of medical problems or other health conditions arising from the pregnancy. In addition to those who develop complications during pregnancy, women who develop these in late pregnancy or during labor should have access to high-risk maternity services. This high-risk population should be followed in a prenatal care center that also has services for the infants of these women. Clearly, some infants will enter the perinatal system without first appearing in the high-risk prenatal group.

Services During the Intrapartal Period

The birth setting, the qualifications of the birth attendants, and the management of the birth and postpartum period are all important determinants of the health of the mother and the infant. The woman in labor needs continuing observation by a trained attendant. Fetal monitoring may be used to augment but not replace the observation of the nurse or physician. Backup services should be available, including transportation to a perinatal center if indicated. The mother and family unit should be provided with optimal privacy and physical and emotional support during this time. Services to assess the newborn's status and to make referrals to a perinatal center, if necessary, are crucial to the health of the newborn. Opportunities to bond with and care for the infant in a "rooming-in" situation should be available to the family, provided the newborn's physical condition does not necessitate transport to a perinatal center. In that instance, supportive care should be given to the family, and visitation with the infant promoted as soon as possible. All families should receive postpartum instruction on recovery and care of the mother and newborn, including breastfeeding and recognition of illness in the newborn. Home visitation services should be made available not only to high-risk families, but also to any family requesting such services. Counseling and legal services for adoption, foster care, or financial support may be indicated. Information on family planning and self-care should be provided before the 6-week postpartum visit.

Newborn Services

The newborn period, particularly the first 7 days of life, is critical in determining the outlook for the infant. A newborn needs immediate evaluation postdelivery, with appropriate treatment to prevent complications from heat loss or respiratory difficulty. Equipment for resuscitation should always be available, even in uncomplicated labors and deliveries. Safe, rapid transportation to a perinatal center should be provided if needed. The normal newborn also needs screening for certain genetic diseases during the neonatal period. Screening for relatively rare diseases, such as phenylketonuria, during the neonatal period benefits the infant, the family, and society. The costs of detection and prevention have been estimated to be only one tenth of the cost of lifetime institutional care. Breastfeeding should be encouraged whenever possible to provide the mother's immunities to the infant during the first months of life. Adequate nutritional services, such as WIC, and education on the infant's nutritional requirements should be available to families who need them. Early and periodic checkups for the newborn should be accessible and encouraged. The importance of infant immunizations should be recognized and provided free of charge to families in need. Nurses should educate parents on the benefits of breastfeeding, the nutritional requirements of infants, and the importance of immunizations. In addition, nurses can provide information on the normal development of infants and changes in family systems that result from the addition of a new family member. Comprehensive anticipatory guidance can reduce the incidence of infant mortality and morbidity.

SUMMARY

A preventive program as described above would lead to a decrease in maternal mortality, particularly in disadvantaged socioeconomic groups, and also a decrease in the incidence of infant morbidity and mortality. Improvements of the health of mothers and infants can only be achieved by focus on each of the following areas:

1. Improving the knowledge of men and women of childbearing age on reproduction and fertility. This would increase the likelihood of more planned and wanted pregnancies in our society.
2. Ensuring that every pregnant woman receives early prenatal care. These services should be available to our entire population, and especially to teenage mothers and economically disadvantaged women.
3. Continuing research on causes of death in women and children, particularly toxemia associated with pregnancy, ectopic pregnancies, congenital malformations, and SIDS.
4. Continuing advancement of knowledge in the areas of prenatal screening, fetal medicine, fetal surgery, and neonatology.
5. Advocating social programs to enhance the quality of life of all people in the United States, but with particular emphasis on women and infants who, although they are the future of any society, are traditionally the weakest members and those most in need of assistance from others.

REFERENCES

Abma J., Chandra A., Mosher W., Peterson L., Piccino L. (1997) Fertility, family planning, and women's health: New data from the 1995 National Survey of Family Growth. National Center for Health Statistics. *Vital Health Statistics, 23,*19.

Centers for Disease Control. (1995b) First 500,000 AIDS cases—United States, 1995. *Morbidity and Mortality Weekly Report, 44,* 46.

Centers for Disease Control. (1995a) Poverty and infant mortality—United States, 1988. *Morbidity and Mortality Weekly Report, 44,* 49.

Centers for Disease Control. (1991) Premarital sexual experience among adolescent women—United States, 1970–1988. *Morbidity and Mortality Weekly Report, 39,* 51–52.

Centers for Disease Control. (1995c) Update: AIDS among women—United States, 1994. *Morbidity and Mortality Weekly Report, 44,* 5.

Chasnoff I. J., Griffith D. R., MacGregor S., Dirkes K., Burns, K. A. (1989) Temporal patterns of cocaine use in pregnancy: Perinatal outcome. *Journal of the American Medical Association, 261,* 1741–1744.

Clayton R. R. (1986) Cocaine use in the U.S.: In a blizzard or just being snowed. *NIDA Research Monograph, 65,* 8–24.

Fisher M. (Ed.). (1989) *Guide to Clinical Preventive Services: An Assessment of the Effectiveness of 169 Interventions.* U.S. Preventive Services Task Force. Baltimore: William & Wilkins.

Hogue C. J. R., Yip R. (1989) Preterm delivery: Can we lower the black infant's first hurdle? *Journal of the American Medical Association, 262,* 548–550.

Hughs D., et al. (1986) *The health of America's children: Maternal and child health data book.* Washington, D.C.: Children's Defense Fund.

Institute of Medicine. (1985) *Preventing low birth weight.* Washington, D.C.: National Academy Press.

Institute of Medicine. (1988) *Prenatal care: Reaching mothers, reaching infants.* Washington, D.C.: National Academy Press.

Kochanek K. D., Hudson B. L. (1995) Advance report of final mortality statistics, 1992. *Monthly Vital Statistics Report, 43,* 6 (suppl.). Hyattsville, Md: National Center for Health Statistics.

La Dou J. (1990) *Occupational medicine.* Norwalk, Conn.: Appleton & Lange.

Lewis C. T., Matthews T. J., Heuser R. L. (1996) Prenatal care in the United States, 1980–1994. National Center for Health Statistics. *Vital Health Statistics, 21,* 54.

McCormick M. C. (1985) The contribution of low birthweight to infant mortality and childhood morbidity. *New England Journal of Medicine, 312,* 82–90.

National Center for Health Statistics. (1990a) Advance report of final natality statistics, 1988. *Monthly Vital Statistics Report, 34,* 4 (suppl.). Washington D.C.: Public Health Service.

National Center for Health Statistics. (1990b) Advance report of final mortality statistics, 1988. *Monthly Vital Statistics Report, 39,* 7 (suppl.). Washington D.C.: Public Health Service.

Office of the Assistant Secretary for Health and the Surgeon General. (1979) *Healthy people: The Surgeon General's report on health promotion and disease prevention, 1979.* (DHEW Pub. No. [PHS] 79–55071). Public Health Service. Washington, D.C.: U.S. Government Printing Office.

Ouellette E. M. (June 30, 1983) *A report on fetal alcohol syndrome.* Waltham, Mass. Testimony before the House Select Committee on Children, Youth and Families.

Roehat R. W. (1981) Maternal mortality in the United States of America. *World Health Statistics, 34,* 2–13.

Rothstein M. A. (1990) *Medical screening and the employee health cost crisis.* Washington, D.C.: Bureau of National Affairs, Inc.

Scott G. B., Fischl M. A., Klimas N., et al. (April 14–17, 1985) *Mothers of infants with the acquired immunodeficiency syndrome: Outcome of subsequent pregnancies.* Atlanta: International Conference on Acquired Immunodeficiency Syndrome.

Serdula M., Williamson D. F., Kendrick J. S., et al. (1991) Trends in alcohol consumption by pregnant women, 1985–1988. *Journal of the American Medical Association,* 265(7);876–879.

Taffel S. M., Ventura S. J., Gay G. A. (1989) Revised U.S. certificate of birth—New opportunities for research on birth outcome. *Birth, 16,* 188–193.

Thiry L., Sprecher-Goldberger S., Jonckheer T., Levy J., Van de Perre P., Henrivaux P., Cogniaux-LeClerc J., Clumeck N. (1985) Isolation of AIDS virus from cell-free breast milk of three healthy virus carriers (Letter). *Lancet, ii,* 891–892.

U.S. Bureau of the Census. (1978) Trends in child-spacing, June 1975. *Current Population Reports,* Series P-20, No. 315. Washington, D.C.: U.S. Government Printing Office.

U.S. Bureau of the Census. (1996) *Statistical abstract of the United States, 1996* (116th ed.). Washington, D.C.: U.S. Government Printing Office.

U.S. Department of Health and Human Services, Vital and Health Statistics. (1996) Supplements to the Monthly Vital Statistics Report, series 24(8): *Compilations of data on natality, mortality, marriage, divorce and induced terminations of pregnancy,* Hyattsville, Md.: DHS Pub. No. [PHS] 96-1958.

U.S. Department of Health and Human Services. (1991) Healthy people 2000: National health promotion and disease prevention objectives for the nation. Washington, D.C.: Public Health Service.

Ventura S. J., Martin J. A., Taffel S. M., et al. (1994) Advance report of final natality statistics, 1992. *Monthly Vital Statistics Report, 43,* 5 (suppl.). Hyattsville, Md.: National Center for Health Statistics.

Ventura S. J., Taffel S. M., Mathews T. J. (1994) Advance report of maternal and infant health data from the birth certificate, 1991. *Monthly Vital Statistics Report, 1994; 42,* 11, (suppl.) Hyattsville, Md.: National Center for Health Statistics.

Patterns of Morbidity and Mortality in Childhood and Adolescence

he health of young people is of crucial importance to any society because children represent the future of a society. As a result of high childhood mortality rates, parents in much of the world have had to produce many children so that a few survive to adulthood. In these countries, children younger than 15 years still constitute most of the population. For the world as a whole, children younger than 15 years comprised 31.7% of the total population in 1996 (U.S. Bureau of the Census, 1996). Because of declining birth rates and declining mortality at older ages, it is projected that by the year 2000, children younger than 15 years will comprise only 30% of the total world population.

In the United States, children younger than 15 years of age comprised 21.9% of the total population in 1996. Maintaining the health of these children, who represent the next generation of workers and parents, must be a national priority. Health status throughout the remainder of the life span depends on the health status and lifestyle established during the childhood years.

This chapter presents major causes of morbidity and mortality among children and adolescents. The first section of the chapter deals with causes of mortality by age, sex, and race. This is followed by presentation of acute and chronic diseases common in children. Factors that contribute to emerging patterns of health and disease through affecting risk status are then introduced. The final section of the chapter is devoted to interventions that are important to maintain good health from 1 year of age through adolescence.

MORTALITY IN CHILDHOOD AND ADOLESCENCE

Variation in Mortality by Age

As might be expected, death rates among children are low in comparison with death rates for older age groups. Under age 15 years, rates are higher from 1 to 4 years than they are from 5 to 14 years (mortality rates for children under 1 year of age are included in Chapter 8). Data for 1995, shown in Table 9–1, indicate mortality rates of 45 per 100,000 for boys between 1 and 4 years of age and 38 per 100,000 for girls of that age. In the 5- to 14-year age group, rates are 27 for boys and 18 for girls. By age 15 to 24 years, rates are 139 for men and 48 for women and continue to increase with each decade of age throughout the remainder of the life span. To some extent, this higher mortality continues to represent exposures *in utero* (eg, deaths from congenital malformations, neoplasms, and heart disease). A high accident rate is the major cause of the remaining deaths. Available 1995 data comparing mortality in the United States by race show higher rates for blacks than for whites of both sexes at all childhood ages. These rates are also listed in Table 9–1 (U.S. Bureau of the Census, 1997).

TABLE 9–1. DEATH RATES PER 100,000 BY AGE, SEX, AND RACE—UNITED STATES, 1992

	RACE AND SEX					
	All Races		White		Black	
AGE CATEGORY (YEARS)	Male	Female	Male	Female	Male	Female
1–4	45	36	39	31	77	63
5–14	27	18	24	17	41	26
15–24	139	48	121	44	247	71

(Compiled from U.S. Bureau of the Census. Statistical Abstract of the United States, 1997 [117th ed.], Washington, D.C., 1997, Table 121.)

Proportionately, there are more boys relative to girls at birth. This situation continues until age 24 years. The male-to-female ratio younger than 14 years was 104.9:100 in the United States in 1996. For the 14- to 24-year age group it was 105.7:100. However, in the 25- to 44-year age group there are fewer men than women (99.4:100). Above that age bracket, the sex ratio continues to decline with increasing age. By 65 years of age, this ratio is 69.5:100. This is due to the higher mortality rates for men compared with women that begin in childhood and continue throughout the life cycle (U.S. Bureau of the Census, 1997).

The major causes of death for three age subgroups, 1 to 4 years, 5 to 14 years, and 15 to 24 years, are shown in Table 9–2. Because most mortality statistics

TABLE 9–2. RATES PER 100,000 FOR TEN MAJOR CAUSES OF MORTALITY UNDER AGE 24 BY SUBCATEGORIES OF AGE—UNITED STATES, 1994

	AGE (YEARS)					
	1–4		5–14		15–24	
RANK	Cause	Rate	Cause	Rate	Cause	Rate
1	Accidents and adverse effects	15.9	Accidents and adverse effects	9.3	Accidents and adverse effects	38.7
2	Congenital anomalies	4.5	Malignant neoplasms	2.8	Homicide and legal intervention	22.6
3	Malignant neoplasms	3.3	Homicide and legal intervention	1.2	Suicide	13.8
4	Homicide and legal intervention	3.0	Suicide	1.5	Malignant neoplasms	4.8
5	Diseases of the heart	1.8	Congenital anomalies	0.9	Diseases of the heart	2.8
6	Human immunodeficiency virus infection (HIV)	1.3	Diseases of the heart	0.9	HIV infection	1.8
7	Pneumonia and influenza	1.1	HIV infection	0.5	Congenital anomalies	1.3
8	Conditions originating in the perinatal period[a]	0.7	Pneumonia and influenza	0.3	Pneumonia and influenza	0.6
9	Septicemia[a]	0.5	Benign neoplasms, carcinoma in situ, and unspecified neoplasms[a]	0.3	Chronic obstructive pulmonary diseases	0.6
10	Anemias[a]	0.4	Chronic obstructive pulmonary disease and allied conditions[a]	0.2	Cerebrovascular diseases	0.5
All Causes of Death		42.9		22.5		98.0

[a]1994 data unavailable, so 1992 data used.

(1995 data compiled from U.S. Bureau of the Census. Statistical abstract of the United States, 1997. [117th ed.]. Washington, D.C., 1997, Table 13.)

include ages 15 to 24 years as one subgroup spanning late childhood and young adulthood and because causes of death in this age group resemble those of ages 5 to 14 years more than those of the age group 25 to 34 years, this age subgroup is included in this chapter. Accidents are the leading cause of death in all three of these age subcategories. In 1994, there were 19,923 accidental deaths, accounting for 39% of all deaths between ages 1 and 24 years. Congenital anomalies at 4.5 per 100,000 are the second leading cause of death in the youngest age category. This cause drops to fifth place in the 5- to 14-year age group and seventh in the 15- to 24-year group. Malignant neoplasms, about half of which are leukemias, are among the top six causes of death in all three age categories, as are homicide and heart diseases. Suicide moves into third place as a cause of death for those in the 15- to 24-year category and ranks fifth for the 5- to 14-year group. Acquired immunodeficiency syndrome (AIDS) did not appear among the top ten causes of death for children until the mid-1980s. By 1994, it was in sixth place among children 1 to 4 years of age, due to maternal transmission, and in seventh place among those 5 to 14 years and in sixth place among those 15 to 24 years. Because this disease has a high case fatality rate, its impact as a cause of death is likely to become more prominent since incidence was rising through the mid-1990s.

The numbers of deaths are relatively small for most individual causes of death (eg, 1,604 for diseases of the heart and 1,611 for congenital anomalies between ages 1 and 24 years in 1994). Nonetheless, many deaths in this age group are theoretically preventable. Since the mid-1950s, mortality from natural causes has been lower than mortality from accidents and violence among children 1 to 19 years of age. Data indicate that in 1994, motor vehicle accidents accounted for more than 17,400 deaths among individuals between 1 and 24 years of age (U.S. Bureau of the Census, 1997). Between ages 1 and 4, motor vehicle accidents represented 34.9% of accidental deaths in 1992. Comparable rates were 56.1% between ages 5 and 14 and 75.4% between ages 15 and 24 (Kochanek & Hudson, 1995). Use of child restraint seats is a proven lifesaver. Accident prevention for children is discussed more fully in the final section of this chapter.

The other major accidental causes of death vary among the three age subcategories. Between 1 and 4 years of age, fatal accidents are mainly caused by fires, burns, and firearms, in that order. Among those 15 to 24 years, the other major accidents are drowning, firearms, and poison.

Of the other nine of the ten major causes of death under age 24, five are clearly candidates for primary prevention: homicide, suicide, pneumonia and influenza, chronic obstructive pulmonary disease, and AIDS. Cancer and congenital anomalies may also be prevented in some instances by eliminating maternal exposure to hazardous substances during pregnancy. Because the cause of these conditions is often unknown, early detection and prompt treatment can reduce the case fatality rates. Heart disease and cerebrovascular disease in this young age group may be inherited or related to maternal diet during pregnancy and compounded by a high fat, high sodium diet, inactivity, and smoking during childhood.

The improvement in childhood mortality in the United States in the 20th century has been dramatic. Elimination of the major childhood infections as causes of death was accomplished during the early part of the century. Major decreases in rates of mortality for accidents, congenital abnormalities, cancer, and diseases of the heart occurred between 1950 and 1992 among children 1 to 14 years of age (Fig. 9–1). These reductions are due to improved survival of children with congenital anomalies, cancer (particularly leukemia), and influenza and pneumonia, which have declined approximately 90% since 1950. Clearly, it is possible to further reduce mortality in this age category.

Variation in Mortality by Sex and Race

Figure 9–2 shows male and female rates of injury in various age groups related to visits to the emergency room. These patterns parallel rates of mortality from

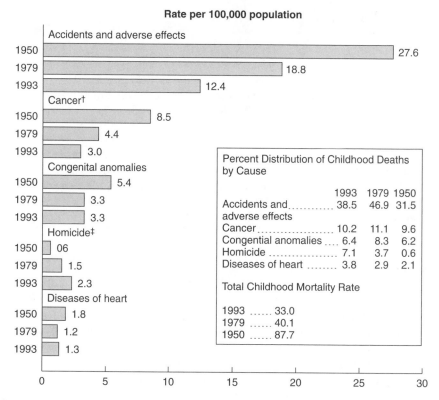

†Cancer = malignant neoplasms, including neoplasms of lymphatic and hematopoietic tissues.
‡Homicide=homicide and legal intevention.

Figure 9–1. Leading causes of childhood (ages 1–14 years) deaths: 1950, 1979, and 1993. (*Adapted from U.S. Department of Health and Human Services.* Prevention 89/90: Federal programs and progress. *Washington, D.C.: U.S. Government Printing Office, 1990; and U.S. Bureau of the Census.* Statistical abstract of the United States, 1996 [116th ed.]. *Washington, D.C.: U.S. Government Printing Office, 1996.*)

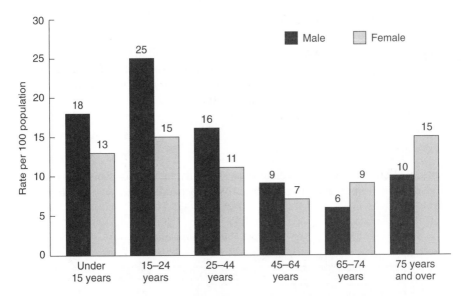

Figure 9–2. Rates of injury related to emergency room visits by age, 1993. (*Adapted from National Center for Health Statistics. Advance data from vital and health statistics: Numbers 261–270. Vital Health Statistics, 1996; 16, 27, Fig. 2. Hyattsville, Md.: National Center for Health Statistics.*)

accidental injury. Variation in mortality rates by sex reflects, to some extent, traditional sex differences in lifestyle, although death rates for boys tend to be higher among all causes including those not related to lifestyle. Greater differences between the sexes are observed, for example, in accidents, homicides, and suicide; these are causes that should be preventable and that are related to lifestyle and societal conditions. Sex differences in rates are greater for nonmotor vehicle accidents than they are for motor vehicle accidents. Excess nonmotor vehicle accidents among boys may reflect the more active and daring play of male children. Reasons for higher rates of homicide and suicide deaths among male children are unclear. Use of alcohol likely plays a role. There have been reports of higher rates of child abuse among male children than among female children. The social and psychological factors contributing to aggression toward male children and self-destructive tendencies among male children need further investigation. Lifestyle differences may also play a role in the higher rate of AIDS deaths among males.

Large racial differences in mortality are observed for nonmotor vehicle accidents, particularly fire and drowning, with black children under 14 years of age nearly twice as likely as whites to die from such accidents (Kochanek & Hudson, 1995). For motor vehicle accidents, death rates for black children are about 20% higher than for white children among those 1 to 14 years of age, but are about 30% lower among those 15 to 24 years of age (34.4/100,000 for whites and 22.4 for blacks in 1992). Whether the higher mortality rates are due to higher accident rates, higher case fatality rates, or both is not entirely clear. Since 1950, however, the racial differences have been narrowing.

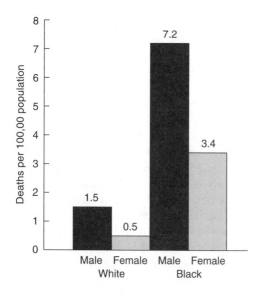

Figure 9–3. Death rates for human immunodeficiency virus infection among persons 15–24 years of age, by race and sex: United States, 1992. (*Adapted from Kochanek K. D., Hudson B. L. Advance report of final mortality statistics, 1992.* Monthly Vital Statistics Report, *1995; 43 [6] [suppl.], 23, Table 6. Hyattsville, Md.: National Center for Health Statistics.*)

A striking excess of AIDS deaths is seen among black males and females compared with whites in the age group 15 to 24 years (Fig. 9–3). Males have higher AIDS mortality than females within both racial groups. Black males under 18 years had a considerably higher rate of homicide than white males, but white males have higher suicide death rates than black males. In 1994, homicide mortality rates per 100,000 were 157.6 for 15 to 24 year old black males, but only 15.4 for white males. Suicide rates in that age group were 9.0 for black males and 23.0 for white males. Rates for females of both races are considerably lower.

Declines in mortality from natural causes occurred fairly equally in both racial groups for congenital anomalies and cancer and slightly faster among white children than black children for influenza and pneumonia. This latter difference could be related, in part, to blacks seeking care at a later stage in the natural history of the illness.

Mortality rates for those younger than age 25 years have been declining much faster for black females than for black males. As a result, among those younger than 25 years of age, gaps in mortality between the races have closed much faster for females than for males. The excess mortality among black males continues to be primarily in the rates of deaths from preventable causes, accidents, homicide, and suicide.

MORBIDITY IN CHILDHOOD AND ADOLESCENCE

In general, childhood is a time of good health in the United States. Children have much less illness than older persons. Data from the National Health Survey for 1988 to 1990 indicate that only about 2.2% of white children younger than 18 years rated their health as fair or poor and 4.9% of nonwhites rated their health fair or poor. All other children of this age group rated their health as good or excellent. This contrasts with approximately 26.9% of whites and 44.1% of blacks older than 65 years of age who rate their health as fair or poor (Collins & LeClere, 1996).

The majority of illnesses among children are acute in nature. Chronic conditions are relatively rare. In the following sections of this chapter, data relating to major causes of acute and chronic illness are presented. One factor that affects rates of these conditions is access to care. Medical care is not equally available for all persons. Differences in access likely contribute to how early illness is diagnosed and, therefore, to prognosis. Lack of care may also lead to underdiagnosis in those subgroups of the population who rarely seek care. Figure 9–4 shows the percentage of children with a regular source of medical care by race and/or ethnicity and family income. In general, whites and non-Hispanic blacks have similar percentages within comparable socioeconomic strata. Hispanics with an annual family income of under $35,000 have substantially fewer children with a regular source of care, but are equivalent to other races when their annual income is higher than $35,000. However, distributions of income vary by race and there are more blacks and Hispanics in the lower strata leading to those races having overall fewer children who receive regular health care. Major reasons given for no regular source of care for children from infancy to age 17 are: (1) does not need to see a doctor (31.8%); (2) cannot afford to see a doctor (34%); and (3) doctor is unavailable or inconvenient to access (17.4%) (Simpson et al, 1997).

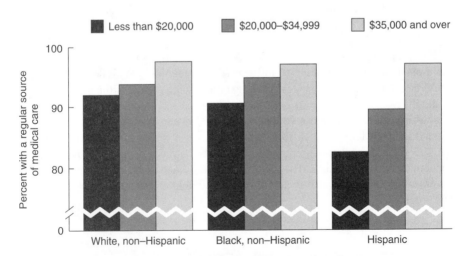

Figure 9–4. Percent of children from infancy to 17 years of age with a regular source of medical care by race and/or ethnicity and family income: United States, 1993. (*Adapted from Simpson G., Bloom B., Cohen R .A., Parsons P. E. Access to health care. Part 1: Children.* Vital Health Statistics, *1997;* 10, 196. Hyattsville, Md.: National Center for Health Statistics.)

Acute Conditions

Acute conditions, as presented in data from the National Center for Health Statistics, generally refer to illness or injury of short duration, typically less than 3 months, that has involved either medical attention or one-half day or more of restricted activity (Adams & Marano, 1995). Acute conditions usually include respiratory conditions, infective and parasitic diseases, injuries, digestive system disorders, and miscellaneous conditions, including diseases of the ear, headaches, skin diseases, genitourinary and musculoskeletal diseases, and disorders of pregnancy or delivery. A classification system for acute disorders is shown in Table 9–3. Acute

TABLE 9–3. CLASSIFICATION OF ACUTE CONDITIONS

I. Respiratory conditions
   A. Upper respiratory
      Common cold
      Other upper respiratory
   B. Influenza
      With digestive manifestations
      Other
   C. Other respiratory
      Pneumonia
      Bronchitis
      Other
II. Infective and parasitic conditions
   A. Common childhood diseases
   B. Virus
   C. Other
III. Injuries
   A. Fractures and dislocations
   B. Sprains and strains
   C. Open wounds and lacerations
   D. Contusions and superficial injuries
   E. Other
IV. Digestive system disorders
   A. Dental conditions
   B. Functional and symptomatic upper gastrointestinal conditions
   C. Other
V. Other
   A. Ear diseases
   B. Headaches
   C. Genitourinary
   D. Deliveries/disorders of pregnancy
   E. Skin diseases
   F. Musculoskeletal diseases

(From Bloom B. Current estimates from the National Health Interview Survey: United States, 1981. Vital and Health Statistics, Series 10, No. 141. [DHHS Publication No. (PHS) 83–1569]. Washington, D.C.: U.S. Government Printing Office, 1982.)

conditions are reported in terms of the annual number of acute conditions per 100 persons (eg, 2.41 per 100 persons). One could think of this figure as an annual average of 2.41 conditions or episodes per person.

Acute conditions are most common in the group younger than 6 years of age, declining continuously as age increases to a low of 109.9 conditions per 100 persons per year for those older than 65 years of age (Adams & Marano, 1995). The incidence of specific acute conditions is shown in Table 9–4 for ages younger than 5 years, 5 to 17 years, and 18 to 24 years of age. In 1994, those younger than age 5 years had an annual incidence of 358.8 acute conditions per 100 persons, compared with 220.1 for the 5- to 17-year group and 175.6 for the 18- to 24-year group. Nearly half of the acute conditions in all three age groups were respiratory conditions. Although the number of acute conditions decreases with age, the duration of restricted activity caused by acute conditions increases with age; in other words, each episode lasts longer in older persons than in children. Acute conditions accounted for an average of 3.3 days of school lost per child per year in 1994; fully 49.8% of these days of school lost per child in the 5- to 17-year age group were attributable to respiratory conditions (Adams & Marano, 1995).

The proportional distribution of conditions seen during visits to physicians' offices has generally reflected the incidence rates for acute conditions, although, as seen in Table 9–4, some conditions are less likely than others to receive medical attention. Visits to the school nurse could be expected to show a similar distribution of conditions.

TABLE 9–4. INCIDENCE OF ACUTE CONDITIONS PER 100 PERSONS BY AGE (YOUNGER THAN 24), AND PERCENTAGE OF THESE MEDICALLY ATTENDED—UNITED STATES, 1994

	YOUNGER THAN 5 YEARS		5–17 YEARS		18–24 YEARS	
CONDITION	Incidence	Percent Attended	Incidence	Percent Attended	Incidence	Percent Attended
Respiratory conditions	153.8	74	103.4	45	82.4	40
Common cold	68.5	68	29.4	33	26.1	29
Other acute upper respiratory	25.1	94	20.3	76	9.9	77
Bronchitis, pneumonia, and other	22.9	91	7.4	83	7.7	90
Influenza	37.3	58	46.3	33	38.7	27
Infective and parasitic conditions	54.7	84	41.9	62	18.5	59
Injuries	25.6	93	26.0	95	32.7	89
Digestive system disorders	10.5	79	8.3	37	7.4	52
All acute conditions	358.8	84	220.1	61	175.6	60

(Adapted from Adams P. F., Marano, M. A. Current estimates from the National Health Interview Survey: 1994. Vital Health Statistics, 1995; 10,193. Hyattsville, Md.: National Center for Health Statistics.)

In general, the annual incidence of all respiratory conditions in children has been decreasing for some time. Infective and parasitic diseases have also been declining over time. Of the defined categories of acute conditions, injury shows the least decline.

For certain of the infective conditions, reporting to public health authorities is mandatory (see Chap. 13, "Disease Control and Surveillance"). The 1995 incidence of the top ten mandatory-notice (notifiable) diseases for subgroups from infancy to age 24 is shown in Table 9–5. Gonorrhea is the most common infection in this age group, although syphilis and AIDS are also among the top ten; all of these conditions could potentially be controlled through early detection, prompt treatment, and follow up of sexual contacts. In the 1950s and 1960s large amounts of money were channeled into venereal disease control programs. The effectiveness of such programs was reflected in decreasing rates of gonorrhea and syphilis during that time. Later, as funds were diverted to other programs, rates of gonorrhea and syphilis began increasing again. This was probably due to a number of factors, including the introduction of the birth control pill which led to greater sexual freedom, and to the evolvement of penicillin-resistant strains of venereal organisms linked to the return of Vietnam veterans, many of whom were infected, as well as to poorer case identification and follow up of contacts as a result of cuts in funding to control programs.

Many cases of tuberculosis today are related to immigrants coming to this country infected with the disease and inadequate public health screening and detection of cases among these populations. Foodborne infections, such as *Escherichia coli* infections are receiving increased attention in recent years, for example, the

TABLE 9–5. RATES PER 100,000 FOR THE TOP TEN NOTIFIABLE DISEASES FOR INFANTS THROUGH 24 YEARS OF AGE—UNITED STATES, 1995

UNDER 5 YEARS		5–14 YEARS		15–24 YEARS	
Condition	Rate	Condition	Rate	Condition	Rate
Salmonellosis	61.8	Gonorrhea	21.8	Gonorrhea	645.0
Shigellosis	46.3	Shigellosis	20.1	Hepatitis A	18.0
Pertussis	13.9	Hepatitis A	18.0	Syphilis	13.7
Hepatitis A	10.4	Salmonellosis	12.1	Salmonellosis	11.3
Meningococcal disease	5.6	Lyme disease	5.4	AIDS	7.5
Tuberculosis	4.0	Pertussis	3.4	Shigellosis	6.7
Lyme disease	3.6	Tuberculosis	1.7	Hepatitis B	5.9
Acquired immunodeficiency syndrome (AIDS)	2.8	*Escherichia coli*	1.7	Tuberculosis	4.8
		Meningococcal disease	1.4	Lyme disease	2.8
Escherichia coli	2.7	Mumps	1.2	Meningococcal disease	1.7
Haemophilus influenzae type B	1.5				

(*Compiled from Centers for Disease Control. Summary of notifiable diseases, United States, 1995. Morbidity and Mortality Weekly Report, 1995; 44[53] 10.*)

publicity attendant upon the 1995 Jack-in-the-Box restaurant outbreak that was traced to contaminated hamburger meat.

Other mandatory-notice conditions are preventable through appropriate schedules of immunization. In the early part of the 20th century before immunizations were available, childhood infections were major killers of children as well as major causes of morbidity. Figure 9–5 shows the dramatic decline since 1950 in childhood infectious diseases for which immunization is available and which have been the focus of mass immunization programs in the past 3 or more decades. Cases of measles and mumps are few in number because most schools require immunization prior to enrollment. Some diseases covered by school immunization requirements have become so rare that they no longer fall among the top ten notifiable conditions (eg, diphtheria, tetanus, and polio). Current recommendations for preventive immunization of children are discussed later in this chapter.

Table 9–6 shows incidence of acute conditions and related activity limitations by sex and race for those younger than 5 years, those 5 to 17 years, and those 18 to 24 years of age using various measures of acute illness commonly found in the National Health Survey. Although boys younger than 5 years have a higher

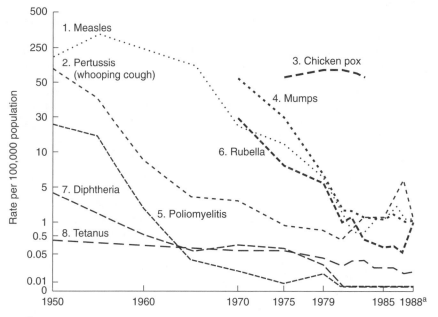

a *Provisional data*

Note: Chicken Pox, which was reported from 1975 to 1983, is no longer a national reportable disease.

Figure 9–5. Trends in reported incidence rates of childhood (aged 1–14 years) infectious diseases: selected years, 1950–1988. (*Adapted from U.S. Department of Health and Human Services,* Prevention 89/90: Federal Programs and Progress, *Washington, D.C.: U.S. Government Printing Office, 1990.*)

TABLE 9–6. INCIDENCE OF ACUTE CONDITIONS AND RESTRICTED ACTIVITY FOR ACUTE CONDITIONS, CHILDREN UNDER 18 YEARS OF AGE BY SEX—UNITED STATES, 1994

	AGE (YEARS)			
	Younger than 5		5–17	
	Male	*Female*	*Male*	*Female*
Acute conditions/100 persons/year	371.3	345.6	209.0	231.8
Restricted activity days/100 persons/year	856.2	897.4	586.3	681.1
Bed disability days/100 persons/year	372.4	383.1	231.2	309.9
School lost days/100 persons/year	—	—	294.9	369.3

(*Data from Adams P. F., Marano, M. A. Current estimates from the National Health Interview Survey: 1994. Vital Health Statistics, 1995; 10,193. Hyattsville, Md.: National Center for Health Statistics.*)

incidence of acute conditions than girls of the same age, they have less restricted activity associated with acute conditions than girls.

Hospitalization

Although 94.8% of children younger than 18 years of age had one or more contacts with a physician in 1994, only 2.3% were hospitalized (Adams & Marano, 1995). Children under 5 years averaged 6.8 physician contacts per year compared with 3.5 for those 5 to 17 years, and 3.9 for those 18 to 24 years. Of these, 4.0, 2.0, and 2.1, respectively, were office visits. The larger number among the younger age group reflects visits for preventive care, including immunizations.

Acute illness, as reflected in 1994 hospital discharge data, is shown in Table 9–7 for the age group younger than 15 years. Consistent with previously presented data on incidence of acute diseases and reasons for physicians' office visits, respiratory diseases top the list. Among the respiratory diseases, pneumonia is the most frequent, followed closely by acute upper respiratory conditions and asthma. Injury and poisoning was the second most frequent set of diagnoses among hospital discharges. Fractures were the most frequent type of injury. Diseases of the digestive system, seventh among diagnoses in physicians' office visits, were the third most frequent hospitalization diagnoses; particularly common in this complex of illnesses were enteritis and colitis, inguinal hernia, and appendicitis. These acute conditions can be life-threatening and therefore usually require hospitalization rather than office treatment. Ear-related problems were the most common of the conditions included under the fourth most frequent diagnostic category, diseases of the nervous system and sense organs. The fifth through seventh most frequent discharge diagnostic categories—congenital anomalies, infectious and parasitic diseases, and diseases of the genitourinary system—have between 28,200 and 13,300 hospitalizations.

Length of hospital stay is generally short in this age group. Among the ten leading diagnostic categories of hospitalizations, the longest length of stay is for

TABLE 9–7. NUMBER (IN THOUSANDS) OF FIRST LISTED DISCHARGE DIAGNOSES FROM SHORT-STAY HOSPITALIZATIONS AND AVERAGE LENGTH OF STAY FOR PATIENTS YOUNGER THAN 15 YEARS OF AGE—UNITED STATES, 1994

DIAGNOSTIC CATEGORY BY RANK OF FIRST LISTED DIAGNOSIS	NUMBER (THOUSANDS)	AVERAGE LENGTH OF STAY
1. Diseases of the respiratory system	131.7	3.2
Acute upper respiratory infections except influenza	(31.6)	(3.3)
Chronic disease of tonsils and adenoids	(23.5)	(1.2)
Pneumonia	(34.7)	(4.6)
Asthma	(31.0)	(2.8)
2. Injury and poisoning	65.6	4.1
Fractures	(20.1)	(5.0)
Intracranial injuries	(8.7)	(2.5)
Lacerations and open wounds	(6.3)	(3.0)
3. Diseases of the digestive system	51.5	3.6
Noninfectious enteritis and colitis	(18.1)	(2.9)
Inguinal hernia	(5.6)	(1.6)
Appendicitis	(9.9)	(4.9)
4. Diseases of the nervous system and sense organs	36.5	3.7
Diseases of the ear and mastoid	(20.0)	(2.1)
Diseases of the central nervous system	(10.8)	(6.5)
5. Congenital anomalies	28.2	5.9
6. Infectious and parasitic diseases	18.4	4.1
7. Diseases of the genitourinary system	13.3	3.9
8. Symptoms, signs, and ill-defined conditions	9.3	2.7
9. Diseases of the blood and blood-forming organs	8.9	4.2
10. Diseases of the skin and subcutaneous tissue	8.6	4.0

(Compiled from Graves, E. J., Gillum B. S. National Hospital Discharge Survey: Annual summary, 1994. National Center for Health Statistics. Vital Health Statistics, 13(128), 1997.)

congenital anomalies at 5.9 days. Injury and poisoning are in second place at 4.1 days (see Table 9–7).

Chronic Conditions

Chronic conditions are not common among children. This is because chronic conditions usually develop over long periods of time after exposure to environmental hazards or an unhealthy lifestyle. The bodies of children have not had a lifetime of exposure to such hazards or to the general stresses and strains of living. Nor has sufficient time passed between any harmful exposure and onset of a chornic condition because latency periods are quite long. Incidence of chronic conditions thus increases with age. Because most children do not have chronic conditions, the vast majority of children younger than 18 years of age (93.3% in 1994) have no activity limitation related to such conditions. Of the 6.7% with activity limitation, about three quarters are limited in major activity. Major activity refers to ability to work or keep house (adults) or engage in school or preschool activities (children). Girls younger than 18 years of age are less often limited in activity than boys, although differences are not striking, 5.6% versus 7.9%, respectively (Adams & Marano, 1995). Data from the 1950s and 1960s showed that the major causes of activity limitations in children younger than 17 years seen by physicians were for asthma or hay fever (affecting 20% of children), impairments of lower extremities and hips (8.3%), paralysis (7.4%), chronic bronchitis and sinusitis (5.5%), mental and nervous conditions (3.8%), and heart conditions (3.7%). Over the years, the ability to treat asthma, bronchitis, and heart conditions has improved and they are now less frequently associated with limitation of activity than in the past. New technology has also improved functional ability in those with orthopedic impairments.

Table 9–8 shows rates for selected common chronic conditions of persons younger than 18 years of age. Of these, the major handicapping conditions in the younger than 18 years of age group include vision, hearing, and speech deficits, crippling emotional disturbance, mental retardation, and learning disability. Clearly, orthopedic impairments, particularly of the lower extremity or hip, and speech, hearing, and visual impairments are the most common of these handicapping conditions that limit function. Equally as important for children as physical function is the ability to function well in school and social settings. Emotional disturbances, mental retardation, learning disability or developmental lag, and speech deficits, as well as vision and hearing deficits, affect function in these circumstances.

TABLE 9–8. REPORTED CHRONIC CONDITIONS PER 1,000 PERSONS, YOUNGER THAN 18 YEARS OF AGE—UNITED STATES, 1994

CONDITION OR IMPAIRMENT	RATE PER 1000
Trouble with acne	29.9
Dermatitis	37.6
Anemias	12.2
Migraine headache	16.1
Heart disease	18.1
Heart rhythm disorders	13.9
Murmurs	12.1
Chronic bronchitis	55.3
Asthma	69.1
Hay fever or allergic rhinitis with asthma	60.5
Chronic sinusitis	65.1
Chronic disease of tonsils or adenoids	23.1
Speech impairment	20.9
Deformity or orthopedic impairment	28.0
Lower extremities	16.5
Back	11.2
Visual impairment	8.7

(*Adapted from Adams P. F., Marano, M. A. Current estimates from the National Health Interview Survey: 1994. Vital Health Statistics, 1995; 10, 193. Hyattsville, Md.: National Center for Health Statistics.*)

RISK FACTORS IN CHILDHOOD

Many of the causes of morbidity and mortality of children and adolescence, even the infectious causes, result from preventable behaviors and social–environmental conditions. It is likely that associations of nonwhite race, male gender, and lower socioeconomic status and educational levels with higher rates of morbidity and mortality reflect, to a large extent, social disadvantage that leads to increased exposure to unhealthy lifestyles. Social disadvantage is probably also reflected in less access to health care services. Changes in society in general also contribute to risky behavior. Widespread television viewing, for example, has been implicated in contributing to obesity among children (Dietz & Gortmaker, 1985) and to violent or antisocial behavior (Gadow & Sprafkin, 1989; Centerwall, 1992). Media emphasis on tall, slender women has contributed to anorexia nervosa and bulemia among female adolescents. Changes in society resulting from the increases in the proportion of mothers who work, single-parent families, urbanization, and social isolation resulting from technological changes all have contributed to a breakdown in social structures that protected children in the past. There is concern that as many as 25% of children in the United States currently between 10 and 17 years of age may not reach their full potential as workers, parents, and individuals; 45% of Hispanic youth, 51% of black youth, and 17% of white youth are considered at risk (U.S. Public Health Service, 1993). This has implications for the health and welfare of these individuals as well as for future generations.

Poverty contributes to low birth weight with its developmental consequences, nutritional inadequacy, and exposure to a variety of stresses and other conditions that increase the likelihood of substance abuse and violent behavior or its consequences. Youth who grow up in poverty live in an environment that often places low value on academic performance and may reward risky behavior. In addition, they experience fewer expectations for achievement from family and teachers and less assistance and support during schooling. They may observe parental or sibling modeling of drug use and deliquency, poor family management, family conflict, community disorganization, and geographic mobility. Access to drugs and guns may be easier (U.S. Public Health Service, 1993). Poverty also increases exposure to toxic chemicals, since poor neighborhoods are more often located near industrial areas. Older housing with lead-based paint is another concern; however, intensive federal and state control programs have reduced the occurrence of this problem over the past 25 years. Between the National Health and Nutrition Examinations II Survey (NHANES) in 1976 to 1980 and the NHANES III Survey in 1988 to 1991, geometric mean blood lead levels decreased from 12.8 mg/dl to 2.9 mg/dl. The percent of individuals with blood lead levels 10 μg/dl or over dropped from 77.8% to 4.4% in the same time period. Both have continued to drop since that time (Centers for Disease Control, 1997).

Risky behaviors of particular concern among America's youth include smoking, drinking, unprotected sexual activity, and violence. Lack of physical activity, inadequate nutritional intake, and running away from home are three additional risk behaviors increasing in frequency. During the 1990s, three trends have been noted that relate to increases in the proportion of youth engaging in risky behaviors:

(1) such behaviors are occurring at progressively younger ages; (2) the younger adolescent population is growing rapidly; and (3) the percent of younger adolescents from socioeconomically disadvantaged groups is growing (U.S. Public Health Service, 1993). Two thirds of high school students have tried illicit drugs, tobacco, alcohol or other drugs before they graduate from high school. The average age of starting use of tobacco products, alcohol, and other drugs has dropped from 17 to 19 years in 1930 to 12 years today (U.S. Public Health Service, 1993). Half of youth between 12 to 21 years of age have smoked a whole cigarette in their lifetime and another 10% have taken a few puffs. Smoking status of youth between 12 and 21 years of age are shown in Figure 9–6.

Approximately two thirds of youth under 21 have had at least one drink of alcohol, 45% have had a drink in the last month. Nearly a third of youth between 12 and 21 have used some type of illegal drug at one time—7.3% of those 12 to 13 years, 25.9% of those 14 to 17, and 49% of those 18 to 21. Six in ten never-married youth between 14 and 21 years of age have had sexual intercourse. About one in seven teens carried a weapon at least one day during the past month (Adams et al, 1995). Figure 9–7 shows the prevalence of selected unhealthy behaviors among adolescents by gender.

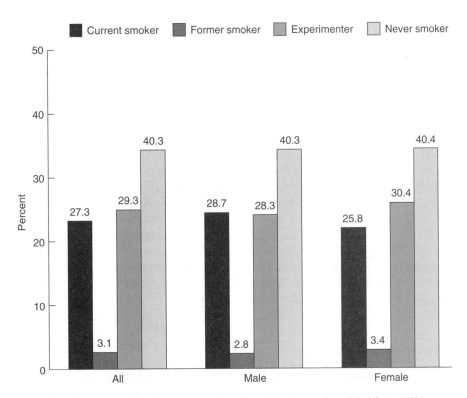

Figure 9–6. Percent of youth 12 to 21 years of age by smoking status and sex: United States, 1992. (*Adapted from National Center for Health Statistics. Advance data from vital and health statistics: Numbers 261–270. Vital Health Statistics, 1996; 16, 27, Fig. 1. Hyattsville, Md.: National Center for Health Statistics.*)

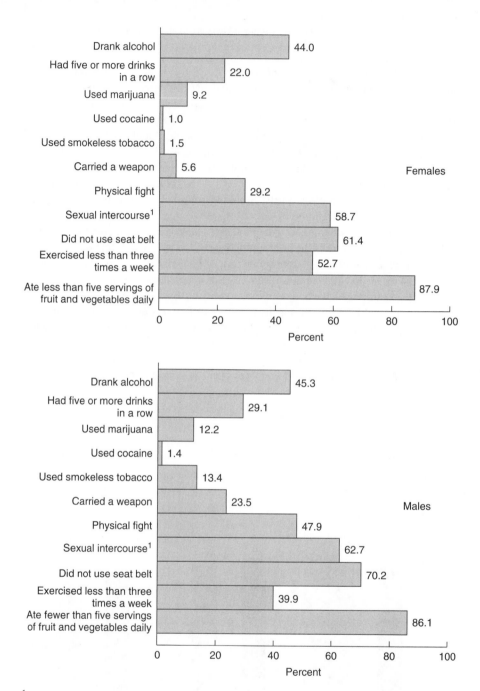

[1]Ages 14–21 years and never married.

Figure 9–7. Prevalence of selected unhealthy behaviors among adolescents by gender: United States, 1992. (*Adapted from National Center for Health Statistics. Advance data from vital and health statistics: Numbers 261–270. Vital Health Statistics, 1996; 16, 27, Figs. 2 & 3. Hyattsville, Md.: National Center for Health Statistics.*)

Male and female adolescents have similar rates of alcohol use, eating fewer than five servings of fruits and vegetables daily, engaging in sexual intercourse, and not using seat belts. However, males are about four times as likely to carry a weapon and twice as likely to have a fight as females. Females are less likely than males to exercise.

Lack of access to medical care represents a risk factor for increased morbidity and mortality of youth in large part because delay in diagnosis and treatment can lead to residual effects, including disability and death from treatable conditions. Lack of preventive services also means more frequent episodes of illness, which may weaken immunological and other body defenses. The third national goal in *Healthy People 2000* was to asssure access to preventive services for all Americans (U.S. Public Health Service, 1991). A strong correlation exists between income and having a regular source of medical care. Race is associated to a lesser extent with having regular care (see Fig. 9–4). In the United States in 1993, over 7.3 million children had difficulty obtaining at least one of the medical servies they needed, 1.3 million were unable to get needed care, and for 2.7 million children, care was delayed because of worry by parent or guardian about the costs of care. The lack of access to care is even worse for dental care; 4.2 million children were unable to get dental care in 1993. Source of coverage (public versus private) is not associated with having an unmet medical need. However, there are nearly three times the percent of children with unmet medical needs among uninsured children as among insured children (Simpson et al, 1997). Education also relates to adequacy of care in that individuals with lower education more often say they do not need to see a doctor for a particular problem than do those with more education.

MAJOR FOCI FOR PREVENTIVE EFFORTS

Because so many of the risk factors associated with the major causes of morbidity and mortality in childhood relate to changing social values and behavioral norms and since children are so desirous of being like their peers, it may be more difficult to change behavior of individuals in this age group than in older individuals. Considerable research has been conducted over the past decade on school-based and community-based approaches to reducing risky behaviors of children. Some of these interventions have been demonstrated to be efficacious. However, to date, few office-based approaches to changing the behaviors of individual children have been tested in clinical settings. Downs and Klein have presented a cost-effectiveness model that argues that it is not feasible from a cost point of view to test office-based interventions for preventing some outcomes, such as deaths from automobile crashes and human immunodeficiency virus (HIV) infection (1995). Public health approaches are needed to effectively prevent these outcomes. Other interventions, such as encouraging use of infant car seats and motorcycle and bicycle helmets to prevent serious injury in the event of an accident, and immunizations against childhood diseases can be effectively delivered in the office-based clinical setting. Still other tactics, such as office-based interventions to prevent children from starting to smoke or to help adolescent smokers to quit, are being tested now.

Prevention of Accidents

Because accidents affect more children than any other cause of morbidity and mortality, they are addressed first. Although changing human behavior has been considered, at times, as a potential method to reduce accidental injuries, this approach is probably less effective than some other strategies because modification of human behavior is expensive, time consuming, and marginally effective. Also, the element of human error still remains. Passive measures requiring no action on the part of the individual are preferred. Airbags and automatic seat belts protect the individual without any action on his or her part. Sprinkler systems that turn on automatically in response to elevated air temperature are another example. A comprehensive approach employing countermeasures aimed at the three phases of the injury control sequence offers the most hope. The three phases are: (1) preventing potentially injurious events, (2) minimizing the chance that injury results when an accident occurs, and (3) reducing unnecessary consequences of injury (Haddon & Baker, 1981). Table 9–9 gives examples of each of these interventions for various types of injuries that commonly affect children.

The measures for primary prevention bypass dependence on the human element of the moment and focus on structuring the environment through safer product design or designing safety features into the environment. For example, better designed cars, mandated use of seat belts, and air safety bags cannot prevent an accident, but may prevent an injury. Fences around swimming pools make unsupervised

TABLE 9–9. STRATEGIES FOR REDUCING INJURIES DUE TO ACCIDENTS AMONG CHILDREN AND ADOLESCENTS

EVENT TYPE	PREVENT PHASE	EVENT PHASE	POSTEVENT PHASE
Electrocution	Covered electric outlets Insulation on electrical tools	Circuit breakers Fuses	Portable defibrillators
Drowning	Fences around pools Stable watercraft Grading slopes of man-made lakes Swimming instruction	Lifelines, poles, rings, jackets	Training public in resuscitation methods
Burns	Elimination of floor heaters Matches that burn with less heat and self-extinguish when dropped	Smoke detectors Flame retardant clothing and furnishings Alternative escape routes	Burn centers Skin grafting Occupational and psychological rehabilitation
Motor vehicle	Road design and maintenance Driver training Drunk driving laws Vehicle design and regular maintenance	Passive seat belts Air bags Paramedic teams	Emergency centers Rehabilitation centers
Poisoning	Childproof caps Locked storage	Poison control center emergency information lines Administration of antidotes	Emergency centers

access difficult. Swimming instruction for children and use of life jackets when boating, although not design features, do reduce the likelihood of drowning because the child is better prepared to cope with water. While these measures do not eliminate the need for adult supervision of children, they do reduce the likelihood of accident when the attention of a supervisory adult is diverted.

Event phase interventions focus on immediate response when an accident occurs. For example, circuit breakers can be activated or fuses can be deactivated to cut off electrical current. Throwing a rope, life line, or other aid to a swimmer in trouble can save a life. Smoke detectors alert occupants of a burning building to danger. Child seats protect the child from serious injury in an automobile accident.

Once an accident has occurred (eg, a child has been burnt or electrocuted), intervention strategies aim at restoring function. Defibrillators can restore the heartbeat of an electrocuted child, emergency transport services can maintain life on the way to the hospital treatment center, and skin grafting and special care procedures at burn centers can save lives and minimize resulting morbidity and disability.

Health education is important to all three phases of injury control. If the general public is unaware of safer products they will not be used. Similarly, the public needs to be aware of behavioral means for reducing the likelihood of accidents; educating parents about growth and development of children gives them a basis for structuring the environment and the child's play activities appropriate to the child's ability. Parents also need to know basic facts that can correct misimpressions (eg, it is possible for a child to drown in even a few inches of water). Instructions on first aid measures and where to call in the event of an emergency are also important.

Prevention of Infection

Prevention of the infectious causes of childhood morbidity and mortality begins with childhood immunizations during infancy and maintenance of booster immunizations during early childhood. Table 9–10 presents the schedule of recommended childhood immunizations. Such artificial, active immunization against communicable disease confers protection directly on the recipient and indirectly on his or her associates by interfering with the chain of disease transmission, thus controlling infection in the community as well as in the individual (herd immunity). In the United States and Canada, routine active immunization of children against pertussis, poliomyelitis, measles, rubella, mumps, tetanus, diphtheria, hepatitis B, and *Haemophilus influenzae* type b is recommended. Active immunization against rabies is advocated after exposure. The rate of case fatality from this encephalitic disease approaches 100%. The frequency of the disease is increasing in wild animals, but decreasing in domestic animals. Although few human cases are reported, more than 30,000 people nationally receive the rabies vaccine each year after possible exposure. Immunization against influenza is recommended in major epidemics and routinely for children who have special health problems likely to make the impact of the disease more severe (eg, children with cystic fibrosis or muscular dystrophy). The Bacillus-Calmette-Guérin (BCG) immunization is sometimes recommended for children with high exposure to

TABLE 9–10. RECOMMENDED CHILDHOOD IMMUNIZATION SCHEDULE[a]—UNITED STATES, JANUARY 1995

VACCINE	BIRTH	2 MONTHS	4 MONTHS	6 MONTHS	12[b] MONTHS	15 MONTHS	18 MONTHS	4–6 YEARS	11–12 YEARS	14–16 YEARS
Hepatitis B[c]	HB-1									
		HB-2			HB-3					
Diphtheria-Tetanus-Pertussis (DTP)[d]		DTP	DTP	DTP	DTP or DTap ≥ at 15 months			DTP or DTaP	Td	
Haemophilus Influenzae type b (Hib)		Hib	Hib	Hib	Hib					
Poliovirus		OPV	OPV	OPV				OPV		
Measles-Mumps-Rubella					MMR			MMR or MMR		

[a]Recommended vaccines are listed under the routinely recommended ages. Shaded bars indicate range of acceptable ages for vaccination.

[b]Vaccines recommended for administration at 12 to 15 months of age may be administered at either one or two visits.

[c]Infants born to hepatitis B surface antigen (HBsAg)-negative mothers should receive the second dose of hepatitis B vaccine between 1 and 4 months of age, provided at least 1 month has elapsed since receipt of the first dose. The third dose is recommended between 6 and 18 months of age. Infants born to HBsAg-positive mothers should receive immunoprophylaxis for hepatitis B with 0.5 ml hepatitis B immunoglobulin (HBIG) within 12 hours of birth, and 5 μg of either Merck, Sharpe & Dohme (West Point, Pa.) vaccine (Recombivax HB®) or 10 μg of SmithKline Beecham (Philadelphia) vaccine (Engerix-B®) at a separate site. For these infants, the second dose of vaccine is recommended at 1 month of age and the third dose at 6 months of age. All pregnant women should be screened for HBsAg during an early prenatal visit.

[d]The fourth dose of DTP may be administered as early as 12 months of age, provided at least 6 months have elapsed since the third dose of DTP. Combined DTP-Hib products may be used when these two vaccines are administered simultaneously. Diphtheria and tetanus toxoids and acellular pertussis vaccine (DTaP) is licensed for use for the fourth and/or fifth dose of DTP in chidlren ≥15 months of age and may be preferred for these doses in children in this age group.

(Adapted from Centers for Disease Control. Recommended childhood immunization schedule—United States, 1995. Morbidity and Mortality Weekly Report, 1995; 44 [No. RR-5], Table 1.)

tuberculosis, particularly repeated household exposures to those with ineffectively treated sputum-positive tuberculosis.

Vaccination coverage among children is less than desired. Table 9–11 shows the coverage levels compared to the desired levels for children 19 to 35 months of age in 1994. Coverage varies by state, with Idaho, Missouri, and Michigan having less than 65% coverage with the 4:3:1 series (four doses of DPT [diphtheria, pertussis, tetanus] vaccine, three doses of poliovirus vaccine, and one dose of measles vaccine) in 1994. In contrast, New Hampshire and Massachusetts had between 85 and 100% coverage (Centers for Disease Control, 1995).

General hygiene measures, including food and water handling practices, maintaining a clean house, teaching children basic hygiene practices such as hand washing, and avoiding contact of infected individuals with children, particularly with a very young child or with ill children, can be helpful in primary prevention of many childhood gastrointestinal and respiratory infections. Plenty of rest and a

TABLE 9–11. VACCINATION COVERAGE LEVELS AMONG CHILDREN AGED 19–35 MONTHS, BY SELECTED VACCINES—UNITED STATES, 1994

VACCINE/DOSE	1996 GOAL	NHIS[a] %	(95% CI[d])	NHIS PROVIDER[b] %	(95% CI)	NIS[c] %	(95% CI)
DTP/DT[e]							
≥3 Doses	90%	89	(±2.4)	93	(±2.2)	93	(±0.7)
≥4 Doses	—	69	(±3.0)	76	(±3.4)	77	(±1.1)
Poliovirus							
≥3 Doses	90%	78	(±2.7)	83	(±3.0)	83	(±1.0)
Haemophilus influenzae type b							
≥3 Doses	90%	73	(±3.1)	89	(±2.6)	86	(±0.9)
Measles-containing (MCV)	90%	91	(±1.8)	88	(±3.8)	89	(±0.9)
Hepatitis B[f]							
≥3 Doses	70%	27	(±3.5)	17	(±2.8)	37	(±1.2)
Combined series							
4 DTP/3 Polio/1 MCV[g]	—	67	(±3.1)	72	(±3.4)	75	(±1.2)

[a]1994 National Health Interview Survey, January–June.
[b]1994 National Health Interview Survey, January–June, with provider data.
[c]1994 National Immunization Survey, April–December.
[d]Confidence interval.
[e]Diphtheria and tetanus toxoids and pertussis vaccine/diphtheria and tetanus toxoids.
[f]The difference between the NIS and NHIS provider estimates for hepatitis B is primarily because of different time periods for the surveys and the rapid improvement in hepatitis B coverage during 1994.
[g]Four doses of DTP/DT, three doses of poliovirus vaccine, and one dose of MCV.
(*From Centers for Disease Control. State and national vaccination coverage levels among children aged 19–35 months—United States, April–December 1994.* Morbidity and Mortality Weekly Report, *1995;* 44, *33; Table 1.*)

well-balanced nutritionally adequate diet can also contribute to primary prevention of childhood infections. Health and sex education programs aimed at young teens can play an important role in preventing venereal diseases and AIDS as well as teenage pregnancies.

Secondary prevention of childhood infections includes screening in high-risk groups for those infections with high prevalence (eg, tuberculosis among inner-city children). Because the incidence of even the most common infections is low in the younger-than-17-year age group, early case finding is often more useful and cost-effective than is population screening. A complete history (including sexual history) and physical examination may be an effective method of detecting conditions such as gonorrhea; diagnosis can be confirmed by testing and treatment promptly instituted.

Prevention of Stress-related Morbidity and Mortality

Included as stress-related conditions in childhood are child abuse, homicide, suicide, alcohol and drug abuse, and mental or emotional problems. Although accidents may, in some instances, be stress-related, they are discussed separately because they often have causes that are clearly not stress-related and because they account for such a large proportion of childhood morbidity and mortality.

Abuse of children is most often inflicted by a parent. Many homicides are also committed by family members. Suicides, alcohol and drug abuse, and other mental or emotional problems often arise out of difficult, unsupportive home environments. Add the pressures of peer relationships, and problems result. Primary prevention should begin before a child is born, perhaps even before a couple marries. Marriage requires maturity, a sense of self, and the ability to deal with the daily pressures of life. It is possible that high school family living courses can help prepare young persons to approach marriage and family with more realistic expectations. More realistic expectations, by leading to a more supportive family environment for future children, could in turn contribute to decreasing the frequency of child abuse and other problems associated with a stressful family environment.

Similarly, pregnant women and their partners should be taught about child growth and development so they are prepared to deal with the demands of a growing child and the pressures on their own relationship that a child can produce. Approaches to maintaining the relationship of the parents can be discussed with the couple at this time. Such preparation can reduce family tension and create a more supportive atmosphere for both parents and children.

Health education programs in schools, on television, and for parents regarding drug, alcohol, and cigarette use and abuse may be of some help to youngsters who are tempted to try these substances. The percentage of high school seniors who perceive great risk in using various substances has increased somewhat in recent years, suggesting that educational efforts may be having some influence on attitudes. Enforcement of laws forbidding sale to and public consumption of these substances by underage children can prevent exposure of their bodies during childhood and thus at least postpone by a few years the onset, in adulthood, of acute and chronic health conditions caused by use and abuse of these substances. If a lifestyle free of use of these substances can be established before 18 years of age, perhaps young adults will be less prone to initiate use. Most adult smokers first tried cigarettes before age 18 and the initiation of smoking among youth under 18 has been increasing, even as smoking rates have declined among older populations. Community programs offering extracurricular activities provide children with opportunities that can build self-esteem and keep them sufficiently busy and involved so that drugs, alcohol, and cigarettes offer little competition. Among 100 such prevention programs reviewed, the most successful shared two characteristics: they provided individual attention and were community-wide, multicomponent, and multiagency (U.S. Public Health Service, 1993).

Secondary prevention of stress-related illness can involve both the parents and a spectrum of health-related professionals. Parents can be taught to watch for early signs of emotional problems and learn what resources are available to treat these problems. When effective communication between parent and child has been established early, the child may come to the parent for help before serious problems develop. Teachers, nurses, and the child's physician are all in a position to detect problems early and to provide the family with a referral for counseling. Unfortunately, this is not an option for those children with no regular source of medical care. Counseling and rehabilitation centers, as well as medical facilities for treatment of physical effects of stress-related illness, are important in tertiary prevention of stress-related conditions.

Prevention of Sports Injuries

Participation in sports involves movements of the body that are exaggerations of those ordinarily performed and those not ordinarily performed, or movements performed in such a way that they place an unusual stress on the affected body parts. They may also call on performance qualities such as strength, speed, flexibility, coordination, agility, balance, or endurance. Although qualities may be essential to the sport, they may be poorly developed in an individual. Thus, physical preparation for any sport must be based on the particular demands and hazards of the sport and sufficient time must be permitted to adequately develop the necessary qualities. Types of potential injuries must be analyzed and equipment and environment structured to minimize injury. Thus, primary prevention involves five strategies: (1) preparticipation evaluation of prospective participants for suitability and documentation of status; (2) preparation of participants through careful training and conditioning; (3) provision of appropriate protective equipment; (4) development of correct participation techniques; and (5) control of the environment in which the sport will be practiced, particularly elimination of physical hazards, careful monitoring of climatic conditions, and control of spectators (Ryan, 1981).

Secondary prevention involves education of coaches and athletes to recognize signs of injury and the importance of reporting injury immediately. Prompt treatment may entail a brief period of disability from the sport, but allowing an injury to go untreated likely will lead to a longer period of disability at a later time. Athletes who have previously suffered an injury are at higher risk for subsequent injury. Treatment for sports injuries must continue over a period of time to allow for healing and rehabilitative measures to restore strength, agility, and endurance must be completed before returning to sports activity to prevent future injury.

Prevention of Dental Diseases

A complete set of healthy teeth is rare in adults. The measure of dental disease most frequently used, the sum of decayed, missing, and filled teeth (DMF), rises steadily with age because of the cumulative nature of the index. However, it is during the years after tooth eruption that susceptibility to dental caries is the greatest; subsequently it declines. Whites experience more dental caries than nonwhites, women slightly more than men. Prevalence of dental caries among children remains above national targets for the year 2000. The good news is that among children under age 15 and among black children and those whose parents have less than 12 years of

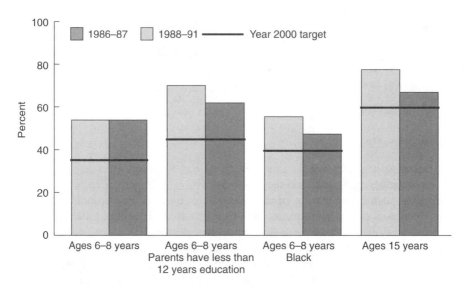

Figure 9–8. Prevalence of dental caries among children: United States, 1986–1987, 1988–1991, and year 2000 targets. (*Adapted from National Center for Health Statistics. Healthy people 2000 review, 1995–1996. Hyattsville, Md.: Public Health Service, 1996, Fig. 14.*)

education, rates have dropped between 1986 and 1987 and 1988 and 1991 (Fig. 9–8) (National Center for Health Statistics, 1996).

Modifiable factors that affect the incidence of dental caries include the gross constituents of the diet, use of cigarettes, and fluoride. Table 9–12 lists the types of dental problems among children and strategies for prevention. Primary and secondary prevention strategies during childhood lead to improved dental health at older ages.

TABLE 9–12. STRATEGIES FOR PREVENTION OF DENTAL DISEASE

DISEASE	STRATEGIES FOR PRIMARY PREVENTION
Dental caries	Appropriate diet
	Rough, fibrous components for mechanical cleansing of tooth surface
	Avoidance of sticky sweets
	Reduction or elimination of refined sugars
	Reducing bacterial population in mouth
	Oral hygiene
	Eliminate smoking
	Minimizing solubility of tooth enamel
	Fluoride
	Good prenatal nutrition
Malposition	Guide teeth into proper position as they erupt
	Prevent spaces from extraction of deciduous teeth
Trauma	Protective mouth guards for sports

Prevention of Problems Associated with Unhealthy Eating Patterns

Nutrition has been mentioned in the previous discussions on prevention of infection and prevention of dental diseases. A good diet is essential to provide the necessary nutrients for general growth and development during childhood and prevention of immediate problems such as iron deficiency anemia, obesity, eating disorders, and dental caries. Poor diet is also associated with specific conditions later in life, including obesity, high blood pressure, osteoporosis, coronary heart disease, stroke, certain types of cancer, and diabetes (Centers for Disease Control and Prevention, 1996). Because the seeds for development of these conditions may originate during childhood, a diet high in saturated fats, salt, sugar, and excess calories is to be avoided. The advent of more highly processed foods in supermarkets and the increasing use of convenience foods or meals in fast-food restaurants, concurrent with the increased number of working women who have children, reduce the likelihood that children will get proper preventive nutrition. Between 1958 and 1978, sales in fast-food restaurants increased by 305% (U.S. Department of Health and Human Services, 1981). From 1980 through 1988, personal consumption expenditures for food eaten away from home has averaged a 5.4 annual increase and other purchased meal expenditures have also increased 7.5% annually (3.4% and 2.6% in constant dollars) (U.S. Bureau of the Census, 1990). Food dollars spent on meals eaten away from home have increased from 29% in 1980 to 57% in 1995 (U.S. Bureau of the Census, 1996). Information on nutrient content of foods and public education regarding healthy diets are imperative. In addition, school lunch programs could help children and adolescents improve their nutrition and foster healthy eating patterns if the quality of meals served is improved and a sequential, coordinated curriculum is included that integrates school food service and nutrition education with appropriate instruction for students, staff training, family and community involvement, and program evaluation (Centers for Disease Control and Prevention, 1996).

SUMMARY AND RECOMMENDATIONS

Many diseases of adulthood have their roots in the health status and ways of living developed during childhood. Arteriosclerotic heart disease and hypertension, for example, are thought to begin with plaque deposition in childhood that continues throughout adult life. Lung cancer and chronic respiratory disease caused by smoking are to some extent time-dependent; the earlier smoking begins, the sooner the disease onset. The minimum latency period is passed at an earlier age because tissues in youngsters are thought to be more susceptible than those of adults and because the number of packs of cigarettes smoked tends to increase over time. Thus, good diet, regular exercise, and obesity control in childhood may contribute to lower adult rates of arteriosclerotic heart disease. Not smoking reduces the risk for lung cancer, heart disease, and chronic respiratory diseases. Similarly, disability resulting from childhood injury will carry over and affect the quality of adult health and life.

For these reasons, efforts toward developing positive health-related behaviors in children are crucial. Health education efforts, however, cannot be limited just to the children. Other sources of influence on a child's health-related behaviors include the family, school, peers, television, and the socioeconomic and political community in which the child lives. Efforts must be made to encourage positive health behaviors in the family and in the community at large. Because of the enormous number of hours of exposure to television experienced by most children, efforts must be directed toward changing the negative images portrayed on television. The average preschooler spends more than 30 hours per week watching television, that equals more than 6,000 hours before starting first grade. By the time of high school graduation, the average child has viewed 15,000 hours of television, about 4,000 hours more than was spent on formal education. Thus, the child is continually exposed to a variety of negative messages. These include advertisements for foods that often offer empty calories or high fat content (Dietz & Gortmaker, 1985), an emphasis on aggressive behavior (Centerwall, 1992; Gadow & Sprafkin, 1989), sex stereotyping, over-the-counter drug use, and drinking (U.S. Department of Health and Human Services, 1981). Television potentially is a medium for promoting positive health messages. Until television provides more positive health emphases though, all other avenues for promoting good health behavior in children must be pursued.

This chapter earlier outlined preventive approaches to some specific childhood health programs. In closing, the author should like to advocate a regular program of preventive care. Pediatricians, school nurses, nurses in well-child clinics, school psychologists, teachers, and others who have regular contact with children should be aware of the recommended components of preventive and health maintenance procedures for children. Recommendations from the U.S. Preventive Services Task Force (1989) are shown in Table 9–13. These recommendations are built on epidemiological evidence of normal growth and development, risk factors, and incidence and prevalence of childhood illness. The author would like to note, however, that she feels certain recommended procedures, for example, counseling as to drug use, smoking, and sexual development and sexual activity, need to begin between the ages of school entry and 11 years rather than beginning at 12 to 15 years as in the original recommendations. Physicians and nurses in clinical practice who follow this basic schedule of primary and secondary prevention can do much to contribute to a society of healthy children and healthy adults. It is particularly important that such programs be readily accessible to disadvantaged groups in our society, those whose children are at higher risk for childhood morbidity and mortality. These same groups, also at higher risk of illness and death at older ages, would derive considerable long-term health benefits from such programs. In conjunction with public health efforts to control environmental hazards and to educate the public about healthful living and social programs in maternal–child health and nutrition, these efforts could do much toward assuring the optimal health of children.

TABLE 9–13. RECOMMENDED PREVENTIVE AND HEALTH MAINTENANCE PROCEDURES FOR CHILDREN BY AGE CATEGORY

AGE	SCREENING	PARENT/PATIENT COUNSELING
1–18 months	Height and weight Hemoglobin and hematocrit Hearing[a] Erythrocyte protoporphyrin[a]	Diet—breastfeeding, nutrient intake Injury prevention—child safety seats; smoke detector; hot water heater thermostat; stairway gates; window guards; pool fence; storage of drugs and toxic chemicals; syrup of ipecac; poison control telephone number Dental health—baby bottle tooth decay Other—effects of passive smoking
2–6 years	Height and weight Blood pressure Eye exam for amblyopia and strabismus Urinalysis for bacteruria Erythrocyte protoporphyrin[a] Tuberculin skin testing (PPD)[a] Hearing[a]	Diet and exercise—sweets and between meal snacks, iron-enriched foods, sodium Injury prevention—safety belts; smoke detectors; hot water heater thermostat; window guards; pool fence; bicycle safety helmets; storage of drugs and toxic chemicals; matches and firearms; syrup of ipecac; poison control telephone number
7–12 years	Height and weight Blood pressure Tuberculin skin testing (PPD)[a]	Diet and exercise—fat (especially saturated), cholesterol, sweets, between-meal snacks, sodium; caloric balance; selection of exercise program Injury prevention—safety belts; smoke detector; storage of firearms, drugs, toxic chemicals, matches; bicycle safety helmets Dental health—regular tooth brushing and dental visits Other—skin protection from ultraviolet light
13–18 years	History—dietary intake; physical activity; tobacco/alcohol/drug use; sexual practices Physical exam—height and weight; blood pressure; complete skin exam; clinical testicular exam[a] Laboratory/diagnostic procedures[a]—rubella antibodies; VDRL/RPR; chlamydial testing; gonorrhea culture; human immunodeficiency virus (HIV) counseling and testing; tuberculin skin testing (PPD); hearing; Papanicolau test	Diet and exercise—fat (especially saturated), cholesterol, sodium, iron, calcium; caloric balance; selection of exercise program Substance use—tobacco: cessation/primary prevention; driving/other dangerous activities while under the influence; treatment for abuse; sharing unsterilized needles and syringes[a] Sexual practices—sexual development and behavior; sexually transmitted diseases: partner selection, condoms; unintended pregnancy and contraceptive options Injury prevention—safety belts; safety helmets; violent behavior; firearms; smoke detector Dental health—regular tooth brushing, flossing, dental visits Other primary preventive measures—discussion of hemoglobin testing;[a] skin protection from ultraviolet light[a]

[a]High-risk persons only.
(*Adapted from U.S. Preventive Services Task Force.* Guide to clinical preventive services: An assessment of the effectiveness of 169 interventions. *Report of the U.S. Preventive Services Task Force. Baltimore: Williams & Wilkins, 1989.*)

REFERENCES

Adams P. F., Marano, M. A. (1995) Current estimates from the National Health Interview Survey: 1994. *Vital Health Statistics, 10,* 193. Hyattsville, Md.: National Center for Health Statistics.

Adams P. F., Schoenborn C. A., Moss A. J., Warren C. W., Kann L. (1995) Health risk behaviors among our nation's youth: United States, 1992. *Vital Health Statistics 10,* 192. Hyattsville, Md.: National Center for Health Statistics.

Centers for Disease Control and Prevention. (1996) Guidelines for school health programs to promote lifelong healthy eating. *Morbidity and Mortality Weekly Report, 45*(No. RR-9), 1–9.

Centers for Disease Control. (1995) Summary of notifiable diseases, United States, 1995. *Morbidity and Mortality Weekly Report, 44,* 53.

Centers for Disease Control and Prevention. (1997) Update: Blood lead levels—United States, 1991–1994. *Morbidity and Mortality Weekly Report, 46*(7), 141–145.

Centerwall B. S. (1992) Television and violence. The scale of the problem and where to go from here. *Journal of the American Medical Association, 267*(22), 3059–3063.

Collins J. G. (1997) Prevalence of selected chronic conditions: United States, 1990–1992. *Vital Health Statistics 10,* 194. Hyattsville, Md.: National Center for Health Statistics.

Dietz W. H., Jr, Gortmaker S. L. (1985) Do we fatten our children at the television set? Obesity and television viewing in children and adolescents. *Pediatrics, 75*(5), 807–812.

Downs S. M., Klein J. D. (1995) Clinical preventive services' efficacy and adolescents' risky behaviors. *Archives of Pediatric and Adolescent Medicine, 149,* 374–379.

Gadow K. D., Sprafkin J. (1989) Field experiments of television violence with children: Evidence for an environmental hazard? *Pediatrics, 83*(3), 399–405.

Haddon W., Jr., Baker S. (1981) Injury control. In D. Clark, B. McMahon (Eds.). *Prevention and community medicine.* Boston: Little, Brown. pp. 109–140.

Kochanek K. D., Hudson B. L. (1995) Advance report of final mortality statistics, 1992. *Monthly Vital Statistics Report, 43,* 6 (suppl.). Hyattsville, Md.: National Center for Health Statistics.

National Center for Health Statistics. (1996) *Healthy people 2000 review, 1995–1996.* Hyattsville, Md.: Public Health Service.

Ryan A. (1981) Prevention of sports injuries. In L. Schneiderman (Ed.). *The practice of preventive health care.* Menlo Park, Calif.: Addison-Wesley. pp. 96–123.

Simpson G., Bloom B., Cohen R. A., Parsons P. E. (1997) Access to health care. Part 1: Children. *Vital Health Statistics, 10,* 196. Hyattsville, Md.: National Center for Health Statistics.

U.S. Bureau of the Census. (1990) *Statistical abstract of the United States, 1990 (110th ed.).* Washington, D.C.: U.S. Government Printing Office.

U.S. Bureau of the Census. (1996) *Statistical abstract of the United States, 1996 (116th ed.).* Washington, D.C.: U.S. Government Printing Office.

U.S. Department of Health and Human Services. (1981) *Better health for our children: A national strategy.* The report of the select panel for the promotion of child health. Vol. III. (DHHS Publication No. [PHS] 79-55071).

U.S. Preventive Services Task Force. (1989) *Guide to clinical preventive services: An assessment of the effectiveness of 169 interventions.* Report of the U.S. Preventive Services Task Force. Baltimore: Williams & Wilkins.

U.S. Public Health Service. (1993) *Healthy people 2000: National health promotion and disease prevention objectives.* Washington, D.C.: U.S. Government Printing Office.

U.S. Public Health Service. *Prevention report.* February–March, 1993. Washington, D.C.: U.S. Government Printing Office.

Patterns of Morbidity and Mortality in Young and Middle Adulthood

*t*he health of young and middle-aged adults is of critical importance, both because of the desire for assuring high quality of life during the adult years and because of society's need to maintain an active and healthy labor force. Because persons 25 to 64 years of age constitute most of the labor force, they provide the economic security base for themselves as well as for dependent children, adolescents, disabled persons, and older adults. This chapter examines the major causes of morbidity and mortality among middle-aged adults and presents recommended strategies for disease prevention and health promotion for this age group.

In 1995, there were approximately 136 million Americans who were 25 to 45 years of age. Of these, approximately 84 million were between the ages 25 and 44 and 52 million were between the ages 45 and 64 (U.S. Bureau of the Census, 1996). These working-age adults accounted for about half of the total U.S. population.

According to the 1994 National Health Interview Survey, most young and middle-aged Americans perceive themselves to be relatively healthy. Ninety-three percent of adults 24 to 44 years of age report "good or excellent" health; only 7% of this age group reports "fair or poor" health. By age 45 to 64 years 83% rate their health status as "good or excellent," and 17% as "fair or poor" (Adams & Marano, 1995). Despite the fact that men in these age groups have much higher rates of mortality from debilitating conditions such as heart disease, cerebrovascular disease, and malignancies, there are no major differences in the self-reported health ratings of men and women. Blacks in young and middle adulthood report "fair or poor" health twice as frequently as do whites (Adams & Marano, 1995), and their higher mortality and morbidity rates correspond to these ratings.

MAJOR CAUSES OF MORTALITY

In the United States, mortality during the young and middle adult years has markedly declined over the decades, from a rate of 1,200 per 100,000 persons in 1900 to 583 per 100,000 persons in 1993 (U.S. Department of Health, Education, and Welfare, 1979; U.S. Bureau of the Census, 1996). Between 1950 and 1993, mortality among young adults between 25 and 44 years of age decreased by more than one third, primarily because of decreasing numbers of deaths caused by cancer and heart disease. For adults in the 45- to 64-year age group, mortality rates declined by more than one fourth during this 43-year period.

Variations in Mortality by Age, Sex, and Race

Age and Mortality.   Current mortality rates for persons in young and middle adulthood are higher than the rates for children and adolescents, but are much lower than the rates for persons 65 years of age and older, since mortality rates consistently increase with age. There were 191.3 deaths per 100,000 for those 25 to 44 years old and 736.9 deaths per 100,000 for those 45 to 64 years old in 1994 (U.S. Bureau of the Census, 1997). The major causes of death for young adults (ages 25–44) and middle-aged adults (ages 45–64) in the United States in 1994 are shown in Table 10–1. Death rates have declined for most of these leading causes of death in adults aged 25 to 64 since 1950. Since 1979, the declines have either continued or stabilized, except for chronic obstructive pulmonary disease, diabetes, and septicemia, which have increased. Human immunodeficiency virus (HIV) has only appeared among the leading causes of death for this age group in the past 10 years.

Differences by Gender.   The comparison of the 1994 mortality rates for young and middle-aged adults given in Table 10–1 shows higher death rates for men than for women. The higher mortality among young adult men is primarily due to excessive deaths from accidents, homicides, suicides, and HIV infection, whereas the higher mortality rates among men in the middle adult years are primarily due to deaths from heart disease, malignancies, especially cancer of the lung, and accidents. Approximately 20% of all heart disease deaths in the United States occur in young and middle adulthood. During these years, men are nearly three times as likely as women to die of heart disease. This gender difference is partly due to the higher levels of smoking, hypertension, and cholesterol among men. Preventive health

TABLE 10–1. DEATH RATES PER 100,000 POPULATION FOR THE TEN LEADING CAUSES OF DEATH IN ADULTS 25–64 YEARS OF AGE—UNITED STATES, 1994

RANK	AGES 25–44 Males		AGES 25–44 Females		AGES 45–64 Males		AGES 45–64 Females	
1	Human immuno-deficiency virus (HIV) infection	62.4	Malignant neoplasm	28.3	Diseases of the heart	295.5	Malignant neoplasm	234.4
2	Accidents and adverse effects	50.2	Accidents and adverse effects	15.1	Malignant neoplasm	289.6	Diseases of the heart	115.3
3	Diseases of the heart	28.8	Diseases of the heart	11.7	Accidents and adverse effects	43.9	Cerebrovascular diseases	25.7
4	Suicide	24.8	HIV infection	11.3	HIV infection	35.2	Chronic obstructive pulmonary disease	23.1
5	Malignant neoplasm	24.4	Suicide	5.9	Cerebrovascular diseases	33.3	Diabetes mellitus	20.8
6	Homicide and legal inter-ventions	21.7	Homicide and legal inter-ventions	5.8	Chronic liver disease and cirrhosis	30.5	Accidents and adverse effects	16.7
7	Chronic liver disease and cirrhosis	7.7	Cerebrovascular diseases	4.0	Chronic obstructive pulmonary disease	28.2	Chronic liver disease and cirrhosis	11.7
8	Cerebrovascular disease	4.5	Chronic liver disease and cirrhosis	3.1	Diabetes mellitus	24.4	Pneumonia and influenza	8.1
9	Diabetes mellitus	3.6	Diabetes mellitus	2.4	Suicide	22.1	Suicide	6.4
10	Pneumonia and influenza	3.1	Pneumonia and influenza	1.9	Pneumonia and influenza	13.7	HIV infection	4.4
All causes		270.8		111.4		942.6		544.8

(*Compiled from U.S. Bureau of the Census. Statistical abstract of the United States, 1997. [117th ed.]. Washington D.C., 1997, Tables 129 and 130*)

programs during the 1970s and 1980s began to lower these risk factors, subsequently reducing mortality from cardiovascular disease (U.S. Department of Health and Human Services, 1990).

Causes of death for young adult women and middle-aged adult women also differ, with accidents, HIV infection, and homicide, legal intervention, and suicide more prominent among the younger women. Among malignancies in women aged 25 to 64, lung cancer is the leading cancer cause of death, followed by breast cancer. In the 45 to 64-year age group, heart disease mortality rates are nearly ten times that of women aged 25 to 44.

Overall, the ten leading causes of death for young and middle-aged adults reflect a combination of acute and chronic illness conditions, with a pattern of increasing chronicity emerging over the 40-year period from age 25 to age 64. From a public health perspective, many of the deaths, including those caused by accidents, homicides, suicides, and acquired immunodeficiency syndrome (AIDS), as well as those caused by chronic illness, are largely preventable. About 50% of the deaths from accidents, for instance, are motor vehicle casualties (U.S. Bureau of the Census, 1996), and approximately half of all motor vehicle deaths are alcohol-related (National Center for Health Statistics, 1990).

Currently, malignancies and heart disease account for about half of all deaths in young and middle adulthood. Mortality from heart disease has steadily decreased since the 1950s because of advances in medical research, diagnoses and treatment, and prevention programs that have focused on the identification and alleviation of chronic disease risk factors (National Center for Health Statistics, 1990). Although the overall cancer death rate in this age group has remained relatively stable since the 1980s, lung cancer rates have increased, especially among women. The increase in lung cancer deaths among middle-aged women is primarily among smokers and ex-smokers. Overall, smoking is responsible for more than 80% of lung cancer deaths (National Center for Health Statistics, 1990).

Fatalities from suicide and homicide during the adult years present a very challenging problem. Better understanding of the direct cause of violence, as well as the possible predisposing factors such as social stressors, mental illness, and childhood abuse, is necessary to plan effective prevention programs. Stronger economic support for mental health and social service programs, as well as legislation to control hand guns and other means of violence, may help to lower the death rates from homicide and suicide.

Differences by Race.   The different mortality patterns of blacks versus whites in young and middle adulthood are as striking as the differences between men and women; black persons have a higher rate of death. Table 10–2 shows the ratio of death rates for the 15 leading causes of death for blacks compared with whites for all ages combined in the United States in 1992. With the exception of chronic obstructive pulmonary disease, suicide, atherosclerosis, and motor vehicle accidents, rates are higher for blacks than for whites. Particularly among young adults (under 45 years of age), violent deaths from homicides and legal interventions account for much of the higher mortality of blacks; black men in this age group are seven times as likely as white men to die from violence, whereas black women are three times as likely as white women to die from violence (National Center for Health Statistics, 1990).

In comparison with white persons, black persons in the middle adult years traditionally have had higher death rates from certain malignancies (eg, stomach and esophogeal), as well as from heart disease, strokes, and cirrhosis of the liver. Fortunately, the death rates for many of these diseases declined in the 1970s and 1980s.

Because both morbidity and mortality rates for many acute and chronic conditions are highest among black Americans and persons of low-income groups, these

TABLE 10–2. BLACK/WHITE RATIO OF AGE-ADJUSTED DEATH RATES[a] FOR THE 15 LEADING CAUSES OF DEATH—UNITED STATES, 1992

RANK[b]	BLACK/WHITE RATIO
1. Diseases of the heart	1:5
2. Malignant neoplasms, including neoplasms of lymphatic and hematopoietic tissues	1:4
3. Cerebrovascular disease	1:9
4. Chronic obstructive pulmonary disease	0:8
5. Accidents and adverse effects	1:3
Motor vehicle accidents	(1:0)
All other accidents	(1:6)
6. Pneumonia and influenza	1:4
7. Diabetes mellitus	2:4
8. Human immunodeficiency syndrome (HIV)	3:7
9. Suicide	0:6
10. Homicide and legal intervention	6:5
11. Chronic liver disease and cirrhosis	1:5
12. Nephritis, nephrotic syndrome, and nephrosis	2:8
13. Septicemia	2:7
14. Atherosclerosis	1:0
15. Certain conditions originating from perinatal period	3:2

[a]Rates per 100,000 population.
[b]Rank based on number of deaths.
(*Adapted from Centers for Disease Control. Monthly Vital Statistics Report, 1995; 43[6] [suppl.], 8, Table D.*)

high-risk groups have been targeted for prevention efforts in the "National Health Promotion and Disease Prevention Objectives for Year 2000" (Centers for Disease Control, 1990a). Although the rates for blacks are still much higher than for whites, preventive programs have begun to demonstrate success in reducing both mortality from chronic conditions and excessive risk factors for chronic disease (eg, high blood pressure and cigarette smoking) among the black population. For example, rates of coronary heart disease among blacks have decreased from 168 per 100,000 population in 1987 (baseline for the "Healthy People 2000" comparisons [Centers for Disease Control, 1990a]) to 154 in 1993, but were still far from the year 2000 target of 115. Rates of lung cancer among black males decreased from 86.1 per 100,000 population in 1990 to 80.7 in 1993 (National Center for Health Statistics, 1996). The prevalence of current cigarette smoking has also declined dramatically over time and has likely contributed to the decline in mortality from heart disease and lung cancer. Cigarette smoking declined for both black and white men (Fig. 10–1). In the mid-1960s, more than half of men aged 25 to 64 were current smokers. In 1993, rates for white men were around 30% and for black men were between 30% and 41%, varying by age subgroup. Rates have also declined for women of both races (U.S. Bureau of the Census, 1996). High blood pressure, more common among blacks than whites, is another risk factor targeted under the "Healthy People

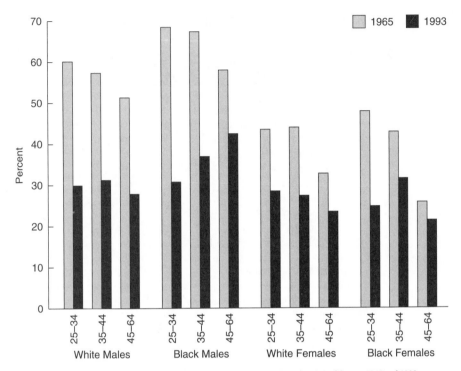

Figure 10–1. Prevalence of current cigarette smoking by race and gender, United States, 1965 and 1993. (*Data from U.S. Bureau of the Census. Statistical abstract of the United States, 1996 (116th ed.). Washington, D.C.: U.S. Government Printing Office, 1996; Table 222, p. 145.*)

2000" initiative. Significant progress has been made, particularly among black males, in achieving control of high blood pressure, although the year 2000 goal has not yet been reached (Fig. 10–2). Other risk factors still require intervention. Blacks are less likely to exercise regularly and black women, in particular, are more likely to be 20% or more overweight.

In 1995, HIV infection accounted for 31,256 deaths in the United States (Table 10–3), down from 41,930 deaths in 1994 (Centers for Disease Control, 1996). Nearly 90% of these HIV-associated deaths occurred among 24- to 49-year-old adults. Beginning in 1993, HIV deaths became the leading cause of deaths for men aged 25 to 44 years. Age-adjusted death rates from AIDS are highest for black men between 35 and 44 years of age (72.9 per 100,000). Rates are much lower for women, although the proportion of new cases among women is rising and is higher for black women than for white women. Of 24,358 new cases diagnosed between 1981 and 1986, only 2,136 were among women. Of the 71,547 new cases identified in 1995, 13,540 were among women. Figure 10–3 shows the increases over time among black and white men and women aged 25 to 44 years between 1982 and 1994. Vaccine development and education efforts to allay the spread of the virus remain high public health priorities.

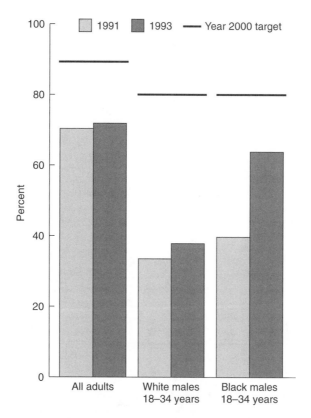

Figure 10–2. Proportion of people with high blood pressure who are taking action to help control their blood pressure, United States, 1991 and 1993, and year 2000 targets for objective 15.5. (*Adapted from National Center for Health Statistics.* Healthy People 2000 Review, 1995–1996. *Hyattsville, Md.: Public Health Service, 1996, Fig. U, p. 18.*)

TABLE 10–3. MORBIDITY AND MORTALITY FROM ACQUIRED IMMUNODEFICIENCY SYNDROME (AIDS) AMONG YOUNG AND MIDDLE-AGED ADULTS, 1995

AGE	NUMBER OF DIAGNOSED CASES	DISTRIBUTION OF CASES (%)	NUMBER OF DEATHS	DISTRIBUTION OF DEATHS (%)
13–29 years	11,612	16.2	5,105	16.3
30–39 years	31,988	44.7	14,083	45.1
40–49 years	19,649	13.5	8,543	27.3
50–59 years	5,604	7.8	2,572	8.3
Total all ages*	71,547	82.8	31,256	97.0

*Includes cases in those older than 59 years of age.

(*Adapted from U.S. Bureau of the Census.* Health United States, 1996 [116th ed.]. *Washington, D.C.: U.S. Government Printing Office, 1996.*)

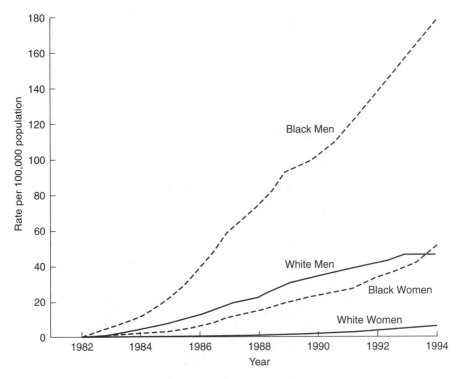

Figure 10–3. Death rates from human immunodeficiency virus (HIV) infection among persons aged 25 to 44 years of age, by sex, race, and year, United States, 1982 to 1994. The national vital statistics are based on underlying cause of death, using final data for 1982–1992 and provisional data for 1993–1994. Data were unavailable for races other than white and black. (*Adapted from Centers for Disease Control. Morbidity and Mortality Weekly Report, 1996; 45(6), 124, Fig. 3.*)

MAJOR CAUSES OF MORBIDITY

Acute Conditions

As noted in the previous chapter, acute conditions refer to illnesses lasting less than 3 months that are serious enough to require medical attention or that result in brief periods of restricted activity. The estimated incidence rates for specific types of acute illness episodes are available from the National Ambulatory Medical Care Survey of the National Health Interview Survey published by the Center for Health Statistics (Adams & Marano, 1995). The classifications of acute illnesses in the National Health Interviews include: (1) respiratory conditions, (2) infectious and parasitic diseases, (3) injuries and poisonings, (4) digestive system disorders, and (5) other miscellaneous conditions.

The number of acute conditions reported by young and middle-aged adults for 1994 is shown in Table 10–4, and the impact of these conditions on activity is shown in Table 10–5. Overall, the highest rates of acute illness episodes among

TABLE 10–4. ACUTE CONDITIONS AND PERCENT MEDICALLY ATTENDED, AGES 18–64—UNITED STATES, 1994

TYPE OF ILLNESS EPISODE	NUMBER PER 100 PERSONS			PERCENT MEDICALLY ATTENDED		
	Ages 18–24	Ages 25–44	Ages 45–64	Ages 18–24	Ages 25–44	Ages 45–64
All acute conditions	175.6	153.5	112.9	60.4	62.9	64.9
Infective and parasitic	18.5	14.6	7.7	58.5	61.0	52.7
Respiratory	82.4	77.1	55.4	39.7	44.7	45.4
Common cold	(26.1)	(22.4)	(16.1)	(29.0)	(31.4)	(36.0)
Influenza	(38.7)	(37.8)	(25.9)	(27.0)	(34.1)	(40.2)
Digestive system	7.4	4.7	4.7	51.6	55.1	78.8
Injuries	32.7	25.0	17.2	88.5	91.0	91.2
Acute musculoskeletal	2.8	3.7	5.6	90.0	88.0	83.9

(*Compiled from Adams P. F., Marano M. A. Current estimates from National Health Interview Survey: 1994.* Vital and Health Statistics, *1995; 10[193], 12, 24,30,42,54, Tables 1, 11, 16, 26, 36. Hyattsville, Md.: National Center for Health Statistics.*)

young to middle-aged adults are among those between 18 and 24 years of age. The rate of acute illness episodes decreases in each of the two subsequent age groups.

Among all the young and middle-aged adult groups, respiratory conditions are the most frequently reported type of acute illness for both men and women. Influenza accounts for an increasing proportion of respiratory conditions in each successive age group. Although these respiratory illnesses rarely have fatal consequences in young adulthood, they do cause much discomfort as well as loss of workdays. In 1994, young adults aged 18 to 24 lost 99 days of work per 100 employed persons because of respiratory illnesses, and those aged 25 to 44 lost 113 days of work per 100 employed persons (see Table 10–5). Injuries accounted for

TABLE 10–5. RESTRICTED ACTIVITY DAYS, BED DAYS, AND WORK LOSS DAYS DUE TO ACUTE ILLNESSES AMONG ADULTS AGED 18–64—UNITED STATES, 1994

TYPE OF ILLNESS EPISODE	RESTRICTED ACTIVITY DAYS[a]			BED DAYS[a]			WORK LOSS DAYS[b]		
	Ages 18–24	Ages 25–44	Ages 45–64	Ages 18–24	Ages 25–44	Ages 45–64	Ages 18–24	Ages 25–44	Ages 45–64
All acute conditions	639	664	630	296	255	250	309	336	283
Infective and parasitic	53	45	28	29	21	14	35	22	16
Respiratory	233	252	231	128	122	110	99	113	99
Common cold	(68)	(51)	(47)	(27)	(19)	(18)	(23)	(18)	(15)
Influenza	(105)	(131)	(106)	(69)	(70)	(54)	(54)	(60)	(52)
Digestive system	30	20	37	11	9	13	19	12	11
Injuries	171	203	187	62	52	59	94	131	105
Acute musculoskeletal	17	32	43	3	9	14	15	14	10

[a]Days per 100 persons per year.
[b]Days per 100 employed persons per year.
(*Compiled from Adams P. F., Marano M. A. Current estimates from National Health Interview Survey: 1994.* Vital and Health Statistics, *1995; 10[193], 12, 24,30,42,54, Tables 1, 11, 16, 26, 36. Hyattsville, Md.: National Center for Health Statistics.*)

nearly as much time lost from work. Injuries are the second most frequently reported acute conditions among young adult men.

Women report greater numbers of acute conditions than men and they lose more workdays because of these conditions compared to their male counterparts. Overall, acute illness episodes among young adults during 1994 resulted in a loss of more than 300 workdays per 100 working persons, or about 3 workdays per person per year.

Although there is often a perception that older workers are sicker and lose more time overall from work than younger persons, adults aged 45 to 64 lose fewer days from work due to acute illnesses than their younger contemporaries. They are, however, more likely than younger adults to have their acute illnesses medically attended (Table 10–4). These illnesses may pose greater risks for older adults than for younger adults because complications are more likely to occur. Table 10–6 shows summary data from the 1993 National Health Interview Survey on all types of physician office visits, excluding contacts during hospitalizations, made by young and middle-aged adults. Women in both young and middle adulthood report more physician contact than do their male counterparts, and whites report more contacts than do blacks and other nonwhites. These black–white differences may relate to income. Individuals with low income (< $10,000/year) are more likely to receive care in hospital settings than those with high income (> $35,000/year) (Adams & Benson, 1990). Black persons are more likely to see physicians in hospital settings than are whites and other nonwhites.

Chronic Conditions

A listing of the most prevalent chronic health problems reported by young and middle-aged adults in the 1994 National Health Interview Survey is shown in Table 10–7. Among 18- to 44-year-old adults, chronic sinusitis, orthopedic impairments, and hay fever were the most prevalent chronic conditions. Migraine headaches, arthritis, and hypertension were the fourth through sixth most prevalent problems. The prevalence rates have increased for most of these conditions since 1979. Heart conditions were the ninth most prevalent type of chronic health problem for young

TABLE 10–6. NUMBER OF PHYSICIAN OFFICE VISITS[a] AMONG ADULTS AGED 25–64 YEARS BY GENDER AND RACE—UNITED STATES, 1993

AGES 18–44		AGES 45–64	
Male	1.6	Male	2.7
Female	3.1	Female	3.7
White	2.5	White	3.3
Black	1.7	Black	1.7

[a]Number per person per year.

(From Woodwell D. A., Schappert S. M. National ambulatory medical care survey: 1993. Advance data from Vital and Health Statistics, 1995; 270, 6, Table 6. Hyattsville, Md.: National Center for Health Statistics.)

TABLE 10–7. RATE OF HIGH PREVALENCE CHRONIC CONDITIONS PER 1,000 PERSONS BETWEEN 18–24 YEARS—UNITED STATES, 1994

CONDITION	AGES 18–44	AGES 45–64
Hypertension	51.3	222.3
Heart disease	37.9	135.7
Chronic sinusitis	153.3	179.9
Hay fever/allergic rhinitis without asthma	123.3	120.8
Migraine headache	62.9	52.5
Diabetes mellitus	12.4	63.1
Chronic bronchitis	46.7	63.9
Asthma	51.7	50.8
Arthritis	52.3	239.0
Intervertebral disc disorders	22.5	50.7
Bursitis	15.7	42.0
Dermatitis	35.7	33.6
Hearing impairment	47.4	137.9
Tinnitis	16.2	46.3
Deformity or orthopedic impairment	142.4	170.0
Frequent indigestion	31.2	40.9
Visual impairment	29.3	45.1

(Compiled from Adams P. F., Marano M. A. Current estimates from the National Health Interview Survey: 1994. Vital and Health Statistics, 1995; 10[193], 81, Table 57. Hyattsville, Md.: National Center for Health Statistics.)

adults in 1979, but by 1994 had dropped to the eleventh most prevalent type of problem (Adams & Benson, 1990; Adams & Marano, 1995).

The 1994 prevalence rates for chronic conditions were generally higher for 45- to 64-year-old adults than for younger adults, with the middle-aged persons having considerably more disabling conditions such as arthritis, hypertension, hearing impairments, heart disease, and diabetes. The most prevalent chronic condition among the middle-aged adults was arthritic diseases with a prevalence rate of 239 cases per 1,000 persons. From 1979 to 1994, there was a decrease in the prevalence rates for chronic sinusitis, heart disease, hypertension, and hearing impairments among adults 45 to 64 years of age, but an increase in the prevalence rates for arthritis, orthopedic impairments, and diabetes. Diabetes mellitus is of particular concern for women, blacks, and Hispanics. Findings from the Centers for Disease Control's 1988–1989 Behavioral Risk Factor Surveillance System surveys show that the prevalence of diabetes is 22% higher for women than men, 91% higher for blacks than whites, and 61% higher for Hispanics than whites (Centers for Disease Control, 1990b). One of the Year 2000 National Health Objectives is to decrease diabetes prevalence to less than 25 per 1,000 persons. The Centers for Disease Control (CDC) has established a national diabetes surveillance system to monitor progress toward this goal (Centers for Disease Control, 1990c). Unfortunately, the Healthy People 2000 review done in

1995–1996 shows an an increasing incidence and prevelance of diabetes for both the total populaton and, in particular, blacks, American Indians and Alaska natives (Fig. 10–4). Related measures of chronic disease impact, such as years of healthy life remaining decreased particularly among targeted subgroups of low-income individuals and minorities (National Center for Health Statistics, 1996).

As with acute conditions, use of medical care services for chronic medical conditions increases with age. Obesity accounted for 8.7% of all medical office visits in 1993 among 25 to 44 year olds and 14.7% among those 45 to 64 years old (Table 10–8). Since obesity is also thought to be a risk factor for diabetes and heart disease, this one condition accounts for a disproportionate share of medical care. Preventing obesity could make a major contribution to improving the health of the population. Asthma is another medical condition that contributes disproportionately to use of medical care services. This disease has been increasing in prevalence in recent years. Research leading to better ways to control asthma is urgently needed. Both of these conditions also eventually relate to functional status.

Data from the National Health Interview Surveys show that functional disabilities related to chronic health problems increase over the decades of adulthood. In

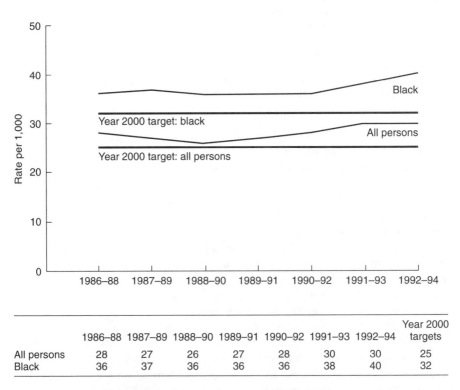

	1986–88	1987–89	1988–90	1989–91	1990–92	1991–93	1992–94	Year 2000 targets
All persons	28	27	26	27	28	30	30	25
Black	36	37	36	36	36	38	40	32

Figure 10–4. Prevalence of diabetes: United States, 1986 to 1988 and 1992 to 1994, and year 2000 targets for objective 17.11. (*Adapted from National Center for Health Statistics.* Healthy People 2000 Review, 1995–1996. *Hyattsville, Md.: Public Health Service, Fig. 18, p.147.*)

TABLE 10–8. NUMBER AND PERCENT OF PHYSICIAN OFFICE VISITS FOR SELECTED MEDICAL CONDITIONS
BY AGE AND SEX—UNITED STATES, 1993

	AGES 25–44		AGES 45–64	
CONDITION	Number[a]	Percent	Number[a]	Percent
Obesity	16,896	8.7	23,508	14.7
Diabetes	4,692	2.4	14,366	9.0
Asthma	8,946	4.6	7,214	4.5
Osteoporosis	399	0.2	2,388	1.5
Human immuno- deficiency virus (HIV) infection	939	0.5	212	0.1
Other	164,988	85.1	120,028	74.9
Total	193,914	100.0	160,146	100.0

[a]Number in thousands.
(*Compiled from Woodwell D. A., Schappert S. M. National ambulatory medical care survey, 1993 Summary. Advanced data from* Vital and Health Statistics, *1995; 27. Hyattsville, Md.: National Center for Health Statistics.*)

1988, 8.4% of adults in the 15- to 44-year age group and 22.4% of the adults in the 45- to 64-year age group reported activity limitations because of chronic illness, and 2.2% of 15 to 44 year olds and 8.6% of 45 to 64 year olds reported that they were unable to perform their major daily activities because of chronic illness (National Center for Health Statistics, 1990). This means that these individuals needed help with at least one basic physical activity such as walking, bathing, dressing, using the toilet, going outside, or eating. Walking was the primary physical activity affected by chronic illness during middle adulthood. About 1.5% of men 45 to 64 years of age and 1.2% of women in this age group needed assistance with walking. Home management activities, especially those activities requiring ambulation, also are difficult for a number of middle-aged adults.

Hospitalization Episodes for Acute and Chronic Illness

The rates of "first listed diagnoses" for adults discharged from short-stay hospitalizations during 1993 are shown in Table 10–9. These diagnoses may represent single, acute illness episodes or recurrent exacerbations of more chronic serious illnesses. Adults in the 15- to 44-year age group were primarily hospitalized for delivery of newborns (women) and for acute illness conditions; genitourinary tract problems, injuries and poisonings, and digestive system disturbances account for most of these hospitalizations for acute conditions. Other problems requiring short-stay hospitalizations in this age group included mental disorders (with 481,000 admissions for psychotic episodes and 144,000 admissions for alcoholism treatment in 1993), complications of pregnancy, and diseases of the musculoskeletal system.

Adults in the 45- to 64-year age group were hospitalized with a variety of acute and chronic illness conditions during 1993 (see Table 10–9). Diseases of the digestive system had the largest number of short-stay hospitalizations in this age group

TABLE 10–9. NUMBERS OF FIRST-LISTED DIAGNOSES FOR YOUNG AND MIDDLE-AGED ADULTS DISCHARGED FROM SHORT-STAY HOSPITALIZATIONS—UNITED STATES, 1993

FIRST-LISTED DIAGNOSES (PRIMARY REASON FOR HOSPITALIZATION)	NUMBER OF PATIENTS DISCHARGED (IN THOUSANDS)		AVERAGE LENGTH OF STAY (IN DAYS)	
	Young Adults (Ages 15–44)	Middle-Aged Adults (Ages 45–64)	Young Adults (Ages 15–44)	Middle-Aged Adults (Ages 45–64)
Infections and parasitic diseases	197	243	7.7	9.5
Neoplasms	295	1178	4.8	7.3
Malignant neoplasms	(154)	(926)	(6.1)	(8.0)
Benign	(142)	(252)	(3.5)	(4.5)
Endocrine, nutritional, and metabolic disorders	218	606	5.2	6.1
Diabetes mellitus	(102)	(298)	(5.0)	(7.3)
Diseases of the blood	85	128	5.3	5.8
Mental disorders	928	758	9.3	10.5
Psychoses	(481)	(479)	(10.9)	(12.4)
Alcoholism	(144)	(125)	(8.4)	(8.5)
Diseases of the nervous system	153	311	5.1	5.2
Diseases of the circulatory system	359	1094	5.3	5.9
Diseases of the respiratory system	399	1165	4.9	6.9
Diseases of the genitourinary system	636	899	3.4	4.0
Complications of pregnancy	504	—	2.0	—
Diseases of the skin	110	213	6.5	7.5
Diseases of the musculoskeletal system	410	874	3.7	4.8
Diseases of the digestive system	749	1636	4.4	5.4
Congenital anomalies	23	20	4.8	4.8
Symptoms, signs, undefined illnesses	114	175	2.4	2.3
Injuries and poisonings	858	1039	4.8	6.3
Women with deliveries	3410	—	2.4	—

(*Compiled from Graves E. J. 1993 summary: National hospital discharge. Advance data from* Vital and Health Statistics, *1995;* 264, 5–6, Tables 5 & 6. Hyattsville, Md.: National Center for Health Statistics.)

with 1,636,000. Other frequent reasons for hospitalization included neoplasms, diseases of the respiratory system, diseases of the circulatory system, and injuries and poisonings.

Comparisons of the hospitalization rates for young and middle-aged adults (see Table 10–9) demonstrate the increasing prevalence of serious chronic conditions with advancing age. Adults in the 45- to 64-year age group accounted for many more of the hospitalizations necessitated by neoplasms, diabetes, and cardiovascular (circulatory) diseases. The difference in the rates of hospitalizations for neoplasms was particularly striking. In comparison with young adults, middle-aged adults had nearly four times as many hospitalizations for all neoplasms and nearly seven times the number of hospitalizations for malignant neoplasms.

The average length of short-stay hospitalizations provides additional data for assessing the relative seriousness of various illness conditions and changes in treatment over time. Both the overall rate of hospitalization and length of stay have been dropping in the past several years. Table 10–9 shows that the conditions requiring the longest hospital stays for young and middle-aged adults in 1993 were the mental disorders, in particular psychoses. Neoplasms required the fourth longest hospitalization, following infections and parasitic diseases and skin diseases. This reflects changes in treatment, including outpatient chemotherapy. Length of stay for neoplasms in 1980 was 7.0 days for 15 to 44 year olds and 10.3 days for 45 to 64 year olds. The 1993 length of stay reflects decreases of 2.2 and 3.0 days, respectively, since 1980. The length of stay for most other conditions also decreased since 1980.

PUBLIC HEALTH AND CLINICAL SERVICES INTERVENTIONS FOR HEALTH PROMOTION

Young and middle adulthood covers a span of approximately 40 years, and it is apparent from the previous discussion that many different types of health problems occur during these years. In young adulthood, acute illnesses, accidents, and violence present the greatest threats to health. By the third and fourth decades, malignancies, AIDS, and other chronic disease conditions have caused many deaths and have left large numbers of Americans permanently disabled. However, most of these conditions are preventable. Interventions for maximizing positive health in the adult years must be broad in scope, yet appropriately targeted toward specific health risks. In the Surgeon General's 1979 report on health promotion and disease prevention, the Secretary of the U.S. Department of Health, Education, and Welfare (1979) summarized the major risks to health and longevity by stating:

> We are killing ourselves by our careless habits; we are killing ourselves by carelessly polluting the environment, and we are killing ourselves by permitting harmful social conditions to persist.

These statements continue to be relevant for health problems of the adult years. Although the etiology of most adult health problems is not perfectly understood, many risk factors and preventive interventions are well known. Some of the major causes of death in young and middle adulthood and both public health and clinical service setting interventions to prevent these are discussed in the following paragraphs.

Diseases of the Heart

Heart disease not only remains the leading cause of death for men older than 40 years of age and the second leading cause of death for women older than 40 years of age, but it is also a major contributor to work disability and activity limitations. Factors long recognized as increasing one's risk for cardiovascular diseases include smoking, hypertension, elevated blood cholesterol, low levels of high-density lipoprotein, and diabetes. Physical inactivity, being overweight, personality factors related to stress, and work overload have also been considered risk factors (Jenkins, 1988; CDC, 1990d). Table 10–10 shows the prevalence of some of these alterable

TABLE 10–10. CORONARY HEART DISEASE (ICD-9-CM 410–414, 429.2) INDICES—UNITED STATES, 1986

MEASURE	NO.	RATE PER 100,000
Mortality (1986)	593,111	246
Prevalence[a]	11,193,000	4,692
Hospitalizations[b]	1,615,320	670
Years of potential life lost before age 65[c]	1,557,041	646

RISK FACTOR	PREVALENCE (%)[d]	CRUDE RELATIVE RISK	POPULATION-ATTRIBUTABLE RISK (%; NONADDITIVE)[e]	ESTIMATED PREVENTABLE DEATHS (NONADDITIVE)[f]
Smoking (current)	26.5[g]	1.7[h]	15.6	92,525
Hypertension				
(>159 mm Hg)	17.7[i]	2.9	25.2	149,464
(140–159 mm Hg)	12.0[i]	1.7	7.7	45,670
Diabetes	2.8[a]	2.9	5.1	30,249
Cholesterol				
(≥240 mg/dl)	24.9	3.0	33.2	196,913
(200–239 mg/dl)	31.1	1.7	17.9	106,167
High-density lipoprotein				
(<35 mg/dl)	11.2	2.4	13.6	80,663
Inactivity	58.8	1.9	34.6	205,216
Overweight				
MRW ≥130	26.6	2.0	21.0	124,553
MRW 110–129	41.4	1.5	17.1	101,422

[a]National Center for Health Statistics. Current estimates from the National Health Interview Survey: United States, 1987. Hyattsville, Md.: U.S. Department of Health and Human Services, Public Health Service, Centers for Disease Control. DHHS Publication no. (PHS) 88-1594. *Vital and Health Statistics,* 1988; *10* (166).

[b]National Center for Health Statistics. National Hospital Discharge Survey, 1987 [machine-readable public-use data tape] (ICD-9-CM 410, 411, 413, 429.2).

[c]Centers for Disease Control. Years of potential life lost before age 65 in 1986. *Morbidity and Mortality Weekly Report,* 1989; *38,* 27-29 (ICD-9-CM 390-398, 402, 404-429).

[d]Prevalences in different studies and samples of the U.S. population.

[e]Population-attributable risk (PAR) = percentage of mortality attributable to the specific risk factor. Because persons may be exposed to more than one risk factor, estimated PAR from different risk factors should not be added. Centers for Disease Control. Chronic disease reports. *Morbidity and Mortality Weekly Report,* 1989; *38*(suppl S-1).

[f]Estimated preventable deaths = PAR × mortality. Because persons may be exposed to more than one risk factor, estimated preventable deaths from different risk factors should not be added.

[g]Data are for adults in 1985. Centers for Disease Control. Cigarette smoking in the United States, 1986. *Morbidity and Mortality Weekly Report,* 1987; *36,* 581-585.

[h]Centers for Disease Control. Reducing the health consequences of smoking: 25 years of progress—A report of the Surgeon General, 1989. Rockville, Md.: U.S. Department of Health and Human Services, Public Health Service, 1989.

[i]Systolic blood pressures, persons age 18–74 years, U.S. population. National Center for Health Statistics. Blood pressure levels in persons 18–74 years of age in 1976–1980, and trends in blood pressure from 1960–1980 in the United States: Data from the National Health Survey. Hyattsville, Md.: U.S. Department of Health and Human Services, Public Health Service. DHHS Publication no. (PHS) 86-1684. *Vital and Health Statistics,* 1986; *11* (234).

(*From Centers for Disease Control. Chronic disease reports: Coronary heart disease mortality—United States, 1986.* Morbidity and Mortality Weekly Reports, *1989; 38 (16), 287, Table 2.*)

risk factors in the total U.S. population, and for each factor, the crude relative risk for coronary heart disease mortality, the population attributable risk, and the estimated number of preventable deaths. Several of these factors are interdependent and many individuals have multiple risk factors. Public health and clinical interventions to reduce the prevalence of these risk factors could further reduce coronary heart disease mortality in the United States.

The risk factors discussed above are the best known risk factors for heart disease. A recent review of the literature has identified a total of 177 risk factors for cardiovascular disease. These were classified into ten categories:

1. Nutrition-related factors (33 factors)
2. Internal cardiovascular risk factors identifiable by laboratory tests (35 factors)
3. Drug, chemical, hormonal, and nutritional supplement intake (34 factors)
4. Signs and symptoms associated with a high incidence of cardiovascular diseases (33 factors)
5. Noninvasively detectable abnormal laboratory findings (13 factors)
6. Hereditary cardiovascular risk factors (5 factors)
7. Environmental cardiovascular risk factors, including air pollution, electromagnetic fields, materials that contact the body surface, poisonous venoms, and insertion of needle into infected body tissue by acupuncture or injection (14 factors)
8. Socioeconomic and demographic risk factors (7 factors)
9. Factors related to medical care (2 factors)
10. Coexistence of multiple factors (1 factor)

Seven factors previously considered as risk factors, for example, use of oral contraceptives, were no longer considered risk factors, either because of new research or, in the case of oral contraceptives, changes in the composition of the drug (Omura et al, 1996). The authors concluded that, except for hereditary factors and inherent characteristics like sex, the risk factors were generally controllable by changing lifestyle, maintaining appropriate dietary intake, and correcting existing abnormalities once they are recognized. Although some of these could be recognized by the individuals, others require physicial examinations and laboratory tests by a trained clinician. Surveillance over time after appropriate baseline values on laboratory tests are established was recommended. Most of these tests and lifestyle interventions are included in the recommended preventive service guidelines of the U.S. Preventive Services Task Force shown in Table 10–11 for individuals aged 19 to 39 years and in Table 10–12 for those aged 40 to 64 years (U.S. Preventive Services Task Force, 1989).

For young adults, prevention should focus on changing the risk behaviors. Because many adults over 40 years of age may already have symptoms of cardiovascular disease, secondary and tertiary interventions that focus on early diagnosis and treatment, and provisions of support for physical and social role functioning become important. Even for this group, changing risk behaviors can reduce long-term disability from cardiovascular disease. Health promotion programs in work settings, health

TABLE 10–11. RECOMMENDED[a] PREVENTIVE SERVICE GUIDELINES FOR INDIVIDUALS 19–39 YEARS OF AGE

SCREENING (EVERY 1–3 YEARS)	COUNSELING		IMMUNIZATIONS

History:
   Dietary intake
   Physical activity
   Tobacco/alcohol/drug use
   Sexual practices
 Physical Examination:
   Height and weight
   Blood pressure
   High-Risk Groups:
     Complete oral cavity examination
     Palpation for thyroid nodules
     Clinical breast examination
     Clinical testicular examination
     Complete skin examination
 Laboratory/Diagnostic Procedures:
   Nonfasting total blood cholesterol
   Papanicolaou smear[b]
   High-Risk Groups:
     Fasting plasma glucose
     Rubella antibodies
     VDRL/RPR
     Urinalysis for bacteriuria
     Chlamydial testing
     Gonorrhea culture
     Testing for human immunodeficiency virus (HIV)
     Hearing
     Tuberculin skin test (PPD)
     Electrocardiogram
     Mammogram
     Colonoscopy
 Remain alert for:
   Depressive symptoms
   Suicide risk factors
   Abnormal bereavement
   Malignant skin lesions
   Tooth decay, gingivitis
   Signs of physical abuse
	Diet and Exercise:
	   Fat (especially saturated fat), cholesterol, complex carbohydrates, fiber, sodium, iron,[c] calcium[c]
	   Caloric balance
	   Selection of exercise program
	 Substance Use:
	   Tobacco cessation/primary prevention
	   Alcohol and other drugs
	     Limiting alcohol consumption
	     Driving/other dangerous activities while under the influence
	     Treatment for abuse
	   High-Risk Groups:
	     Sharing/using unsterilized needles and syringes
	 Sexual Practices:
	   Sexually transmitted diseases (partner selection, condoms, anal intercourse)
	   Unintended pregnancy and contraceptive options
		Injury Prevention:
		   Safety belts
		   Safety helmets
		   Violent behavior[d]
		   Firearms[d]
		   Smoke detector
		   Smoking near bedding or upholstery
		   High-Risk Groups:
		     Back conditioning exercises
		 Dental Health:
		   Regular tooth brushing, flossing, and dental visits
		 Other Primary Preventive Measures:
		   High-Risk Groups:
		     Discussion of hemoglobin testing
		     Skin protection from ultraviolet light
			Tetanus-diphtheria booster[e]
			 High-Risk Groups:
			   Hepatitis B vaccine
			   Pneumococcal vaccine
			   Influenza vaccine[f]
			   Measles-mumps-rubella vaccine

[a]The recommended schedule applies only to the periodic visit itself. The frequency of the individual preventive services listed in this table is left to clinical discretion, except as indicated in other footnotes.

[b]Every 1–3 years.

[c]For women.

[d]Especially for young men.

[e]Every 10 years.

[f]Annually.

Examples of target conditions not specifically examined by the Task Force include: Chronic obstructive pulmonary disease, hepatobiliary disease, bladder cancer, endometrial disease, travel-related illness, prescription drug abuse, occupational illness and injuries.

(*Adapted from U.S. Preventive Services Task Force. Guide to clinical preventive services: An assessment of the effectiveness of 169 interventions. Baltimore: Williams & Wilkins, 1989.*)

TABLE 10–12. RECOMMENDED[a] PREVENTIVE SERVICE GUIDELINES FOR INDIVIDUALS 40–64 YEARS OF AGE

SCREENING (EVERY 1–3 YEARS)	COUNSELING	IMMUNIZATIONS

SCREENING (EVERY 1–3 YEARS)

History:
  Dietary intake
  Physical activity
  Tobacco/alcohol/drugs
  Sexual practices
Physical Examination:
  Height and weight
  Blood pressure
  Clinical breast examination[b]
  High-Risk Groups:
    Complete skin examination
    Oral cavity examination
    Auscultation for carotid bruits
    Palpation for thyroid nodules
Laboratory/Diagnostic Procedures:
  Nonfasting total blood cholesterol
  Papanicolaou smear[c]
  Mammogram[d]
  High-Risk Groups:
    Fecal occult blood/colonoscopy
    Fasting plasma glucose
    VDRL/RPR
    Bacteriuria urinalysis
    Bone mineral content
    Chlamydial testing
    Gonorrhea culture
    Counseling and testing for human immunodeficiency virus (HIV)
    Tuberculin skin test (PPD)
    Hearing
    Electrocardiogram
    Fecal occult blood/sigmoidoscopy
Remain alert for:
  Depressive symptoms
  Suicide risk factors
  Abnormal bereavement
  Signs of physical abuse or neglect
  Malignant skin lesions
  Peripheral arterial disease
  Tooth decay, gingivitis, loose teeth

COUNSELING

Diet and Exercise:
  Fat (especially saturated fat), cholesterol, complex carbohydrates, fiber, sodium, calcium[e]
  Caloric balance
  Selection of exercise program
Substance Use:
  Tobacco cessation
  Alcohol and other drugs
    Limiting alcohol consumption
    Driving/other dangerous activities while under the influence
    Treatment for abuse
  High-Risk Groups:
    Sharing/using unsterilized needles and syringes
Sexual Practices:
  Sexually transmitted diseases (partner selection, condoms, anal intercourse)
  Unintended pregnancy and contraceptive options

Injury Prevention:
  Safety belts
  Safety helmets
  Smoke detector
  Smoking near bedding or upholstery
  High-Risk Groups:
    Back conditioning exercises
    Falls in the elderly
Dental Health:
  Regular tooth brushing, flossing, dental visits
Other Primary Preventive Measures:
  High-Risk Groups:
    Skin protection from ultraviolet light
    Discussion of aspirin therapy
    Discussion of estrogen replacement therapy

IMMUNIZATIONS

Tetanus-diphtheria booster[f]
High-Risk Groups:
  Hepatitis B vaccine
  Pneumococcal vaccine
  Influenza vaccine[g]

[a]The recommended schedule applies only to the periodic visit itself. Frequency of the individual services listed in this table is left to clinical discretion, except as indicated in other footnotes.
[b]Annually for women.
[c]Every 1–3 years for women.
[d]Every 1–2 years for women beginning at age 50 years (age 35 years for those at increased risk).
[e]For women.
[f]Every 10 years.
[g]Annually.

Examples of target conditions not specifically examined by the Task Force include: Chronic obstructive pulmonary disease, hepatobiliary disease, bladder cancer, endometrial disease, travel-related illness, prescription drug abuse, occupational illness and injuries.

(*Adapted from U.S. Preventive Services Task Force.* Guide to clinical preventive services: An assessment of the effectiveness of 169 interventions. *Baltimore: Williams & Wilkins, 1989.*)

care settings, and in the community can be very helpful in supporting healthy lifestyles as well as by providing opportunities for early detection and control of risk factors. Such programs should also maximize the effectiveness of clinical health services because they encourage early diagnosis and better regimen adherence.

Primary prevention efforts during the past few decades have been somewhat successful in reducing cardiovascular risks, especially for young adults. Smoking cessation was a major focus of prevention effort since it is a risk factor not just for heart disease, but for lung and other cancers as well as other diseases. One study estimated that 18% of mortality among men and 12% among women is directly attributable to smoking (Centers for Disease Control, 1989). By 1990, half of all living adults in the United States who ever smoked had quit, and it was estimated that smoking cessation had resulted in avoidance of 789,000 deaths (Centers for Disease Control, 1990). Unfortunately, millions of Americans, particularly blacks, blue-collar workers, and less educated persons continue to smoke cigarettes. The decline in smoking is slower among women than men. Prevention programs need to focus on these high-risk groups and on strategies for preventing smoking initiation among young people (Centers for Disease Control, 1990).

Reduction of other risk factors for cardiovascular disease, however, has not been as successful as efforts in smoking cessation. Reducing the percentage of the population that is overweight is another intervention targeted by national goals for the year 2000. Unfortunately, the prevalence of this risk factor has increased rather than decreased. Similarly, daily servings of grains and fruits and vegetables fall well below the goal. Only 29% of Americans eat the recommended five servings of fruits and vegetables and 40% eat the recommended six servings of grains (National Center for Health Statistics, 1996). Additional interventions that have been recommended for heart disease prevention include long-term estrogen replacement therapy for postmenopausal women (Pines et al, 1997; Langer & Barrett–Connor, 1994) and giving aspirin in daily small doses to reduce risk of ischemic heart disease (Maron, 1996).

Control of hypertension is one effective prevention approach for reducing death rates from heart disease. In the mid-1980s, half of the U.S. population aged 25 to 74 years had borderline or elevated blood pressure and 15% to 30% had definite elevated blood pressure (National Center for Health Statistics, 1988). Since then, the prevalence of hypertension has declined for all gender, age, and race groups, largely because of national hypertension control programs. Nine of the 1990 National Health Objectives addressed hypertension control, and seven of the objectives were met (Centers for Disease Control, 1990f). Year 2000 National Health Objectives give priority to hypertension programs targeted for blacks, who experience rates of hypertension 45% higher than whites (Centers for Disease Control, 1990a).

Reducing hypercholesterolemia is another approach to intervention that has received considerable attention in recent years. This measure can both prevent or slow the process of atherogenesis that leads to thrombotic complications and can also reduce plaque instability (Henderson, 1996). Other interventions aimed at high-risk individuals include use of aspirin to prevent thromboembolic events, regular exercise, and estrogen replacement therapy for postmenopausal women. Genetic stratification of risk is a realistic possibility in the not too distant future. This would allow more cost-effective intervention targeted at truly high-risk individuals.

Early detection and treatment of angina, unstable coronary syndrome, and other physiological states associated with higher risk for coronary heart disease offer opportunities for secondary prevention. New noninvasive tests for endothelial dysfunction are in experimental phases (Henderson, 1996). Finally, providing effective therapy for symptomatic coronary heart disease offers the potential to prevent disability and mortality.

Strokes

Strokes or "cerebrovascular accidents" continue to be major health hazards of the middle adult years. Although most of the deaths from strokes occur after age 65, these conditions nevertheless are a leading cause of death for adults in the 25- to 64-year age group. Disability from strokes imposes tremendous physical, emotional, and economic burdens on families and society. Because atherosclerosis is the underlying disease process for both heart disease and cerebrovascular accidents, the major risk factors for strokes are those previously discussed. Control of hypertension is the most crucial preventive activity. Well-designed and well-implemented prevention programs can be very effective in controlling hypertension and its potential harmful effects.

Early detection and treatment of diabetes may help to prevent strokes because diabetics have about twice as many strokes as nondiabetics. This may be partially because diabetics are more likely to be hypertensive and overweight (Chen & Lowenstein, 1986). Elimination of smoking is also very important for these individuals, both for controlling their primary disease process and for decreasing the risk of strokes and heart attacks. Preventive therapy with aspirin is becoming more accepted. Research is currently exploring the effectiveness of antioxidant therapies in prevention of stroke.

Malignancies

Malignancies are the leading cause of death for both young and middle-aged women, and they are only surpassed by heart disease as the major cause of death among men 45 to 64 years of age. The most prevalent malignancies among adult women are lung cancer and cancer of the breast. Lung cancer is also the most common cause of cancer mortality among men (Parker et al, 1997). For each decade of adulthood, blacks have higher mortality from malignancies than whites, with the rate differential increasing for each decade.

Malignancies are a group of many different diseases, each with its own unique etiology and developmental history. Risk factors that have been identified as potential contributors to cancer development include cigarette smoking and excessive alcohol intake, high fat diet, occupational exposures to carcinogenic agents, water and air pollution, overexposures to radiation and sunlight, heredity factors, and other predisposing medical conditions. At the present time, the most effective prevention efforts against malignancies include smoking cessation, limitation of exposures to known carcinogenic substances, screening, and prompt diagnostic followup testing, so treatment can be initiated while the tumor is still in its early stages (U.S. Department of Health and Human Services, 1990).

Of all the risk factors, cigarette smoking is responsible for more malignancies and cancer deaths than any other known carcinogenic agent. To date, 43 chemicals in tobacco smoke have been identified as carcinogens. Smoking is responsible for an estimated 30% of all cancer deaths, including 87% of lung cancer (Centers for Disease Control, 1989). The risk of dying from cancer quickly multiplies when an individual smokes and is exposed to other carcinogens in the living environment or work setting. The combination of cigarette smoking and exposure to asbestos, for example, increases lung cancer risk 90 times (U.S. Department of Health and Human Services, 1979).

Efforts to decrease the prevalence of cigarette smoking include educational programs to motivate and assist individuals and groups to quit smoking as well as legislative sanctions against smoking. Broad-based educational programs focus on instructing the public about the hazards of smoking and provide the impetus for current anti-smoking programs. During the 1980s, efforts were directed toward providing individuals with behavioral skills for long-term smoking cessation. Health promotion programs in industry, schools, and other community settings played an increasingly important role in assisting persons to gain these behavioral skills as well as to develop more healthy lifestyles. Physicians, nurses, and other health practitioners will continue to have a major responsibility for encouraging smoking cessation because persons may have stronger motivation for smoking cessation when a message is delivered in a health care setting (Hollis et al, 1991) or when they are first diagnosed with a life-threatening illness. If feasible, behaviorally oriented smoking cessation guidance should be offered in the clinical setting. If not, appropriate referrals to community-based educational programs should be made.

Legislative efforts to influence smoking behaviors began in the 1980s. By 1988, 320 local communities had adopted laws or regulations restricting smoking in public places (Centers for Disease Control, 1989). Ongoing efforts target increasing the federal tobacco excise tax, banning cigarette vending machines in areas that are accessible to minors, and promoting clean indoor air acts in all 50 states and the District of Columbia (National Center for Health Statistics, 1996). An important consideration supporting the reasonableness of smoking restrictions in public areas is the effect of smoking on nonsmokers. Given the overwhelming evidence concerning the health hazards of smoking, higher taxes on tobacco products also seem warranted. Finances from increased taxation could be channeled into covering costs of publicly funded medical care programs or health education. Recent efforts of the Clinton administration to keep cigarette advertising away from children, if successful, could, in the future, decrease the burden of illness among middle-aged adults due to tobacco.

Establishing and enforcing appropriate environmental controls on water and air pollution as well as on direct occupational exposures are also critical for preventing malignancies. Most Americans live in urban areas where toxic gases or particulate matter produced by automobiles and industrial exhausts pollute the air. The

National Institute of Occupational Safety and Health estimated that nine of ten American industrial workers are exposed to at least one common hazardous industrial chemical (U.S. Department of Health, Education, and Welfare, 1979). Others are exposed because of the amount of toxins released into the atmosphere by industry (Fig. 10–5). Additional research is needed to better understand the relationship between environmental exposures and adverse health outcomes. Determining the toxic and ecological effects of fossil fuels and synthetic chemicals used in modern society is a difficult challenge (U.S. Department of Health and Human Services, 1990). Noise is another occupational hazard. Figure 10–6 shows the percentage of U.S. civil and military employees exposed to noise levels exceeding 85 dBA. The percentage of individuals exposed has increased since 1989, rather than decreased, and is well above the year 2000 goal (National Center for Health Statistics, 1996).

Responsibility for improving the quality of the environment must be shared by individuals, health professionals, and community groups as well as by industry and governmental agencies. On the individual level, cooperative attitudes toward legislated standards such as those for automobile emissions and waste disposal is critical. Educational messages that focus on both the personal and social consequences of sabotaging environmental control efforts are needed, as are stronger penalties for infringements. Industry can be expected to continually challenge regulations, especially when such regulations increase an industry's immediate financial burden. Increased public demand for industrial controls as well as improved public awareness

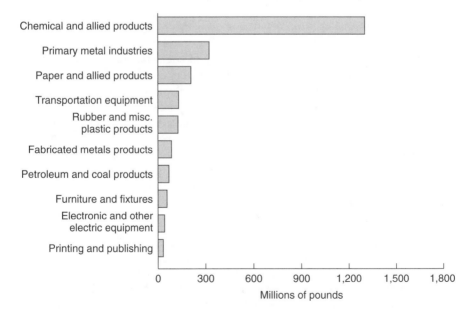

Figure 10–5. Toxic releases by the top ten industries in the United States, 1993. (*Adapted from U.S. Bureau of the Census. Statistical abstract of the United States, 1996* [116th ed.]. *Washington, D.C.: 1996, p. 224, Fig. 6.2.*)

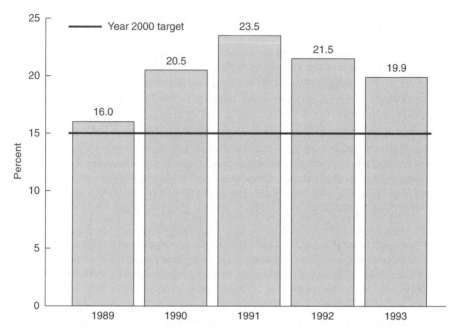

Figure 10–6. Proportion of U.S. civilian and military employees exposed to average daily noise levels that exceed 85 dBA, United States, 1989 to 1994, and year 2000 target for objective 10.7. (*Adapted from National Center for Health Statistics.* Healthy People 2000 Review, 1995–1996. *Hyattsville, Md.: Public Health Service, 1996, p. 96, Fig. 11.*)

of legislative and lobbying skills are necessary to counteract organized efforts of special interest groups that attempt to thwart regulatory controls.

Specific risk factors for some malignancies are unknown. In such cases, secondary preventions that focus on early diagnosis and treatment are the most effective intervention strategies. For example, most breast cancers are found by women themselves rather than by physician examinations, making monthly breast self-examination the key to enhancing early detection. Other effective screening procedures include the Pap smear for detection of cervical cancer, rectal examination for detection of prostate cancer, mammography for detection of breast cancer, and occult blood testing for detection of colorectal cancer.

Accidents and Acts of Violence

Motor vehicle casualties and other accidents such as falls, burns, and poisonings account for most of the deaths among young American adults in the 25- to 34-year age group and continue to cause many unnecessary deaths and permanent injuries throughout the middle adult years. An effective program for preventing accidents must be successful in motivating individuals to take more protective measures as well as in effecting better control of hazards in the environment. Nearly half of the deaths for accidental injuries in the adult years are caused by motor vehicle accidents. Prevention strategies for these were discussed in Chapter 9.

Other accidents and violent acts that result in homicide or suicide are serious problems in the young and middle adult years. Firearms present an especially serious problem in young adulthood. Preventive measures that could reduce the risk of firearm injuries range from encouraging safer storage to a complete ban on ownership. Evidence from studies in England suggest that prohibiting possession of hand guns is effective in reducing firearm injuries in noncriminal assaults (U.S. Department of Health, Education, and Welfare, 1979). Many of the homicides in the United States involve family members, close friends, or acquaintances. Better firearm control would probably help to reduce the high incidence of homicides and accidental shooting deaths among young black men, and it might also curtail those impulsive suicides and homicides related to firearms that are prevalent among young white men. Laws to require a waiting period before purchase of firearms have been passed, but most legislative efforts to control firearms have been unsuccessful. A new Healthy People 2000 goal was added in 1995 aimed at enacting in all 50 states and the District of Columbia laws that would require proper storage of firearms to minimize access to and accidental discharge by minors. These types of laws were nonexistent in 1991, but by 1995, 14 states had enacted such laws (National Center for Health Statistics, 1996). Enforcement of these laws, however, is difficult and public health education efforts to alert parents to the risks associated with the all too common practice of storing loaded firearms where they can be accessed by children must also be implemented.

Primary prevention for acts of violence will necessitate a much stronger emphasis on correcting harmful social conditions that contribute to stress and loss of control (eg, unemployment and economic strain, overcrowded living conditions, unplanned pregnancies, especially among the very young, and lack of opportunity to achieve personal goals). Although alcohol abuse and illicit drug use definitely contribute to loss of control and violence, they are also a symptomatic warning of underlying stress and discontent. Although prevention of substance abuse is certainly a worthwhile goal, it alone is not the solution for violence. Although crisis hotlines have been very beneficial in preventing suicides, they cannot replace needed structural changes in society.

Mental Illness and Substance Abuse

Mental health problems cause much disability and suffering in young and middle adulthood and also substantially contribute to deaths from accidents, suicides, and homicides. Depression and manic depressive disorders are the most prevalent mental illnesses, and they have the most serious consequences in terms of mortality. The psychoses, although less prevalent, are extremely destructive to individuals and families. They often necessitate long-term institutionalizations. Untreated acute psychoses may precipitate acts of violence.

Although many of the biological determinants of mental illness are unknown, it is nevertheless possible to exert much control over acute illness episodes with well-organized and well-funded prevention programs. Persons who have experienced early childhood deprivation or abuse, those living under ongoing acute environmental stress, and those with a generational family history of mental illness are most vulnerable. Prevention programs that identify high-risk groups and offer acceptable supportive interventions may be most successful in preventing or controlling mental illness, for example, crisis counseling, organization of self-help support groups, stress management training, or ongoing institutional consultation. Early diagnosis and treatment can also be very effective in controlling the symptoms of most acute mental illnesses as well as in curtailing or postponing chronicity and its associated disabilities.

Substance abuse (particularly alcohol abuse) continues to be a serious health problem throughout the adult years and is associated with substantial premature mortality. Specific diagnoses that account for alcohol-related mortality include motor vehicle accidents, homicide, suicide, cirrhosis of the liver, and esophogeal cancers (National Center for Health Statistics, 1996). Fortunately, alcohol consumption rates in the United States have been slowly declining since the early 1980s, with corresponding declines in the numbers of cirrhosis deaths and alcohol-related motor vehicle accidents (U.S. Department of Health and Human Services, 1990).

Major preventive interventions for alcohol and drug abuse include educational programs for youths and adults, various attempts to alter social mores and reduce individual and social stress factors, and law enforcement. Preventive education programs that build on peer group counseling and support to resist drinking are generally more successful than programs that merely warn about the hazards of alcohol. Programs that use role playing and other behavioral techniques to teach problem-solving and coping skills are particularly helpful for assisting individuals to resist social pressure to experiment with alcohol or other drugs. Self-help groups such as Alcoholics Anonymous and Alanon are also a good source of support for families already attempting to cope with alcoholism. Because children of alcoholics are at a much greater risk for alcoholism than those in the wider population, their involvement in preventive programs such as Alanon is strongly encouraged.

The role of unmanageable social stress as a risk factor for mental illness and substance abuse, as well as for physical illness in adulthood, cannot be overemphasized. Domestic violence is an increasing problem often related to both social stress and alcohol or drug use. Physical abuse against women by male partners nearly doubled between 1987 and 1992, but appears to have leveled off at 9.3 cases per 1,000 women (National Center for Health Statistics, 1996). While the increase could be due in part to better reporting as the problem gained public attention and help was made available for women in need, it is thought that reported cases represent only a portion of the prevalence. Preventive strategies that are directed toward reducing environmental stressors as well as those that focus on improving individuals' coping skills are needed (U.S. Department of Health and Human Services, 1990). Education on parenting skills, communication, and strategies for anger management could be helpful and might contribute to decreasing second generation problems. Efforts to reduce social environmental stressors might include improving the work climate in institutional settings, strengthening neighborhood networks, creating better community support services, and fostering more healthy racial and ethnic attitudes. Because stressful events are not always preventable, individuals must be better prepared to cope with stress at an early age. School-based educational programs that focus on teaching problem-solving coping skills for stressful situations would be helpful as would stress management programs in work settings. Screening for domestic violence in the clinical setting with referral to appropriate services is also recommended.

REFERENCES

Adams P. F., Benson V. (1990) Current estimates from the National Health Interview Survey: 1989. *Vital Health Statistics, 10,* 176. Hyattsville, Md.: National Center for Health Statistics.

Adams P. F., Marano M. A. (1995) Current estimates from the National Health Interview Survey: 1994. *Vital Health Statistics, 10,* 193. Hyattsville, Md.: National Center for Health Statistics.

Centers for Disease Control. (1990e) Alcohol-related mortality and years of potential life lost—United States, 1987. *Morbidity and Mortality Weekly Report, 39,* 11.

Centers for Disease Control. (1990d) Coronary heart disease attributable to sedentary lifestyle—Selected states, 1988. *Morbidity and Mortality Weekly Report, 37,* 32.

Centers for Disease Control. (1990a) Healthy people 2000: National health promotion and disease prevention objectives for year 2000. *Morbidity and Mortality Weekly Report, 39,* 39.

Centers for Disease Control. (1990c) Prevalence and incidence of diabetes mellitus—United States, 1980–1987. *Morbidity and Mortality Weekly Report, 39,* 45.

Centers for Disease Control. (1990f) Progress toward achieving the 1990 high blood pressure objectives. *Morbidity and Mortality Weekly Report, 39,* 40.

Centers for Disease Control. (1990b) Regional variation in diabetes mellitus prevalence—United States, 1988 and 1989. *Morbidity and Mortality Weekly Report, 39,* 45.

Centers for Disease Control. (1989) Smoking-attributable mortality, morbidity, and economic costs—California, 1985. *Morbidity and Mortality Weekly Report, 38*(16), 273–275.

Centers for Disease Control. (1989) The Surgeon General's 1989 report on reducing the health consequences of smoking: 25 years of progress: Executive summary. *Morbidity and Mortality Weekly Report, 38,* 5–20.

Centers for Disease Control. (1990) The Surgeon General's 1990 report on the health benefits of smoking cessation: Executive summary. *Mordibity and Mortality Weekly Report, 39,* RR-12.

Centers for Disease Control. (1996) Update: Mortality attributable to HIV infection among persons aged 25–44 years—United States, 1994. *Morbidity and Mortality Weekly Report, 45*(6), 121–124.

Chen M. K., Lowenstein F. W. (1986) Epidemiology of factors related to self-reported diabetes among adults. *American Journal of Preventive Medicine, 2*(1), 14.

Henderson A. (1996) Coronary heart disease: An overview. *Lancet. 348*(suppl.), 51–56.

Hollis J., Lichtenstein E., Mount K., Vogt T. M., Stevens V. J. (1991) Nurse-assisted smoking counseling in medical settings: Minimizing demands on physicians. *Preventive Medicine, 20,* 497–507.

Jenkins C. D. (1988) Epidemiology of cardiovascular diseases. *Journal of Consulting and Clinical Psychology, 56*(3), 324–332.

Langer R. D., Barrett–Connor E. (1994) Extended hormone replacement therapy: who should get it, and for how long? *Geriatrics, 49*(12):20–29.

Maron D. J. (1996) Nonlipid primary and secondary prevention strategies for coronary heart disease. *Clinical Cardiology, 19*(5):419–423.

National Center for Health Statistics. (1990) *Health United States, 1989.* Hyattsville, Md.: Public Health Service.

National Center for Health Statistics. (1996) Health United States, 1987. (DHHS Publication No [PHS] 88-1232). Washington, D.C.: Public Health Service, 1988.

National Center for Health Statistics. (1996) *Healthy people 2000 review, 1995–96.* Hyattsville, Md., Public Health Service.

Omura Y., Lee A. Y., Beckman S. L., Simon R., Lorberboym M., Duvvi H., Heller S. I., Urich C. (1996) 177 cardiovascular risk factors, classified in 10 categories, to be considered in the prevention of cardiovascular diseases: An update of the original 1982 article containing 96 risk factors. *Acupuncture and Electrotherapy Research, 21*(1), 21–76.

Pines A., Mijatovic V., van der Mooren M. J., Kenemano P. (1997) Hormone replacement therapy and cardioprotection: basic concepts and clinical considerations. *European Journal of Obstetrics and Gynecology and Reproductive Biology, 71*:193–197.

U.S. Bureau of the Census. (1996) *Statistical abstract of the United States, 1996 (116th ed.).* Washington, D.C.: U.S. Government Printing Office.

U.S. Department of Health, Education, and Welfare. (1979) *Healthy people: The Surgeon General's report on health promotion and disease prevention, 1979.* (DHEW Publication No. [PHS] 79–55071). Washington, D.C.: U.S. Government Printing Office.

U.S. Department of Health and Human Services. (1990) Healthy People 2000. *National health promotion and disease prevention objectives.* (DHHS Publication No. [PHS] 91-50212). Hyattsville, Md.

U.S. Department of Health and Human Services. (1990) *Prevention 89/90: Federal programs and progress.* Washington, D.C.: U.S. Government Printing Office.

U.S. Department of Health and Human Services. (1979) *Smoking and health: A report of the Surgeon General.* (DHHS Publication No. [PHS] 79-50066). Washington, D.C.: U.S. Government Printing Office.

U.S. Preventive Services Task Force. (1989) *Guide to clinical preventive services: An assessment of the effectiveness of 169 interventions.* Baltimore: Wilkins & Wilkins.

U.S. Bureau of the Census. (1997) *Statistical abstract of the United States, 1997* (117th ed.). Washington, D.C.: U.S. Government Printing Office.

Patterns of Morbidity and Mortality Over Age 65

*p*ersons aged 65 years and older represent a growing proportion of the total world population. This growth is particularly dramatic in developed countries. In the United States between 1960 and 1995, the proportion of the total population older than 65 years of age grew from 9.2% to 13.1%. This represents an increase from 16.9 million persons in 1960 to 33.9 million in 1995. By the year 2000, it has been projected that there will be 34.7 million persons older than 65 years in the United States (U.S. Bureau of the Census, 1996). A change in the age distribution of older Americans is also projected. The number of people 75 years or older in the United States is expected to increase to 6.1% of the population by the year 2000 and to 7.9% by 2025 (U.S. Bureau of the Census, 1996). These older populations consume a disproportionate share of health care dollars and these expenditures have fueled governmental concerns for how to fund health care for older Americans in the future. The attendant discussion has also contributed to various changes in care delivery aimed at controlling costs of care.

This chapter presents the major causes of morbidity and mortality in persons over 65 years of age. Prevention of illness and maintenance of function remain important goals and can contribute to quality of life for older persons. Planning the most effective and comprehensive care for elderly patients, including primary, secondary, and tertiary prevention activities, requires familiarity with the major health problems experienced by elderly persons, the effects of particular illnesses on function, and the relationship of specific illnesses to mortality. These are discussed in the context of the physiological changes of aging and changes in society.

OVERVIEW

As mentioned in Chapter 5, several major factors are contributing to the growth in the proportion of older persons in modern societies:

1. High birth rates. During the first decades of the 1900s, high birth rates were accompanied by lower infant, childhood, and young adult mortality rates so that large cohorts of births survived to old age.
2. High immigration rates. Between 1880 and 1910, many immigrants, including many young children, came to the United States. Additionally, young immigrant families had more children after their arrival. Both the young immigrants and the children of young immigrants are now older than or are approaching 65 years of age.
3. Longer life spans resulting from improvements in public health, nutrition, disease prevention, and treatment.

Continued growth in the elderly population in the United States is expected well into the 21st century because of the aging of the baby boomers. It is projected that the median age of the U.S. population will rise from 33 years in 1990 to 36 years in 2000 and 43 years by 2050 (U.S. Department of Health and Human Services, 1991). Many other developed countries are also experiencing growth in the percentage of their population that is elderly and the annual growth rates of the elderly population in the United States are relatively modest compared with that of countries such as Japan, Canada, France, Germany, and Italy. The projected average annual growth rates from 1990 to 2005 for the United States are 0.30% for persons aged 65 to 69 years and 2.7% for those over 80 years of age. Comparable rates in other countries are France—1.3% and 1.3%, respectively; Germany—1.9% and 0.8%, respectively; Italy—1.5% and 3.1%, respectively; Canada—1.6% and 3.8%, respectively; and Japan—3.0% and 4.3%, respectively (U.S. Department of Health and Human Services, 1991). A few developed countries seem to have peaked in growth for the 65- to 69-year age group; Sweden's projected growth rate is –0.6% and that for the United Kingdom is –0.01%. The rates for growth in these countries among those 80 years and older, however, are 2.0% and 2.1%, respectively.

Shifts in longevity have not been equal for all segments of society. Table 11–1 shows the 1990 and projected 2025 sex ratios for the total population, for those 65 years and older, and those 85 years and older for the countries discussed above. Women clearly predominate in the older age groups. In the United States in 1995, men older than 65 years (13.7 million) represented 10.7% of the male population,

TABLE 11–1. SEX RATIO[a] OF THE POPULATION, BY AGE IN SELECTED COUNTRIES—1990 AND PROJECTIONS FOR 2025

COUNTRY	1990			2025		
	All Ages	65–84 Years	85 Years- and Older	All Ages	65–84 Years	85 Years and Older
Canada	97.2	71.9	52.4	95.7	77.4	59.4
France	95.1	64.4	44.3	95.6	74.0	55.0
Germany	92.7	50.5	39.0	96.5	76.0	52.9
Italy	94.4	67.1	49.5	95.4	75.3	56.1
Japan	96.7	67.6	55.1	96.1	78.5	61.6
Sweden	97.3	74.1	53.7	97.3	79.6	61.2
United Kingdom	95.3	66.3	42.4	97.1	77.7	57.8
United States	95.4	68.7	47.1	95.5	77.1	53.8

[a]Number of men per 100 women in the age group.
(*Adapted from U.S. Department of Health and Human Services.* Aging America: Trends and projections *(1991 ed.). [DHHS Publication No. (FCoA) 91-29001]. Washington, D.C.: U.S. Government Printing Office, 1991, Table 9–6, p 259.*)

whereas women older than 65 (20.8 million) represented 15.6% of the female population. The female-to-male ratio is 53:1. The much higher number of women is due to the continuing differential in life expectancies between men and women, although life expectancy has been increasing for both. A white man who had reached age 65 years in 1991 had an average expectation of 15.4 years of life remaining; a white woman aged 65 years in 1991 had an average expectation of 19.2 years of life remaining. The parallel figures for black men and women were 13.4 and 17.2 years, respectively (Cohen & Van Nostrand, 1995).

While a large proportion of the difference in life expectancy for men versus women prior to 65 years of age is accounted for by excess deaths from accidents, suicide, and homicide among men younger than 35 years of age and by heart disease and lung cancer during the middle years (see Chap. 10), different factors are responsible for the difference among those reaching 65 years of age. Diseases in which older men show an excess over women predominate as causes of mortality, whereas diseases in which older women show an excess over men are predominately causes of morbidity. Women also experience higher rates of disability when ill. The divergence of mortality rates by sex is greater among whites than among nonwhites.

Overall, mortality rates for whites are substantially lower than those for nonwhites in the 65-year and older age group, as in younger age groups. In 1995, whites older than 65 years of age represented 14.7% of the total U.S. white population. Blacks older than 65 years constituted only 8.5% of the total black population. Racial distributions of the over 65-year-old population for three age groups are shown by race in Table 11–2.

Although there are many older adults who experience good health and freedom of activity, in general, the population older than 65 years of age is at higher risk of disease and death and is more likely to require medical services than are younger persons. Older individuals make more visits per person to physicians and use hospital facilities more frequently than any younger age group. In the National Health

TABLE 11–2. PERCENT OF TOTAL POPULATION IN AGE GROUPS OVER 65 YEARS OF AGE BY RACE—
UNITED STATES, 1995

	RACE			
AGE GROUP	Hispanic	White	Black	Native American, Eskimo, Aleutian Islander
65–74 years	3.5	8.1	5.0	4.0
75–84 years	1.6	5.0	2.6	2.0
85 years and older	0.5	1.6	0.9	0.7

(*Compiled from United States Bureau of the Census.* Statistical abstract of the United States, 1996 [116th ed.]. *Washington, D.C.: U.S. Government Printing Office, Table 23, p 24.*)

Survey, persons 65 years and older accounted for 24% of all visits to office-based physicians, 34% of all days used in short stay hospitalizations, and constituted the majority of all residents in nursing homes (Cohen & Van Nostrand, 1995). Among those 75 years and older in 1992, 8.3% experienced limitation in personal care activities, 12% in routine care activities, and 19% in other activities. Over 85 years of age, the parallel figures are 20%, 22%, and 14%, respectively; only 43% were not limited. A smaller percentage of males than females are limited. This older population also accounts for nearly one third of monies spent on personal health care.

Assisting older citizens to adapt to life with a chronic illness has increasingly become a responsibility of the family. But support from the health care system and community are crucial. Nurses, in particular, have responsibility in many health care settings to assist in the care of the elderly.

MAJOR CAUSES OF MORTALITY

Rates in Age Subgroups

The ten leading causes of death in the United States in 1992 for the 65 and older age groups are shown in Table 11–3 and are compared with causes for the total U.S. population. Coronary heart disease is the leading cause of death for both sexes within the total U.S. population and in all the older age subgroups. Coronary heart disease mortality rates tend to increase with age; the crude rate for the total U.S. population in 1992 was 281.4 deaths per 100,000 persons. In the 65- to 74-year age group, heart disease mortality rates were 847.9 per 100,000. Rates for those aged 75 to 84 and those 85 and older were 2,147.5 and 6,513.5, respectively. Deaths from heart disease accounted for 37.8% of deaths in those older than 75 years of age (Kochanek et al, 1995).

Malignant neoplasms are the second most frequent cause of death among older Americans, except in the 85 and older age group where it drops to third place, superseded by cerebrovascular disease, which is the third most frequent cause of death in both of the two younger age groups (65 to 74 years and 75 to 84 years) and

TABLE 11–3. RATE PER 100,000 FOR THE TEN LEADING CAUSES OF DEATH FOR TOTAL U.S. POPULATION BY 10-YEAR AGE GROUPS OVER 65 YEARS, 1992

RANK	1992 TOTAL U.S. POPULATION		AGE (YEARS)					
			65–74		75–84		85 and Older	
	Cause of Death	Rate	Cause of Death	Rate	Cause of Death	Rate	Cause of Death	Rate
1	Heart disease	281.4	Malignant neoplasms	873.4	Heart disease	2,147.5	Heart disease	6,513.5
2	Malignant neoplasms	204.1	Heart disease	847.9	Malignant neoplasms	1,350.9	Malignant neoplasms	1,787.3
3	Cerebrovascular disease	56.4	Chronic lung disease	155.5	Cerebrovascular disease	468.2	Cerebrovascular disease	1,566.0
4	Chronic lung disease	36.0	Cerebrovascular disease	135.3	Chronic lung disease	326.5	Pneumonia and influenza	1,022.8
5	Accidents and adverse effects	34.0	Atherosclerosis	93.1	Pneumonia and influenza	227.1	Chronic lung disease	460.9
6	Pneumonia and influenza	29.7	Diabetes mellitus	75.7	Diabetes mellitus	142.9	Atherosclerosis	278.1
7	Diabetes mellitus	19.6	Pneumonia and influenza	55.3	Accidents and adverse effects	96.3	Accidents and adverse effects	254.8
8	Human immuno-deficiency virus (HIV) infections	13.2	Accidents and adverse effects	44.2	Nephritis and nephrosis	70.4	Diabetes mellitus	253.8
9	Suicide	12.0	Chronic liver disease/cirrhosis	33.9	Septicemia	58.5	Nephritis and nephrosis	207.0
10	Homicide and legal interventions	10.0	Nephritis and nephrosis	24.6	Atherosclerosis	46.5	Septicemia	178.5

(Compiled from Kochanek D., Kochanek M. A., Hudson B. L. [1995] Advanced report of final mortality statistics, 1995. Monthly Vital Statistics Report, 43, 6 [suppl.]. Hyattsville, Md.: National Center for Health Statistics.)

in the total U.S. population. Malignant neoplasms account for 26% of male deaths among those older than age 75 and 20% of female deaths in that age group; cerebrovascular disease accounts for 9% and 6.3%, respectively, among those older than age 75 (Kochanek et al, 1995).

Although six of the same causes of death appear among the fourth through tenth causes for the three age groups older than 65 years, the order differs in the three age categories. Chronic liver disease and cirrhosis, the ninth most frequent cause of death among 65 to 74 year olds, is not among the top ten causes in the other two age groups. Septicemia, the tenth leading cause of death for the two older age groups is not among the top ten causes of death for those 65 to 74 years of age.

It should be noted that, except for accidents and adverse effects and for pneumonia and influenza, the remaining eight leading causes of death among the elderly all directly reflect the result of the aging process and long-term lifestyle patterns. Consider cardiovascular disease as an example. It has been documented that the effects of the common cardiovascular risk factors are approximately the same in all age groups (Shurtleff, 1974). Because the prevalence of most of these risk factors, including elevated blood pressure and elevated blood cholesterol, increase with age, the elderly are at high risk for mortality from cardiovascular disease. The one risk factor that is of lower prevalence among those older than 65 years is cigarette smoking. Only 13.5% of men over 65 were current smokers in 1993 compared with 29.2% of men aged 45 to 64. Among females, 10.5% over 65 years were current smokers versus 23.4% of females aged 45 to 64 years. It is generally too late for primary prevention of cardiovascular disease in this age group because most persons are well into the natural history stage of pathogenesis. It is possible, however, to intervene at the stage of secondary prevention. Early detection of risk factors and risk factor reduction through programs of supervised aerobic exercise regimens, modification of diet, and reduction or cessation of smoking is feasible, as is prompt treatment with medication or even surgery when indicated. Such measures can be lifesaving. Counseling elderly persons against unusual exertion, such as snow shoveling, can also prove lifesaving. In colder parts of the country, heart attack deaths are higher during winter months.

Tertiary programs of rehabilitation for patients with existing cardiac disease can still improve the quality of life. For the eight chronic diseases that are among the ten leading causes of death among those older than 65, secondary and tertiary prevention must be the general focus of efforts at intervention.

In the case of accidents and adverse effects and of pneumonia and influenza, even primary prevention may be possible because these diseases generally represent sudden, acute events rather than a lifetime process, although aging changes may contribute to onset. Immune status changes may increase susceptibility to pneumonia and influenza. The high incidence of accidents may also be a result of the aging process in that a decrease in physical strength, flexibility or mobility, vision, hearing or other sensory deficits, poorer balance, and slower reflexes may all contribute to an increased probability of accident. Because of circumstances such as brittle bones, diabetes, or cardiovascular disease, the impact of an accident on the individual may be more severe in this age group. There is less ability to recover without complication. A higher rate of complication may be a factor in the higher case fatality rate associated with accidents among the elderly. Similarly, immobility or limitation of activity caused by chronic illness and already impaired lung function may contribute to higher mortality from influenza or pneumonia. Annual influenza and pneumococcal vaccines are recommended for individuals over age 65 for prevention of these illnesses. Safer cars, well-maintained roadways, adequate lighting at night, and traffic lights at busy intersections may improve the safety of driving for older persons. Measures aimed at improving pedestrian safety are also needed.

Changes in Rates over Time

Rates of death for the ten leading causes of death among those older than 65 have generally been decreasing for some decades. Between 1978 and 1992, rankings of the five leading causes of death changed little among persons older than 65 years of age, although some rates, particularly for heart disease and cerebrovascular disease, declined substantially (Fig. 11–1). In contrast, cancer, chronic obstructive lung disease, and pneumonia/influenza rates have recently been increasing.

The decrease in diseases of the heart actually began in 1963. Although there is some question about why this decrease has occurred, national emphasis by the medical care system, drug companies, and public education programs on risk factor intervention has probably had a major impact on both incidence and mortality. Unfortunately, general population incidence data are unavailable (Blackburn & Luepker, 1992). Behavioral intervention efforts have been directed at diet modification to control fat, cholesterol, and calorie intake; regular exercise; stress reduction; hypertension control; weight control; and smoking cessation. Because all these were attacked more or less simultaneously, we may never know with certainty the relative contribution to the observed decline in U.S. mortality. Other simultaneous factors that are likely to have affected mortality rates are the development of emergency teams for dealing with heart attack victims before they get to the hospital, thus preventing many deaths from myocardial infarction, new drugs for treatment of heart disease and hypertension control, and possibly new surgical techniques.

Some of the above efforts at primary and secondary prevention of heart disease should also have contributed to decreases in mortality between 1968 and 1978 for cerebrovascular disease, atherosclerosis, cancer, and chronic lung disease because they share some common risk factors. For example, cigarette smoking is a risk factor not only for heart disease but also for lung cancer and chronic lung disease. A high fat diet is associated with heart disease, breast and colon cancer, and

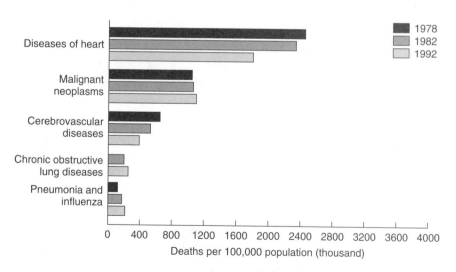

Figure 11–1. Five leading causes of death among persons 65 years of age and older: United States, 1978, 1982, and 1992. (*Adapted from National Center for Health Statistics. Health, United States, 1989. Hyattsville, Md.: Public Health Service, 1990; and Kochanek D., Kochanek M. A., Hudson B. L. Advanced report of final mortality statistics, 1995. Monthly Vital Statistics Report, 1995; 43 [6] [suppl.]. Hyattsville, Md.: National Center for Health Statistics.*)

atherosclerosis. Improvements in detection and management of these other diseases could also have contributed to their decline. Despite this, since 1978, death rates for malignant neoplasms, chronic obstructive lung disease, and pneumonia and influenza have been rising for reasons that are unclear.

Very few renal diseases are preventable. Preventable renal diseases are associated with infections, drug- or chemical-induced disease (which could result from treatment of some other disease condition or from occupational exposures), obstructive or neurological causes, and kidney stones. New drugs, like lisinopril, for control of hypertension are expected to lead to decreasing incidence rates of renal disease in the future, especially among diabetics (Jerums et al, 1995; Goa et al, 1997). Although a huge medical care industry for treatment of those with chronic renal failure has evolved, including dialysis and transplantation, access to these services is variable, expensive, and inconsistent as to effectiveness.

Mortality by Sex

In general, female mortality is lower than male mortality (Table 11–4). Differences between the sexes in rates of mortality from specific causes are observed. In 1992, heart disease rates for white men over age 65 were 2,084.0 per 100,000 population and for white women, 1,690.3. The discrepancy is greater for men compared with women close to 65 years of age than among those over 75 years of age. Lower rates of heart disease among women throughout early life have been attributed in part to protection by female hormones. After menopause, this protection ceases and rates begin to climb toward the levels of mortality present among men. In the past,

TABLE 11–4. RATES OF DEATH PER 100,000 FOR THE TEN LEADING CAUSES OF DEATH OVER 65 YEARS OF AGE[a]
BY RACE AND GENDER—UNITED STATES, 1992

CAUSE OF DEATH	WHITE MALES	WHITE FEMALES	BLACK MALES	BLACK FEMALES
Heart diseases	2,084.0	1,690.3	2,284.2	1,838.1
Malignant neoplasms	1,440.5	891.0	1,940.1	954.2
Cerebrovascular diseases	349.7	407.9	477.8	460.3
Chronic obstructive lung diseases	340.2	194.0	253.3	93.8
Pneumonia and influenza	233.1	198.1	243.6	156.0
Diabetes mellitus	108.7	106.4	181.1	233.8
Accidents and adverse effects	100.6	70.1	125.1	63.5
Nephritis and nephrotic conditions	63.9	47.7	117.1	95.8
Atherosclerosis	—[b]	53.6	—[b]	—[b]
Septicemia	45.4	46.1	101.2	88.2
Rate of Total Deaths	5,598.2	4,376.3	6,727.0	4,757.9

[a]Listed causes of death are the top ten for the total population over age 65.
[b]Rates for this condition not among the top ten for this subgroup. Number 9 cause of death for white males is chronic liver disease (45.6); hypertension is number 9 for black males (60.3) and black females (62.4).
(Compiled from Kochanek D., Kochanek M. A., Hudson B. L. Advanced report of final mortality statistics, 1995. Monthly Vital Statistics Report, 1995; 43 [6] [suppl.], 23-33, Table 6. Hyattsville, Md.: National Center for Health Statistics.)

however, women smoked less than men and were thought to have less stress because they did not work outside the home. Similar patterns are seen for cerebrovascular disease and for atherosclerosis.

For malignant neoplasms, chronic pulmonary disease, pneumonia and influenza, and accidents and adverse effects, mortality rates among women remain considerably lower than those for men throughout all ages older than 65 years for both whites and blacks. Differences observed for the first three of these causes of death may relate to effects of smoking; among the current elderly population, men smoke with much greater frequency than do women. Diabetes mellitus, although showing similar frequency of mortality for the sexes from age 65 through 74 years of age, increases more rapidly in women than in men above that age range and is considerably more frequent among black women than among black men. Although reasons are unknown, it has been postulated that the higher percentage of body fat in women may be a factor.

Mortality by Race

Racial differences in mortality are also observed. For heart disease, malignant neoplasms, cerebrovascular disease, accidents and adverse effects, diabetes mellitus, nephritis and nephrotic conditions, and septicemia, nonwhites, both male and female, have higher mortality rates than do their white counterparts (see Table 11–4) until about 80 years of age. Beginning with the 80- to 84-year age group, rates are higher for some of these causes of death among whites than among nonwhites. However, all death rates for nonwhites in the oldest age groups must be viewed with caution as they are based on small numbers.

The higher mortality rates among nonwhites, particularly blacks, is a continuation of higher rates for blacks at younger ages. Reasons for these differences have not been well investigated, although studies of racial differences in cancer survival have shown that blacks are likely to be diagnosed at a later stage of the disease and are generally in poorer health at diagnosis than are whites. There have also been reports of histological differences in tumor type and racial differences in hormone receptor status; some histological types are more lethal than others, and hormone receptor status relates to whether hormone treatments can be used effectively. Blacks and whites also vary in their rates of incidence for cancer of particular sites—whites have higher rates of breast and colorectal cancers, which are associated with good survival rates. Blacks have higher incidences of stomach and esophageal cancers, which have poorer survival rates. All these factors contribute to the overall differences in the mortality picture for cancer.

Racial differences in constitution, general health status, and lifestyle could affect the other conditions for which nonwhites have higher mortality—heart disease, cerebrovascular disease, diabetes mellitus, and accidents and adverse effects. Differences between the racial groups in promptness of seeking care, quality of care received, compliance with treatment, or quality of the home environment could also influence likelihood of mortality after onset of these conditions.

MAJOR CAUSES OF MORBIDITY

In general, the elderly view themselves as reasonably healthy despite a high frequency of chronic disorders; 71.3% of respondents older than 65 years of age in a national survey of households rated their health as excellent or good. Only 9.1% rated their health as poor. Even among those 85 years of age and older, only 12.6% rated themselves in poor health. Although a slightly higher proportion of men than women rate themselves in good to excellent health, a higher percentage of men also rate themselves as in poor health; women more often specify good or fair health (Cohen & Van Nostrand, 1995). Whites generally rate their health more favorably than do nonwhites, particularly blacks. Such ratings are consistent with higher rates of morbidity and mortality among nonwhites.

Of all the age groups, those older than 65 years have the lowest overall incidence of acute conditions. You will recall from previous chapters that acute conditions were defined by the National Center for Health Statistics as illness or injury of short duration, typically less than 3 months and involving either medical attention or 1 day or more of restricted activity. By type of acute condition, those older than 65 years have the lowest rates of infective and parasitic conditions and respiratory conditions. Their rates of injuries are lower than those of persons younger than 45, but higher than those of persons 45 to 64 years. Rates of digestive system disorders are intermediate between rates for those under 24 years and those between 25 and 64 years (U.S. Bureau of the Census, 1996). However, those older than 65 years of age have the highest prevalence of chronic conditions. Even so, being elderly does not necessarily equate with being ill and debilitated. Nineteen percent of men and 10% of women older than 80 years of age report having none of nine common chronic conditions: arthritis, hypertension, cataracts, heart disease, varicose veins, diabetes, cancer, osteoporosis or hip fracture, or stroke. The elderly do, however, experience more limitation in their activity and more days of disability than do younger persons, and the degree of limitation is related to the number of chronic conditions. Some of these chronic conditions also contribute to high rates of injuries and accidents. The elderly also have the highest rates of hospitalization.

Functional decline represents a major health problem for very elderly persons. A longitudinal study of decline reported an annual incidence of functional decline of 11.9% among previously stable subjects 75 years and older. Risk of decline was reported to double every 5 years (Hebert et al, 1997). Declines in function, shown in Figure 11–2, were also observed in the United States Longitudinal Study of Aging. Functional status is strongly associated with need for hospitalization and nursing home stays (Fig. 11–3). Among those surviving the 6-year followup period, only half as many of those needing no assistance with one or more activities of daily living (ADLs) at baseline were hospitalized as were those needing assistance. Conversely, of those needing assistance with one or more ADL at baseline, more than twice as many needed nursing home care and three times as many required both hospital and nursing home care compared with those needing no ADL assistance.

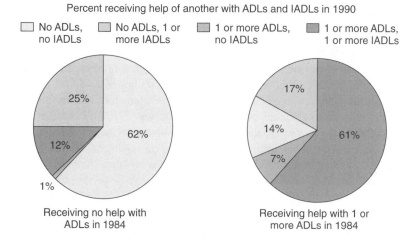

Percent receiving help of another with ADLs and IADLs in 1990

☐ No ADLs,   ☐ No ADLs, 1 or   ▨ 1 or more ADLs,   ▨ 1 or more ADLs,
  no IADLs   more IADLs   no IADLs   1 or more IADLs

Receiving no help with
ADLs in 1984

Receiving help with 1 or
more ADLs in 1984

NOTES: ADL is activity of daily living. IADL is instrumental activity of daily living. ADLs include bathing, dressing, toileting, walking, getting in and out of bed or chair, and eating. IADLs include preparing meals, shopping, managing money, using the telephone, doing light housework, and doing heavy housework. Persons reported as not performing an ADL were classified with those reported as receiving help of another with that ADL. Persons reported as not performing an IADL were not classified with those receiving help of another. Excludes persons whose ADL status was unknown in 1984. Excludes those for whom ADL and/or IADL status was unknown in 1990. Elderly persons are those 70 years of age and over in 1984. Percents may not add to 100 because of rounding.

Figure 11–2. Percent distribution of elderly persons by activity limitation at 1990 recontact, according to receiving help of another person with activities of daily living: United States, 1984. (*Adapted from Cohen R. A., Van Nostrand R. F. Trends in the health of older Americans: United States, 1994. Vital Health Statistics, 1995; 3 [30], 9, Fig. 3. Hyattsville, Md.: National Center for Health Statistics.*)

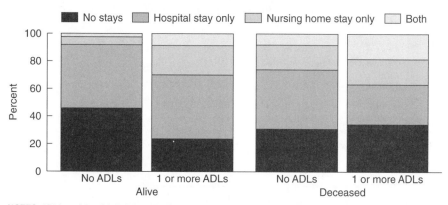

NOTES: ADL is activity of daily living. ADLs include bathing, dressing, toileting, walking, getting in and out of bed or chair, and eating. Persons reported as not performing an ADL were classified with those reported as receiving help of another with that ADL. Excludes persons whose ADL status was unknown in 1984. The alive status excludes those persons for whom no interview was conducted in 1990 and their living arrangement was unknown. Elderly persons are those 70 years of age and over in 1984.

Figure 11–3. Percent distribution of elderly persons by hospital and nursing home stay, according to receiving help of another person with activities of daily living in 1984 and vital status as of 1990 recontact: United States. (*Adapted from Cohen R. A., Van Nostrand R. F. Trends in the health of older Americans: United States, 1994. Vital Health Statistics, 1995; 3 [30], 9, Fig. 4. Hyattsville, Md.: National Center for Health Statistics.*)

Acute Conditions

As in previous chapters, data presented here on acute conditions are based on published data from the National Health Survey. The principal diagnosis and principal reason for visits to physicians' offices probably reflect primarily acute illness, or acute episodes of chronic conditions, and are thus included in this discussion of acute conditions. These acute conditions have implications for the daily activities of the elderly. Clinical personnel working in physicians' offices, outpatient departments, and other settings where these older individuals are treated need to assess the patients' general functional ability and their living arrangements so they can assist these patients to plan modifications of their home environment to preserve safety of function and to obtain necessary services that they may be unable to perform for themselves.

Upper respiratory conditions are the most frequent acute illness among persons older than 65 years of age, with an incidence of 30.6 per 100 population in 1994 for all respiratory conditions (Fig. 11–4). Of the upper respiratory conditions, influenza accounted for 18.3 cases per 100 population, while the common cold accounted for 12.3. Injuries were the other major cause of acute illness, with an incidence of 19.6 per 100 (U.S. Bureau of the Census, 1996). Both of these conditions show some seasonal fluctuation in rates, with highest rates during the winter months. Winter is usually when influenza rates rise in the total U.S. population. Ice and snow increase the probability of injury both from falls and from automobile and pedestrian accidents.

Not surprisingly, elderly persons have more contact with physicians than do younger persons and, as in other age groups, use of ambulatory care increased between 1990 and 1993. For individuals over 75 years of age, the increase was

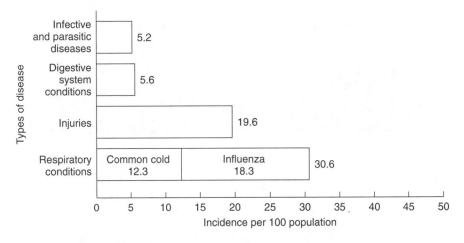

Figure 11–4. Incidence of acute conditions (medically attended) in persons aged 65 years and older: United States, 1994. (*Data from U.S. Bureau of the Census.* Statistical abstracts of the United States, 1996 [116th ed.]. *Washington, D.C.: U.S. Government Printing Office, 1996, Table 218, p 143.*)

2.2 contacts (Adams & Marano, 1995). Results from the National Health Survey indicate that persons between 65 and 74 years of age averaged 9.9 physician contacts per year in 1993 compared with 7.1 for those in the next younger age group (45 to 64 years) and 12.3 for those 75 years and older (Adams & Marano, 1995). These contacts included office visits, telephone contact, and urgency care and emergency room contacts. Elderly people have a higher rate of emergency room visits than younger persons. In 1992, persons over 75 years of age averaged 557.6 visits per 1,000 persons compared with 357.1 for all ages combined (Schappert, 1997). The major reasons for emergency room visits and percentage of visits accountable to each cause for those 65 to 74 years of age were chest pain and related symptoms (11.3%); shortness of breath (8.4%); stomach and abdominal pain, cramps, and spasms (5.1%); labored or difficulty breathing (dyspnea, 4.4%); vertigo-dizziness (2.9%); and back symptoms, headaches, vomiting, general weakness, or abnormal pulsations and palpitations (each 2% or less). Major reasons for visits to the emergency room among those over 75 years of age were chest pain (11.1%); shortness of breath (6.6%); stomach and abdominal pain (5.2%); unconscious on arrival (3.4%); general weakness (3.1%); and labored or difficulty breathing, vertigo-dizziness, back symptoms, hip symptoms, or fever (each 2.8% or less) (Schappert, 1997).

The average number of physician office visits is shown in Table 11–5. These display a similar pattern by age with more visits among the older elderly than the younger elderly. Women have more visits than men and whites more than blacks among those aged 65 to 74, but the male/female visits are similar in number after age 75 (Woodwell & Schappert, 1995). Somewhat over half (55.6%) of visits by the elderly are symptom-related. Another 22.7% comprise initiation and followup treatment for a particular disease condition. Diagnosis, screening, and preventive reasons account for only a small percent of office visits. Among those over age 65, circulatory disease, respiratory system disorders, cerebrovascular disease, and neoplasms—the major causes of morbidity and mortality—result in a large number of physician office visits. However, almost 30% of physician office visits are accounted for by four additional diagnoses: diabetes, obesity, osteoporosis, and asthma. Among those 65 to 74 years of age, 13.3% of physician office visits were for diabetes, 11.9% were for obesity, 6.3% were for osteoporosis, and 4.5% were for asthma. Corresponding percentages of visits among those

TABLE 11–5. AVERAGE NUMBER OF PHYSICIAN OFFICE VISITS PER YEAR PER PERSON BY AGE GROUP— UNITED STATES, 1993

AGE GROUP	MALE	FEMALE	WHITE	BLACK	TOTAL OVER 65 YEARS
65–74 years	4.6	5.4	5.2	3.2	5.0
75 years and older	6.2	6.1	6.3	4.8	6.1

(Compiled from Woodwell D. A., Schappert S. M. National Ambulatory Medical Care Survey: 1993 summary. Advance data from Vital and Health Statistics, No. 20. Hyattsville, Md.: National Center for Health Statistics, 1995.)

75 years and older were 10.1%, 6.8%, 11.3%, and 3.7%, respectively (Woodwell & Schappert, 1995).

Persons over 65 years of age were more likely than younger persons to have a regular source of medical care (94%), largely related to having insurance coverage. Ninety-six percent of the elderly have Medicare and many have additional, supplementary insurance (Cohen et al, 1997). Reasons given by the 6% without a regular source of care for not having such coverage are given in Figure 11–5. The most frequent reason, given by 47% of these individuals, is that they do not need a doctor.

Chronic Conditions

Table 11–6 lists selected chronic conditions reported by persons older than 65 years in the United States for three age subgroups, those 65 to 74 years of age, those 75 to 84 years of age, and those older than 85 years of age. Of the six most prevalent of these conditions affecting those between 65 and 74—heart conditions, hypertension, arthritis, hearing impairments, deformities or orthopedic impairments, and chronic sinusitis, all but heart disease and hypertension increase in prevalence from this age group to the next. Hypertension decreases in prevalence for both men and women, while heart disease prevalence increases for men in the 75 to 84-year age group, then declines, while prevalence for women continues to increase. Cataracts and chronic constipation are two other conditions that show a consistent increase in prevalence with aging. Bronchitis and diabetes, however, show a decrease in preva-

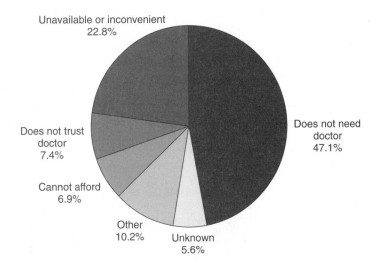

Figure 11–5. Reason for no regular source of care for persons 65 years of age and over: United States, 1993. (*Adapted from Cohen R. A., Bloom B., Simpson G., Parsons P. E. Access to health care. Part 3: Older adults. Vital Health Statistics, 1997; 10 [198]. Hyattsville, Md.: National Center for Health Statistics.*)

TABLE 11–6. PREVALENCE PER 1,000 PERSONS OF SELECTED CHRONIC CONDITIONS FOR U.S. POPULATION AGED 65–74, 75–84, AND 75 YEARS AND OLDER, BY SEX—1990–1992

	AGE (YEARS)					
	65–74		75–84		85 and Older	
CONDITION	Male	Female	Male	Female	Male	Female
Heart conditions	178	94	222	139	161	155
Hypertension	316	403	300	417	330	390
Arthritis	358	493	423	610	440	671
Hearing impairments	334	204	438	222	549	550
Cataracts	100	140	167	259	218	265
Deformities or orthopedic impairments	159	171	157	212	167	267
Tinnitus	105	81	103	82	27	65
Frequent constipation	24	46	47	94	100	102
Varicose veins of lower extremities	37	103	44	106	49	64
Hemorrhoids	63	68	40	67	43	62
Chronic bronchitis	65	75	48	62	22	59
Chronic sinusitis	125	181	130	164	69	115
Diabetes	106	107	101	100	52	69
Glaucoma	45	42	67	57	64	106
Abdominal hernia	52	57	68	70	61	53
Cerebrovascular disease	70	48	83	72	127	84

(*Compiled from Cohen R. A., Van Nostrand R. F. Trends in the health care of older Americans: United States, 1994.* Vital and Health Statistics, 1995; 3 [30], 69, 130, Tables 8 & 31. Hyattsville, Md.: National Center for Health Statistics.)

lence with age. Some of these patterns may reflect not only frequency of the disease, but also, case fatality rates. Heart disease has both high incidence and high case fatality rates. Although digestive diseases and orthopedic impairments are common, they are rarely fatal. This fact contributes both to them ranking higher as a cause of morbidity than as a cause of mortality and, in part, to the increasing prevalence with age.

Alzheimer's and other demential diseases, while not among the leading chronic conditions in terms of numbers, are important because of their impact on the individual and family. Increased attention has been focused on Alzheimer's disease in recent years because of the announcement in 1996 of President Ronald Reagan's diagnosis with the condition. Alzheimer's disease is increasing in incidence concurrent with the aging of the population. Annual deaths from Alzheimer's disease, the easiest way to monitor frequency, increased 16-fold between 1967 and 1991 (Hoyert, 1996). Alzheimer's disease is thought to be substantially underreported on death certificates. The condition can be a major contributor to limitation of activity because of the necessity of sedating persons with the disease due to safety concerns and limited social interaction due to withdrawal of persons in the patient's social systems. Limitation of activity subsequently leads to functional limitation beyond that due to the mental capacity limitations brought on by the disease.

Limitation of Activity

An important reflection of the impact of disease in a population group is how much it interferes with normal activity. Table 11–7 shows the percentage of persons with activity limitations due to chronic disease for males and females older than 70 years of age living in the community in 1992. A slightly higher percentage of women have general limitation of activity than do men; women also have more limitation of major activity such as ability to work or keep house, which are included under the category of routine care activities. Whites have less limitation of activity than blacks. The overall rate of 60% of elderly persons who have no activity limitation is contrary to the popular image of the incapacitated elderly person, although it should be noted that the 40% of persons older than 70 years of age who do have such limitations represents a substantial increase over the percentage of those 45 to 64 years of age who have activity limitation (Cohen & Van Nostrand, 1995). The number of restricted activity days experienced by persons older than 65 years of age dropped to 30.3 days per person in 1987 from a high of 41.9 days per person in 1979 (National Center for Health Statistics, 1990). The 1992 rate remained at 30.2 for persons aged 65 to 74 years of age, but was 41.5 for those aged 75 to 84 and 49.6 for those 85 and older. Of these restricted activity days, among those aged 65 to 74 years, 11.8 (39%) were bed disability days, days when the individual was restricted to bed. The respective figures for the two older groups were 17.5 days (42%) and 25.3 days (50%).

In addition to the activity limitations brought on by the major causes of mortality, such as heart disease, cerebrovascular disease, diabetes, cancer, and chronic obstructive pulmonary disease, activity limitations are common among this age group because of problems with vision, hearing, mental status, musculoskeletal impairment, and incontinence. Women have a striking excess of activity limitation associated with the second-ranked chronic cause of activity limitations, arthritis and rheumatism. The percentage of women reporting activity limitation imposed by

TABLE 11–7. PERCENTAGE OF PERSONS OLDER THAN 70 YEARS OF AGE WITH LIMITATIONS OF ACTIVITY CAUSED BY CHRONIC CONDITIONS BY SEX AND RACE—UNITED STATES, 1992

TYPE OF LIMITATION	AGE 70 YEARS AND OLDER					AGE 85 YEARS AND OLDER			
		White		Black			White		Black
	Total	Male	Female	Male	Female	Total	Male	Female	Male & Female[a]
Personal care activity	8.3	6.7	8.6	10.7	15.6	20.0	13.9	20.1	37.1
Routine care activity	12.3	8.8	14.2	10.9	18.1	22.3	18.4	24.6	18.4
Other activity	19.1	22.9	16.9	23.6	15.4	14.3	17.8	13.6	9.3
Not limited	60.3	61.6	60.3	54.8	50.9	43.4	49.9	41.7	35.2

[a]Males and females are combined for blacks over age 85 due to small numbers.
(Compiled from Cohen R. A., Van Nostrand R. F. Trends in the health care of older Americans: United States, 1994. Vital and Health Statistics, 1995; 3 [30]. Table 3, pp 54–56. Hyattsville, Md.: National Center for Health Statistics.)

arthritis and rheumatism is nearly twice that of men (29.4% versus 15.6%), consistent with the higher prevalence of arthritis and rheumatism among women. Women have higher rates of fractures than do men, probably related to osteoporosis; this could contribute to the higher frequency of musculoskeletal-related limitations of activity.

Many older persons have several of these chronic conditions. It is probable that an individual who has multiple chronic conditions associated with limitation of activity is more likely to experience activity limitation than is an individual with only one condition. Nurses are most often the health care personnel who are in a position to assess the patient's lifestyle and resources and to plan adaptation of the environment and the individual's mode of functioning to minimize the impact of the illness on ADLs. But any clinical personnel who encounter elderly persons in a health care setting need to be alert to the necessity for such assessment and intervention. Maintaining independent function is a high priority for most older persons. Limitation of activity is further discussed in the section of this chapter on home care.

Hospitalization

Hospital discharges among the elderly often relate to chronic conditions or acute episodes of chronic conditions. Data on inpatient hospitalization come from the National Hospital Discharge Survey, conducted by the National Center for Health Statistics since 1965. Data from the most recent survey in 1993, show that, as with other age groups, the rate of hospitalization for those older than 65 years of age (based on the hospital discharge rate) has been declining (Graves, 1995). Rates for those older than 65 years peaked between 1980 and 1983 and have declined since (Fig. 11–6). This reflects in part a shift of a number of procedures to outpatient settings as a result of improved technology and treatment procedures and evidence from research that some procedures formerly done in hospitals could be done safely in ambulatory settings.

The most frequent primary diagnosis associated with discharges from short-stay hospitalizations is circulatory disease, particularly heart disease. The rate of discharge of those older than 65 years of age in 1993 was 1,093.9 per 10,000 population for all circulatory diseases; of this 771.3 per 10,000 was due to heart disease. Respiratory system disorders are the second most frequent primary discharge diagnosis, at 436.2 per 10,000 population, with the major contributing disorder being pneumonia. In third place are digestive system disorders. Neoplasms are fourth; malignant neoplasms account for 247.4 per 10,000 and benign *in situ* and other neoplasms for another 22.7 per 10,000. These data and the frequency of discharges for other major systems are shown in Table 11–8.

Nurses, physicians, and other health care personnel working in hospital inpatient units may develop biased views of the elderly if they base their impressions of the health of the older population on the patients for whom they care. Practitioners in these settings see elderly persons who are generally sicker and more disabled than the elderly population as a whole. This population of hospitalized elderly

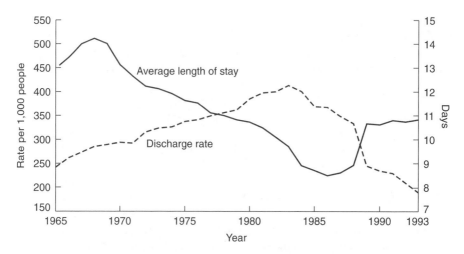

Figure 11–6. Trends in hospital usage by persons over 65 years of age: United States, 1965–1993. *(Adapted from U.S. Department of Health and Human Services.* Aging America: Trends and Projections *[1991 ed.]. [DHHS Publication No. (FCoA) 91-28001.] Washington, D.C.: U.S. Government Printing Office, 1991, Chart 4–8, p 125 [for years 1965–1988]; Gillum B. S., Graves E. J., Kozak L. J. Trends in hospital utilization: United States, 1988–1992.* Vital Health Statistics, 1996; *13 [124], 24–25, Tables 3 & 4. Hyattsville, Md.: National Center for Health Statistics; and Graves E. J. 1993 summary: National Hospital Discharge Survey. Advance data from* Vital and Health Statistics, 1995; *16(27) No. 264, 2, Tables 2 and 3. Hyattsville, Md.: National Center for Health Statistics.)*

requires careful discharge planning to enable them to function in the home and community and to obtain followup care after discharge.

Some of the discharge diagnoses could be iatrogenically caused during hospitalization. To avoid preventable iatrogenic disease, practitioners in hospital inpatient settings need to practice primary prevention. Effects of immobility, strange surroundings, new medications, and so on may have serious consequences for individuals of older ages. They are at higher risk for muscle atrophy, impairment of joint mobility, development of decubitus ulcers, and pneumonia. Appropriate nursing care can prevent these conditions from developing. Mental confusion caused by the strange, perhaps fearful surroundings and new medications also is a risk. Efforts to orient these patients to surroundings and events can decrease the risk. Monitoring for mentation changes that could be drug-related may permit early detection of such effects so that dosage can be adjusted or the medication changed.

Quality of care has a major impact on another measure, the length of hospital stay. This measure is used increasingly as a result of the diagnostic-related group (DRG) regulations passed by Congress. Average length of hospital stay declined steadily from the early 1970s until the early 1980s partly in response to utilization review procedures and payment criteria implemented by the federal government in relation to Medicare reimbursement (see Fig. 11–6). The decline was particularly steep for those over 65 years of age and length of stay varies considerably from one region of the country to another (Gillum et al, 1996). Because of shorter lengths of

TABLE 11–8. RATE OF DISCHARGES (PER 10,000 POPULATION) FROM SHORT-STAY HOSPITALIZATIONS FOR SELECTED FIRST-LISTED DIAGNOSES AND AVERAGE LENGTH OF STAY IN DAYS FOR PATIENTS 65 YEARS AND OLDER—UNITED STATES, 1993

CATEGORY OF DIAGNOSIS[a]	RATE PER 10,000	AVERAGE DAYS OF STAY
1. Diseases of the circulatory system	1,094	7.2
Heart disease	(771.3)	(6.8)
Cerebrovascular disease	(192.0)	(8.4)
2. Diseases of the digestive system	361.2	7.1
3. Neoplasms	270.0	8.4
Malignant	(247.4)	(8.6)
Benign, *in situ*, other	(22.7)	(6.6)
4. Diseases of the respiratory system	436.2	8.6
5. Diseases of the genitourinary system	201.8	6.1
6. Injury and poisoning	292.3	8.1
Fractures, all sites	(150.7)	(9.4)
Intracranial injury, lacerations, and open wounds	(10.7)	(10.5)
7. Diseases of the nervous system and sense organs	76.9	6.3
8. Diseases of the musculoskeletal system and connective tissue	186.3	8.2
9. Endocrine, nutritional, and metabolic diseases and immunity disorders	171.9	7.8
Diabetes	(55.4)	(9.6)
10. Mental disorders	87.7	12.5

[a]Diagnostic categories are based on the ninth revision, International Classification Disease.
(*Compiled from Graves E. J. 1993 summary: National Hospital Discharge Survey. Advance data from* Vital and Health Statistics, *No. 264. Hyattsville, Md.: National Center for Health Statistics, 1995, Tables 5 & 6, pp 5-6.*)

stay, patients hospitalized today are more acutely ill than in previous years and need more support services when they leave the hospital. In the western part of the country, where length of stay is generally shorter than in the rest of the country, planning for discharge often needs to begin almost as soon as hospitalization begins. Table 11–8 shows average length of hospital stay for common diagnoses among those over 65 years of age. Patients with mental disorders have the longest hospital stays at 12.5 days. Those with intracranial injuries, lacerations, and open wounds, a subcategory under injury and poisoning also have a long length of stay, with an average hospitalization of 10.5 days. Fractures, neoplasms, and cerebrovascular disease result in intermediate lengths of stay. Under the DRG system, hospitals are reimbursed for each patient based on a predetermined "usual and reasonable" length of stay for patients in that category of diagnosis (eg, fracture). These averages are determined from past data such as that shown in Table 11–8. If a patient stays less time than usual and the care while hospitalized is less costly than that of the average patient's used for determining a reimbursement figure, the hospital will make money; if a patient's costs are higher, then the hospital loses money. Quality of nursing care can have a major impact on how long a patient needs to remain in the hospital. Prevention of complications is essential.

Patients in Home Health, Hospice, and Nursing Homes

Those over 65 years of age represent 72% of hospice admissions and 75% of those admitted to home health services (Fig. 11–7). The former reflects the high rate of cancers in this age group and the latter the functional impairments. Nationally, this represented 1.38 million patients over 65 years of age in 1994. Almost 20% of home health patients were over 85 years of age. Only about 40% of those over 65 years of age receiving home health care lived alone. Spouses were the primary caregivers for those aged 65 to 74. Among those aged 75 to 84, caregiving was provided for about half by a spouse, and by a child or other relative for the rest. Over age 85, caregivers were most likely to be a child (54%), followed by a spouse (30%) or another relative (18%).

Functional status, as might be expected was better for the young elderly (65–74 years) than for older persons receiving home health services. Thirty-one percent of those aged 65 to 74 received no help in either ADLs or Instrumental Activities of Daily Living (IADLs) and only 30.3% received help in three or more

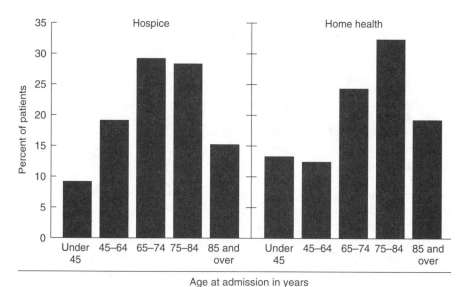

Agency	Under 45 years	45–64 years	65–74 years	75–84 years	85 years and over
Hospice	9	19	29	28	15
Home health	13	12	24	32	19

Figure 11–7. Hospice patients and home health care patients by age at admission: United States, 1993. Percent distribution of nursing home residents by morbidity status, age, and sex. (*Adapted from Cohen R. A., Van Nostrand R. F. Trends in the health of older Americans: United States, 1994.* Vital Health Statistics, 1995; 3 [30], Fig. 14, p 28, Hyattsville, Md.: National Center for Health Statistics.)

ADLs (Jones & Strahan, 1997). Among those over 85 years, only 25% received no help in ADLs or IADLs and 43% received help in three or more ADLs. Table 11–9 shows the percentage of patients in the three age groups that received assistance with particular ADLs and IADLs. For all elderly patients receiving help from home health, bathing and dressing were the individual ADLs for which the largest percentage required assistance (40–65%, depending on age). Light housework was the IADL requiring the most assistance. Meal preparation and medication dispensing also were required by about one quarter of service recipients.

Hospice offers a full range of services at the end of life, including personal care, social services, counseling, medications, physical therapy, homemaker/companion services, respite care (inpatient), referral services, dietary and nutritional services, physician services, high-tech care, and dental treatment services. Most frequently used services in all age groups are personal care, social services, counseling, and physical therapy. Hospice services are relatively less common for persons under 65 years of age; this age group accounted for only 27% of all hospice discharges. Of the hospice care among those over age 65 years, individuals 65 to 74 years accounted for 27.8%, those 75 to 84 years for 27.9%, and those 85 years and over the remaining 17.2%. Circulatory system diseases accounted for 40.5%, 32.3%, and 22.3%, respectively of discharges in the three age groups. For those 65 to 84 years, malignant neoplasms accounted for 28% of discharges versus 15% for those over 85 years.

TABLE 11–9. PERCENTAGE OF CURRENT HOME HEALTH PATIENTS RECEIVING HELP WITH SPECIFIC ADLs[a] AND IADLs[b] BY AGE—UNITED STATES, 1994

	AGE		
	65–74 Years	75–84 Years	85 Years and Older
ADL Help Provided			
Bathing	47.8	51.7	65.0
Dressing	40.0	43.4	55.9
Eating	7.8	9.3	10.5
Transferring	31.0	29.4	35.7
Walking	27.2	28.3	32.8
Using toilet	22.2	22.3	30.1
IADL Help Provided			
Light housework	37.2	39.9	46.7
Managing money	1.9[c]	2.1[c]	[c]
Shopping	15.8	17.5	22.5
Preparing meals	20.4	27.6	28.0
Taking medications	24.8	24.1	25.5

[a]ADL = activities of daily living.
[b]IADL = instrumental activities of daily living.
[c]Data does not meet standard of reliability or precision and is therefore not reported (sample size < 30) or if reported with a number may not be reliable because of small sample size (30–59) or standard error is > 30%.
(*Adapted from Jones A., Strahan G. The National Home and Hospice Care Survey: 1994 summary. Vital Health Statistics, 1997;* 13 *[126], 22, Table 12. Hyattsville, Md.: National Center for Health Statistics.*)

Congestive heart failure represented 27.3% and 24.4% of hospice discharges among those 75 to 84 years and 85 years and over (Jones & Strahan, 1997).

Admission to a nursing home implies a need for skilled nursing care, usually accompanied by activity limitation requiring assistance in ADLs for at least a period of time. Many residents of nursing homes require close supervision that cannot be easily provided at home or personal care that may be awkward or uncomfortable for family members. Incontinence is a frequent cause of nursing home placement and is present in nearly 50% of nursing home residents of all ages. Depression is present among approximately one quarter of nursing home patients and abusive behavior or wandering accounts of another 25 to 30%, depending on age group. The mean age of nursing home admission based on analysis of data from the 1995 National Nursing Home Survey was 75.8 years for men and 80.2 years for women (Murtaugh et al, 1997). Overall, 91% of all nursing home first admissions were among individuals over 65 years of age.

Heart disease, stroke, organic brain syndrome, arthritis/rheumatism, and diabetes are the five major diseases among nursing home discharges for women. Among men, heart disease, stroke, and organic brain syndrome are also the top three, but chronic obstructive respiratory disease and other psychoses are fourth and fifth. Senility is the only diagnosis found in common to both sexes among the sixth through tenth discharge diagnoses.

MAJOR FOCI OF PREVENTIVE EFFORTS

The leading causes of morbidity and mortality among those older than 65 years are, by and large, chronic diseases. In general, these develop over a long period of time either subsequent to a specific hazardous exposure, as with many cancers, or from long-term exposure to high-risk lifestyles, as with heart disease.

The concept of health held by the elderly appears to be a functional one—if they are able to carry out activities of daily living, they are likely to perceive their health as good. If they are functionally impaired, they perceive their health as fair or poor. Seeking health care is usually motivated by an actual or perceived dysfunction in health rather than preventive services, as evidenced by the 56% of physician office visits that are symptom-related and the additional 15% of visits related to initiation of treatment for a particular disease condition. These trends may result, in part, from a health care system that has had primarily a disease focus. Thus, interactions of persons in this age group with nurses, physicians, and other health care personnel are largely for purposes of treating acute symptoms, including acute exacerbations of chronic conditions, or for ongoing supervision and control of these conditions. Persons with worsening symptoms who have not previously been in the medical care system are likely to seek out necessary services to enable them to retain functional ability. Thus, the morbidity statistics for this age group largely reflect services for a tertiary level of intervention—diagnosis, treatment, and rehabilitation. Primary and secondary prevention receive much less emphasis.

This emphasis on illness care for the elderly is a function both of the aging process and of social circumstances. The elderly may wait longer to seek care, thinking that "nothing can be done," that they will be told they are terminally ill, that they can no longer live alone, or that it is too difficult or expensive to seek care unless the illness is serious. Also, health care professionals, who think of the aged as sick, are less likely to think in terms of primary and secondary prevention when dealing with this age group. The all-too-frequently heard statements of nurses or physicians, "What do you expect at your age?" or "You're in pretty good shape considering your age," reflect an expectation that the old will be sick. This expectation is bound to affect the elderly and their perceptions of which illnesses and symptoms are worth bothering to treat. Thus, the statistical picture of morbidity among the elderly may be as much a reflection of effects of the distribution of services, what Medicare and Medicaid will pay for, and attitudes of health care practitioners and society toward health and illness in old age as it is a reflection of the health status and needs of the elderly. For these reasons, rather than focusing this discussion of prevention only on the diseases of high statistical frequency, the author has chosen to discuss preventive efforts by focusing on the aging process and the special needs that arise as a result of this process. It is hoped that this approach will alert care providers to the potential benefit of considering primary and secondary prevention for the older population.

Physiological Effects of Aging

In many ways, older persons are physiologically different from their younger counterparts. They have a decreased capability for adaptation to physiological and psychological challenges or stresses. Aging is associated with altered immune responses to specific antigens, altered physiological responses to exercise, stress, administration of hormones, drugs, nutrients, and so on (Adelman, 1980). Although age is useful as an index representing the processes that causally underlie the universal, progressing, and deleterious changes we call aging, it is, at best, a rough approximation; individuals may be physiologically and psychologically younger or older than their years in a variety of respects, showing a range of individual performance on age-related functions within any single age cohort. For purposes of research on aging, some more precise measure that classifies the psychophysiological level of function for each individual may be important and could potentially be developed. It currently appears that chronological age is still the best predictor of changes in physiological and functional status.

Because of the physiological differences of the elderly resulting from aging, it must be recognized in the process of assessment that the same definition for normality versus abnormality used in younger populations may not be applicable. The physiological differences of the elderly must be considered in decisions of whether to treat or not to treat and how to treat if treatment is given. The amount and kind of drugs appropriate for the elderly may be quite different from those for younger persons. It has been recognized, for example, that adult-onset diabetes diagnosed in those older than 65 years of age often can benefit from treatment with insulin or insulin combined with oral hyperglycemic drugs, but using very low doses of insulin. Because insulin treatment can—on the positive side—induce antiatherogenic changes in serum lipids and lipoproteins and enhance general well-being, but have the negative effect of increasing body weight and risk of hypoglycemia, individualization of therapy is essential (Niskanen, 1996). Because the distribution of blood sugar values in the elderly population differs substantially from that in younger populations, questions have arisen about the appropriate definition of normal, ie, what values should be used to represent a diagnosis for diabetes? Blood sugars tend to increase as a normal part of the aging process. Is this increase in blood sugar at older ages associated with the same harmful effects as at younger ages? If not, then is treatment necessary? Such questions remain to be answered, but point out some of the special problems in managing disease in elderly patients.

Treatment with medication often can create new problems because of the high sensitivity of the elderly patient to drugs. Not only must physicians concern themselves with adjusting dose to account for this sensitivity, but both physicians and nurses must be alert to unexpected physiological or psychological changes in a patient that might reflect a drug response. Drug treatment should be considered as a source of sudden mentation changes in elderly patients.

Physiological changes of aging may also affect patterns of sleep and rest, elimination, and nutrition. Sensory function often decreases slowly but steadily; visual, auditory, taste, tactile, and temperature senses may all be affected. These changes, in turn, affect the individual's perceptions of the immediate environment, often leading to a sense of isolation or loss of control at a time when physical disability or disruptions in roles and relationships caused by death or illness of a spouse or friends interfere with existing social networks and available human resources. If psychological adaptation is also impaired or decreased during the aging process, then ability to tolerate or cope with stress is impaired. Therefore, assessment of an older client must consider habitual patterns of functioning, methods of communicating, likes and dislikes, thoughts and feelings, beliefs and values, and resources so that any response to a new illness or disability helps the patient comply with treatment and maintain as much as possible of what is important to him or her. Furthermore, such background factors are important baseline information in plans for primary and secondary intervention.

Accidents and the Elderly

The primary prevention activities with perhaps the greatest potential among the elderly relate to accident prevention. Accidents and injuries are among the ten leading causes of mortality and are major causes of morbidity and disability for those over 65 years of age. More than half of accidental deaths in this age group are due to falls that may occur in the place of residence. Seventy-five percent of all injury deaths among the elderly are due to falls, fires and contact with hot substances, and vehicular crashes, including those involving pedestrians. As Hogue points out in an excellent discussion of the epidemiology of injury in older age groups, existing data indicate that accidents, like diseases, are not random events; they should be preventable if causes are known (Hogue, 1980).

Physiological factors that are known to contribute to an increased risk of injury among the elderly are listed in Table 11–10 along with interventions that decrease the likelihood of accidental injury. Optimizing available sensory function is crucial.

TABLE 11–10. SOME PHYSICAL FACTORS CONTRIBUTING TO AN INCREASED RISK OF INJURY AMONG THE ELDERLY AND POTENTIAL INTERVENTIONS

PHYSICAL FACTOR	SPECIFIC CONSIDERATIONS	APPROACHES TO PREVENTION OF INJURY
Vision	Decreased visual acuity	Use of vision aids
	Increased sensitivity to light and glare	Homemaking adaptations such as nonglare utensils; wearing of sunglasses, hats with brims to reduce glare outside
	Slower adaptation to darkness	Use of night lights; waiting for eyes to adjust before moving from place to place
	Blurring of contrast sensitivity	Use of contrasting colors to enhance visibility
	Alterations in visual field	Placement of objects at eye level; looking to sides before moving; colored tape on edges of steps
	Decreased spatial ability	Orientation instruction
		Hearing aid
Hearing	Decreased threshold sensitivity	Hearing aid; leaving car window open when driving so warning signals (eg, sirens) can be heard
	Decreased loudness perception	
Sensory-motor function	Decreased reaction time	Anticipating events
	Loss of balance ⎫ Gait changes ⎭	Proper shoes; slower rate of walking with maximum width of base; lifting feet off the ground; nonslip floor surfaces; walking aids (eg, cane)
	Coordination impairment	Larger handles on cooking utensils, canister lids, and other household implements
	Decreased tactile sensitivity	Use of bath thermometers to assess water temperature; daily assessment of extremities for undetected injuries
Musculoskeletal	Decreased muscle strength	Lighter cooking utensils and other household implements
	Decreased bone density	Avoiding falls by maintaining clear walkways; no throw rugs
	Decreased agility ⎫ Postural flexion ⎭	Structural changes (eg, stall showers rather than step-over tubs), rubber mats, grab bars
	Decreased endurance	Frequent rest periods
	Joint deformity or change in range of motion	Long-handled implements; adjusting placement of objects
	Pain	Medication
Circulatory system	Altered cerebral function with tendency toward confusion	Avoiding change of environmental arrangements (eg, furniture placement)
	Orthostatic hypotension	Changing position slowly (eg, sitting before standing when rising from recumbent position); avoiding sudden movements

Any functional deficit can be compensated to some extent by adjustments in the physical environment that enable the individual to function safely with their handicap. Making such adjustments in the home environment is usually feasible. Making changes in the environment outside of the home is more difficult and probably requires intervention by public policy makers. Heavy traffic, bustling crowds in public places, and public transportation may all be difficult for a person with sensory or musculoskeletal impairments. It may be unsafe for some elderly persons to drive, and it may be necessary periodically to screen elderly individuals for adequacy of vision, hearing, and reaction time for renewal of driver's licenses. Alternative sources of transportation may have to be provided to such elderly individuals as a public service so they can maintain a degree of independence. Many forms of public transportation currently available are physically challenging to the elderly. The high steps on buses and crowded vehicles that may require the elderly to stand are difficult for a young person with excellent balance but almost impossible for many elderly persons. More readily available seating in public places where the elderly can rest would be helpful. Public education programs could sensitize the public to the special needs of the elderly.

Health care providers must also be aware of the likelihood that once an injury occurs, the effects on the older person are likely to be more serious than on a younger person. Because of osteoporosis, fractures are more likely to occur. Injuries resulting in breaks in the skin are more likely to produce infection because of decreased immune response. Activity restrictions imposed by the injury may contribute to permanent effects on physical mobility because of a loss of muscle tone, balance, and so on during the period of recuperation. Also, preexisting musculoskeletal conditions may be aggravated contributing to the injury and producing a permanent musculoskeletal impairment.

Fear of a future accident may also lead older persons to limit their activity. Caregivers must plan ways to minimize these effects and to provide active rehabilitation once an initial injury has healed. This is particularly important in view of the link of an older person's self-perception of health to functional ability. Furthermore, many of the chronic conditions associated with morbidity and mortality in the elderly may be exacerbated by the inactivity associated with accidental injury. Regular exercise may contribute to maintaining physical as well as social and emotional health. Cardiovascular function is enhanced by regular exercise; a lack of such activity may contribute to lower cardiopulmonary efficiency. Some gastrointestinal conditions may also be affected; inactivity may contribute to decreased motility of the intestines leading to constipation and can affect appetite and eating patterns. Older persons are more prone to respiratory infection as a result of decreased adaptive response of the immune system; inactivity may increase the risk. Because regular exercise also contributes to better oxygen uptake from the blood into the heart and musculoskeletal system and increased glucose tolerance, such enforced inactivity may have implications for diabetic control. Exercise, with its cardiopulmonary benefits, may also contribute to reducing the severity of effects in the event of respiratory infection. Research has demonstrated that regular excercise can increase muscle strength, endurance, and organ function even in older persons (McCartney et al, 1996; Fielding, 1996; Nieman, 1997). It can also result in an improved social life, fewer physician visits, and fewer medications required (Singh et al, 1997).

Chronic Illness Prevention and Management in Older Persons

Heart disease, cerebrovascular disease, cancer, arthritis, and chronic dementia lead to much disability and often institutionalization among the population older than 65 years of age. Risk factors and causes of many of these conditions have been discussed in earlier chapters. By age 65, it is often too late for primary prevention of these diseases. Secondary prevention, particularly risk factor identification and treatment, may still be appropriate.

A major goal for those older than 65 years of age is to prevent disability from chronic diseases and to maintain maximum independence in the activities of life. This requires thorough evaluation and diagnosis, appropriate vigorous therapy of treatable conditions, and a comprehensive rehabilitative approach. Conditions such as thinning of bones in postmenopausal women, if detected early, can be treated by administration of additional estrogen, calcium/vitamin D, or alendronate. Vitamin supplements may be appropriate, particularly for those on limited or unbalanced diets because of restrictions ordered for certain diseases (eg, cardiovascular or gastrointestinal disease) or because of dietary limitations imposed by dental problems. The U.S. Preventive Services Task Force recommends the screening, counseling, and immunization services listed in Table 11–11 for persons older than age 65 years (U.S. Preventive Services Task Force, 1989). Many of these target diseases and delivery of screening procedures, counseling, and intervention efforts relate to goals identified under the Surgeon General's Healthy People 2000 report (U.S. Department of Health, Education, and Welfare, 1979), where the main goals for elderly persons were directed toward improvement in health and quality of life, particularly the reduction of restricted activity resulting from chronic conditions.

The presence of multiple chronic illnesses often leads to multiple physicians, each treating their own specialty disease. Patients may accumulate a wide spectrum of drugs over the years, some of which should not be taken in conjunction with others and some of which are outdated, but that the patient may still use as self-treatment for particular symptoms. Inappropriate use of drugs may exacerbate existing chronic conditions and precipitate new health problems. Mentation changes, cardiac irregularity, and dizziness are some of the problems that may arise. Periodic review of all drugs taken by older patients is useful. The Healthy People 2000 goals encourage giving written information when drugs are prescribed so that patients will use drugs more appropriately.

We know that some conditions of aging can be helped through appropriate dietary intervention. Common gastrointestinal maladies of older persons, such as constipation, can be helped by high fiber diets and adequate hydration. Aging is accompanied by a decrease in lean body mass and an increase in the proportion of adipose tissue. Age-related degenerative changes in body composition also include

TABLE 11–11. PREVENTIVE SERVICES RECOMMENDED FOR PERSONS 65 YEARS AND OLDER[a]

SCREENING	COUNSELING	IMMUNIZATIONS	WATCH FOR

History:
  Prior symptoms of transient
    ischemic attack
  Dietary intake
  Physical activity
  Tobacco/alcohol/drug use
  Functional status at home
Physical Examination:
  Height and weight
  Blood pressure
  Visual acuity
  Hearing and hearing aids
  Clinical breast examination
  High-Risk Groups:
    Auscultation for carotid
      bruits
    Complete skin examination
    Complete oral cavity exami-
      nation
    Palpation of thyroid nodules
Laboratory/Diagnostic Procedures:
  Nonfasting total blood choles-
    terol
  Dipstick urinalysis
  Mammogram
  Thyroid function tests
  High-Risk Groups:
    Fasting plasma glucose
    Tuberculin skin test (PPD)
    Electrocardiogram
    Papanicolaou smear
    Fecal occult blood/sigmoi-
      doscopy
    Fecal occult blood/colonoscopy
	Diet and Exercise:
	  Fat (especially saturated fat),
	    cholesterol, complex carbohy-
	    drates, fiber, sodium, calcium
	  Caloric balance
	  Selection of exercise program
	Substance Use:
	  Tobacco cessation
	  Alcohol and other drugs
	    Limiting alcohol consumption
	    Driving/other dangerous
	      activities while under the
	      influence
	    Treatment for abuse
	Injury Prevention:
	  Prevention of falls
	  Safety belts
	  Smoke detector
	  Smoking near bedding or uphol-
	    stery
	  Hot-water heater temperature
	  Safety helmets
	Dental Health:
	  Regular dental visits, tooth
	    brushing, flossing
	Other Primary Preventive Measures:
	  Glaucoma testing by eye
	    specialist
	  High-Risk Groups:
	    Discussion of estrogen
	      replacement therapy
	    Discussion of aspirin therapy
	    Skin protection from ultravi-
	      olet light
		Tetanus-diphtheria
		  booster
		Influenza vaccine
		Pneumococcal vaccine
		High-Risk Groups:
		  Hepatitis B vaccine
			Depression symptoms
			Suicide risk factors
			Abnormal bereavement
			Changes in cognitive
			  function
			Medications that increase
			  risk of falls
			Signs of physical abuse or
			  neglect
			Malignant skin lesions
			Peripheral arterial disease
			Tooth decay, gingivitis,
			  loose teeth

[a]This list of services reflects only topics reviewed by the U.S. Preventive Services Task Force. Conditions not specifically examined by the Task Force include chronic obstructive pulmonary disease, hepatobiliary disease, bladder cancer, endometrial disease, travel-related illness, prescription drug abuse, and occupational illness and injury.

(*Adapted from The U.S. Preventive Services Task Force.* Guide to clinical preventive services: An assessment of the effectiveness of 169 interventions. *Baltimore: Williams & Wilkins, 1989.*)

a loss of muscle mass, motor function, and bone tissue, leading to fragile, easily fragmented bones. Whether such age-related decreases in muscle fiber and bone density can be prevented or stabilized by eating more foods with amino acids, protein, and calcium is unknown (Evans & Campbell, 1997).

Maintaining adequate nutrition in the elderly poses a challenge. Many older persons report a loss of appetite. For many others, the dietary restrictions imposed for treatment of chronic conditions such as diabetes or heart disease make food less interesting; and it is difficult to break eating habits of a lifetime. Many medications used in treating chronic diseases may have gastrointestinal side effects. Dental disease may contribute to limited food intake. Depression that may follow loss of a spouse or friends may lead to anorexia. Eating is often a social event and when one becomes isolated, whether because of deaths, physical incapacity, or limited economic resources, poor nutrition may follow. A well-balanced diet and adequate hydration, however, are essential to maintenance of health. Ingenuity is required when working with older patients to tempt finicky appetites and provide access to nourishing meals and social settings that facilitate maintenance of nutrition.

Keeping older patients in familiar surroundings by adapting their environment to physical limitations can help maintain independence and can help prevent the depression and withdrawal that often accompany relocation. Involuntary relocation, in particular, often challenges the older person's adaptive abilities and may contribute to symptoms resembling senility. Illness often necessitates such relocation, whether to an acute care setting or to a long-term care facility. Visual and verbal reminders to elderly patients of where they are and why as well as how they can obtain desired services (ie, "press the call button if you need the nurse") may help. Appropriate architectural features to minimize barriers and hazards to independent function may also help prevent mental and emotional difficulties. This is important in the home as well as in care facilities. Appropriate changes in the home physical environment can facilitate maintaining independent function for a longer time.

The goal of less dependency for the elderly benefits both older citizens and society in general. Society benefits through reduced costs. Older citizens benefit from increased self-esteem and quality of life.

REFERENCES

Adams P. F., Marano M. A. (1995) Current estimates from the National Health Interview Survey, 1994. *Vital Health Statistics, 10,* 193. Hyattsville, Md.: National Center for Health Statistics.

Adelman R. (July 1980) *Definitions of biological aging.* In S. Haynes, M. Feinleib (Eds.). Second Conference on the Epidemiology of Aging. (DHHS Publication No. [NIH] 80-969). Bethesda, Md.: U.S. Department of Health and Human Services, pp 9–14.

Blackburn H., Luepker R. (1997). Heart disease. In J. Last (Ed.). *Maxcy-Rosenau-Last Public Health and Preventive Medicine.* Appleton-Century-Crofts, New York: 1980, pp 1168–1201.

Cohen R. A., Bloom B., Simpson G., Parsons P. E. Access to health care. Part 3: Older adults. *Vital Health Statistics, 10,* 198. Hyattsville, Md.: National Center for Health Statistics.

Cohen R. A., Van Nostrand R. F. (1995) Trends in the health of older Americans: United States, 1994. *Vital Health Statistics, 3,* 30. Hyattsville, Md.: National Center for Health Statistics.

Evans W. J., Cyr-Campbell D. (1997) Nutrition, exercise, and healthy aging. *Journal of the American Dietetic Association 97*(6), 632–638.

Fielding R. A. (1996) Effects of exercise training in the elderly: Impact of progressive resistance training on skeletal muscle and whole-body protein metabolism. *Proceedings of the Nutrition Society, 54*(3), 665–675.

Gillum B. S., Graves E. J., Kozak L. J. (1996) Trends in hospital utilization: United States 1988–1992. *Vital Health Statistics, 13,* 124. Hyattsville, Md.: National Center for Health Statistics.

Goa K. L., Haria M., Wilde M. I. (1997) Lisinopril. A review of its pharmacology and use in the management of the complications of diabetes mellitus. *Drugs, 53*(6), 1081–1105.

Graves E. J. (1995) National Hospital Discharge Survey: Annual summary, 1993. *Vital Health Statistics, 13,* 121. Hyattsville, Md.: National Center for Health Statistics.

Hebert R., Brayne C., Spiegelhalter D. (1997) Incidence of functional decline and improvement in a community-dwelling, very elderly population. *American Journal of Epidemiology, 145*(10), 935–944.

Hogue C. (July 1980) *Epidemiology of injury in older age.* In S. Haynes, M. Feinleib (Eds.). Second Conference on the Epidemiology of Aging. (DHHS [NIH] Publication No. 50-9691). Bethesda, Md.: U.S. Department of Health and Human Services.

Hoyert D. L. (1996) Mortality trends for Alzheimer's disease, 1979–1991. *Vital Health Statistics, 20,* 28. Hyattsville, Md.: National Center for Health Statistics.

Jomes A., Strahan G. (1997) The National Home and Hospice Care Survey: 1994, summary. *Vital Health Statistics, 13,* 126. Hyattsville, Md.: National Center for Health Statistics.

Jerums G., Allen T. J., Gilbert R. E., Hammond J., Cooper M. E., Campbell D. J., Faffaele J. (1995) Natural history of early diabetic nephropathy: What are the effects of therapeutic intervention? Melbourne Diabetic Nephropathy Study Group. *Journal of Diabetes Complications, 9*(4), 301–314.

Kochanek D., Kochanek M. A., Hudson B. L. (1995) Advanced report of final mortality statistics, 1995. *Monthly Vital Statistics Report, 43,* 6 (suppl.). Hyattsville, Md.: National Center for Health Statistics.

McCartney N., Hicks A. L., Martin J., Webber C. E. (1996). A longitudinal trial of weight training in the elderly: Continued improvements in year 2. *Journals of Gerontology, Series A, Biological Sciences and Medical Care Services, 51*(6), B425–433.

Murtaugh C. M., et al. (1997) The National Nursing Home and Hospice Care Survey: 1994 summary. *Vital Health Statistics, 13,* 126. Hyattsville, Md.: National Center for Health Statistics.

Nieman D. C. (1997) Exercise immunology: Practical applications. *International Journal of Sports Medicine, 18* (suppl. 1): S91–100.

Niskanen L. (1996) Insulin treatment in elderly patients with non-insulin-dependent diabetes mellitus. A double-edged sword? *Drugs and Aging, 8*(3), 183–192.

Shappert S. M. (1997) National hospital ambulatory medical care survey: 1992 emergency department summary. *Vital Health Statistics, 13,* 125. Hyattsville, Md.: National Center for Health Statistics.

Shurtleff D. (1974) *Some characteristics related to the incidence of cardiovascular disease and death.* The Framingham Study, Section 30 (U.S. Department of Health, Education, and Welfare Publication No. [NIH] 74-599). Washington, D.C.: U.S. Government Printing Office.

Singh N. A., Clements K. M., Fiatarone M. A. (1997) A randomized controlled trial of progressive resistance training in depressed elders. *Journals of Gerontology, Series A, Biological Sciences and Medical Sciences.* 52(1), M27–35.

U.S. Bureau of the Census. (1996) *Statistical abstract of the United States, 1996 (116th ed.).* Washington, D.C.: U.S. Bureau of the Census.

U.S. Department of Health and Human Services. (1991) *Aging America: Trends and Projections.* (DHHS Publication No. [FCoA] 91-28001). Washington, D.C.: U.S. Government Printing Office.

U.S. Department of Health, Education, and Welfare. (1979) *Healthy people 2000: The Surgeon General's report on health promotion and disease prevention.* (DHEW Publication No. [PHS] 79-5507). Washington, D.C.: U.S. Government Printing Office.

U.S. Preventive Services Task Force. (1989) *Guide to clinical preventive services: An assessment of the effectiveness of 169 interventions.* Baltimore: Williams & Wilkins.

Woodwell D. A., Schappert S. M. (1995) National ambulatory medical care survey: 1993 summary. Advance data from *Vital Health Statistics,* No. 270. Atlanta: Centers for Disease Control and Prevention.

Applications of Epidemiology

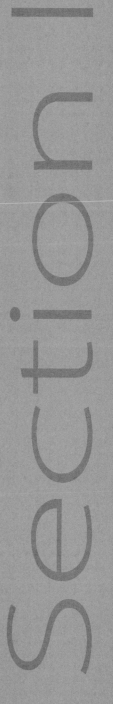

Etiology and Natural History

*i*ntervention in the disease process is aimed at halting, reversing, or minimizing the process of pathological change. In general, the earlier in the disease process an intervention occurs, the easier it is to prevent or minimize damage. The natural history of a disease provides a description of the process by which the disease occurs and progresses in humans. Knowledge of the natural history of a disease and ability to relate the stage of disease progression to the event of diagnosis allows a clinician to choose the appropriate treatment for each patient. To plan and evaluate public health and clinical interventions, it is necessary to know the natural history of the disease.

This chapter includes general concepts that are of importance in understanding the natural history of a disease and a description of the type of knowledge about the natural history of a specific disease that is needed by the clinician. Applications of natural history to health care administration and patient management are integrated throughout. Finally, issues relating to studying the natural history are discussed.

GENERAL CONCEPTS

The topics discussed in this section are included because they provide important concepts for understanding the remainder of the chapter, and because they have a significant impact on the choice of intervention. Understanding these concepts also should enable the health professional to critically review the literature on the natural history of a disease. One important concept, the levels of prevention—primary, secondary, and tertiary—were presented in Chapter 2 as they apply to each period or stage of a disease. Reviewing Table 2–1 and the Prevention section of Chapter 2 before reading this chapter would be helpful.

Natural History: A Continuum

As previously stated, there are two aspects to the natural history of a disease. One aspect is the process by which the disease occurs and the other is the process of disease progression. To describe the natural history is to describe the changes that lead from health to disease. Progression means to move forward, usually in a continuous, connected manner. To describe the progression of a disease, then, is to describe its movement from one stage to another along the natural history continuum, beginning where the individual is healthy and totally free of any abnormal or pathological condition to the opposite end of the continuum where frank pathology and clinical findings are present and death may occur. To understand the process, researchers attempt to identify significant phases along the continuum. These phases are divided into two periods which are subdivided into stages. The two periods are called prepathogenesis and pathogenesis.

Prepathogenesis.   As discussed in Chapter 2, the first period before initiation of any changes at the cellular level is prepathogenesis. This period includes two stages, *susceptibility* and *adaptation*. Susceptibility represents a time of vulnerability when the ground work has been laid for development of disease through presence of factors favoring its occurrence. Susceptibility is followed by the stage of adaptation. Adaptation is the time when intracellular or intercellular reactions to some agent or stimulus may be occurring, but the reactions reflect the normal adaptation response of the cell or the functional system (eg, the immune system).

Pathogenesis.   The second period is pathogenesis. The first stage in this period is *early pathogenesis,* a phase of subclinical cellular and tissue changes that represent the failure of the cell, tissue, or system to continue to adapt to or cope with the presence of a noxious agent or stimulus. The difference in response between prepathogenesis and early pathogenesis is determined by whether the response represents normal adaptation or a breakdown in the ability to adapt. A breakdown of normal adaptive response thus represents the beginning of the pathogenesis period, which extends from the earliest pathological changes to death. *Latency,* or *induction,* is the time between exposure to a disease-producing agent and presence of unequivocal disease. The period of latency includes prepathogenesis and at least part of the early pathogenesis stage.

Symptoms appear in some diseases during early pathogenesis, before any available technology can identify the presence of early pathogenesis. For example, altered emotional responses may occur in the early pathogenesis period for some brain tumors. In other instances, symptoms do not appear until late pathogenesis. A lump detectable by physical examination of the breast, nipple retraction, orange skin appearance of the breast, and nipple discharge are considered by most clinicians to be symptoms that are very late in the natural history of breast cancer. In such cases, where detection through symptoms occurs late in the natural history, early detection may be possible by laboratory or other technological procedures. In the case of breast cancer, mammography can detect the disease before onset of symptoms.

Figure 12–1, which represents the natural history continuum as a straight line, illustrates the relationship of the stages of prepathogenesis and pathogenesis to one another. At the left end of the line, points between *a* and *b* represent complete health with no abnormalities, even at the intracellular level. This is the period of prepathogenesis during which the individual may be susceptible but has not had contact with the agent. At the right end of the line is the worst stage of illness, or death, point *e*. The period of intracellular changes occurs from *b* to *c,* beginning when an agent has contact with a susceptible host and the first intracellular changes occur. This is also the beginning of pathogenesis. Pathogenesis extends from *b* to *e*.

In many diseases it is only with the identification of substages within the stages of pathogenesis that it is possible to study and understand the onset of a disease and how and why the disease progresses. Cancer of the uterine cervix is one disease for which the natural history and its stages are reasonably well defined. The development of cervical cancer is believed to involve passage from normal cervical epithelial tissue to a dysplastic stage, to carcinoma *in situ,* to invasive carcinoma of the cervix, and then to death. There are five stages of cancer of the cervix, beginning with carcinoma *in situ* (stage 0) and extending to stage IV—spread beyond the true pelvis or with clinical involvement of the bladder and rectum. Stages I through IV each have several substages (Nelson et al, 1989). Identification of these stages, which describes the process of the natural history, is the first step in understanding the progression of the disease. How or why it progresses through these stages may be studied once the stages are identified. Risk factors for the disease are important in determining how and why the process begins and progresses. Risk factors are discussed further in the following paragraphs.

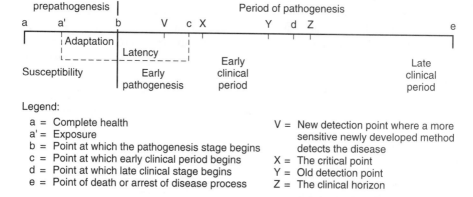

Figure 12–1. Detection point, critical point, and natural history of a disease.

Multifactorial Diseases and Stage-specific Risk Factors

As stated in Chapter 2, multiple factors are generally involved in the onset and progression of a given disease. Several agents may interact in initiating the first stage of pathogenesis, whereas others may promote the development of subsequent stages. Still others may affect the rate at which the stages of the disease progress. Cancer, for example, is believed to result from a series of steps that include an initiation phase and a promotion phase (Pitot, 1981). One specific agent may produce an initial change in deoxyribonucleic acid (DNA). A second factor may prevent or prolong the repair of DNA, producing multiple cells with abnormal DNA. A third agent may stimulate nucleic acid synthesis, which may lead to abnormal cells. Whether these abnormal cells are destroyed or whether they progress to malignancy may be dependent on yet another factor, and whether the growth and multiplication of malignant cells continues unchecked may depend on still other factors. In this scenario, a cancer could be broken down into these stages: normal cellular DNA, abnormal cellular DNA, abnormal cells, malignant cells, malignant neoplasm, and invasive malignant neoplasm.

After stages in the natural history have been identified, research focuses on identifying the factors associated with each stage of the natural history and how they relate to progression or transition between stages. Diabetes may serve as an example to further emphasize this point. Insulin-dependent diabetes mellitus (IDDM) has been associated with a genetic predisposition (although there is a lack of good concordance between identical twins); environmental factors (beta-cell cytotoxic virus and beta-cell cytotoxic chemicals), presence of autoimmune phenomena in pancreatic islands of Langerhans, seasonality, a temporal relationship to mumps, and the presence of neutralizing antibodies to Coxsackie B_4 virus (Nerup, 1981). Attempts to understand what causes IDDM must consider logical relationships between these multiple factors, including potential biological mechanisms. A natural history that could be hypothesized as a sensible explanation for these associations is shown in Figure 12–2. The finding of genetic association that does not exhibit good twin concordance may reflect that only one twin was exposed to the viral agent and developed the infection. Seasonality and temporal associations may reflect the role of the viral agent in the disease; presence of viruses in the environment may fluctuate with time and by season, thus explaining the seasonality in the onset of IDDM. The presence of autoimmune phenomena and neutralizing antibodies may reflect beta-cell destruction as a result of autoimmune processes or lack of regeneration

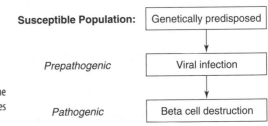

Figure 12–2. Hypothesized relationships in the natural history of insulin-dependent diabetes mellitus.

after damage by the virus. Beta-cell destruction may also occur as a direct result of viral infection in susceptible individuals. However, additional risk factors must also be fit into the picture, including obesity, particularly excess intraabdominal fat; activity level; diet; and smoking (DeFronzo, 1997). These characteristics could affect response to a viral infection or operate independently on beta-cell destruction. Alternatively, obesity could result from an inherited defect that produces insulin resistance associated with an abnormality in the glycogen synthesis pathway in muscle (DeFronzo, 1997).

Viral infection is a stage-specific risk factor in this hypothesized natural history of IDDM; it is not a risk factor for development of a genetic predisposition in the hypothesized natural history. Risk factors associated with only one stage in the natural history of a disease may be considered *stage-specific risk factors*.

Once the stages of a disease and the corresponding specific risk factors have been identified, methods of intervention at each stage can be studied. For IDDM, this may mean genetic manipulation (a method of primary prevention currently being investigated), immunization of genetically susceptible individuals (also primary prevention), medical treatment to eliminate or reduce beta-cell destruction (secondary and tertiary prevention), or medical treatment with insulin to control hyperglycemia (tertiary prevention). It is not mandatory to prove that a factor causes a stage-specific reaction before doing a randomized trial to determine if an intervention method is effective. In fact, many hypothesized causal factors are verified as causal factors only through the process of a randomized intervention trial. For instance, if vaccination for Coxsackie B_4 virus in genetically susceptible individuals was found in a randomized trial to eliminate the bulk of IDDM cases, then the hypothesized series of events is validated.

Unfortunately, many diseases are not understood well enough to identify stage-specific risk factors. Of course, the stages of a disease must be known or hypothesized before stage-specific risk factors may be studied. Fortunately, stages for most diseases are known or hypothesized; stage-specific risk factors may then be hypothesized from the risk factors known to be associated with the disease. Findings of research on stage-specific risk factors will have a major impact on intervention techniques used in health care practice in the future.

Technology and Detection of Disease

The concept of the clinical horizon, which was first presented in Chapter 2, is a direct result of the status of research on stages of the natural history and is a function of available methods of detection. As previously stated, the *clinical horizon* is an imaginary line dividing the point where there are detectable signs and symptoms from where none are detectable. Detectable is the key word in this statement. Complete cell death or significant aberrant cellular changes are usually required to produce clinically recognizable disease. Although signs of early pathogenesis may be present, they are usually not measurable. Cell death and significant morphological cellular changes reflected in clinical disease are extremely late effects in the natural history of most diseases.

Scientists may be able to describe the mechanisms of prepathogenesis and pathogenesis of some diseases at the intracellular or tissue level. Thus, stages of change in the cell may be known by research scientists. But until these changes can be detected by tests with proven predictive validity for clinical disease, early detection is not possible and diagnosis cannot be made until symptoms have been present for some time; until nonspecific symptoms become more specific to the particular disease in process, it cannot be diagnosed and treated.

An improvement in diagnostic technology will frequently change the stage at which diagnosis is possible and, therefore, the clinical horizon. Before x-rays were available, tumors were usually very large, causing severe symptoms prior to diagnosis. Better quality x-rays and computer enhancement made it possible to detect changes when symptoms are milder or absent and thus to diagnose the disease earlier in its natural history. This point is demonstrated graphically in Figure 12–1. In the past, cancer was detected between points *d* and *e*. The clinical horizon was extremely late. Now, cancers can be detected in the earlier clinical period of pathogenesis between *c* and *d*. The advent of electron microscopy, nuclear magnetic resonance, and other methods may move the clinical horizon farther toward the left of the period of prepathogenesis, *b* to *c*. Stages that precede the clinical horizon can only be hypothesized before more sensitive methods of detection are developed. Therefore, knowledge about the natural history of a disease is limited by our detection methods. To reiterate, the clinician should keep abreast of changes in diagnostic techniques and how they affect our knowledge of the natural history of a disease. Such knowledge may have profound effects on application of secondary prevention activities and on the survival associated with a disease.

The Critical Point in Relation to the Detection Point

The *critical point* is a theoretical time in the natural history that is crucial in determining whether there will be major or severe consequences of the disease. Examples of major consequences are serious disabilities, birth defects, coma, and death. If the point of detection is at point *Y* (see Fig. 12–1) and the critical point is at point *X*, then no method of secondary prevention will be available. Cancer again serves as an example. Until recently, a breast cancer of sufficient size to be detected by x-ray was considered to be in a late stage of pathogenesis; the neoplasm had existed for some time before detection was possible and was often associated with metastasis. Treatment of breast tumors at this stage was not very successful. Let us say the detection point was at point *Y* during the invasive stage of pathogenesis. Because treatment of tumors (tertiary prevention) at this point was not very successful, the critical point was probably farther to the left in the continuum, say point *X*. A new method of detection must be capable of detecting the tumor to the left of this critical point if survival from breast cancer is to be improved. Current methods of mammography appear to detect breast cancers before this critical point for women older than 50 years of age. Significant improvement in survival (a 30% decrease in mortality) of such women with breast cancer was demonstrated in a 1973 randomized trial of 62,000 women aged 40 to 64 years (Shapiro, 1977). This increase in survival was not found for breast cancer in the younger women studied. It might be presumed that the type of breast cancer affecting younger women has a critical point earlier in the natural history of the disease than does breast cancer affecting women past the age of 50 (this age difference may reflect premenopausal- versus postmenopausal-type breast cancers).

Unfortunately, this was the only randomized trial of mammography ever conducted in the United States. Subsequent trials in other countries involved inadequate numbers of women between the ages of 40 and 49 to examine effects of mammography on mortality in this age group (Mettlin & Smart, 1994), so screening mammograms for women under 50 years remains controversial. In fact, the National Institutes of Health consensus panel concluded that data do not warrant a universal recommendation for screening mammography for all women in their 40s, although a minority report disagreed (National Institutes of Health, 1997).

The improved detection techniques for breast cancer have moved the detection point toward the left to an earlier point in the natural history for women over 50 years of age. When the detection point shifts to where it precedes the critical point, then significant opportunities for secondary prevention become available. Screening for breast cancer was once not an effective method of prevention for breast cancer because screening had no impact on survival. Now that the detection point has changed and appears to precede the critical point for most breast cancers in older women, screening is an efficacious method of secondary prevention for women older than 50.

Efficacy is the extent to which a specific intervention (procedure, regimen, or service) produces a beneficial result under ideal conditions. Ideally, the determination of efficacy is based on the results of a randomized controlled trial. The objective of the intervention is to minimize or prevent damage.

The question of whether a particular intervention actually minimizes or prevents damage is an important one. The answer requires knowledge about a disease's natural history. Minimizing or preventing damage means that the natural history will be changed or altered in some way by the intervention. Changes or alterations considered beneficial are elimination of the disease, minimization of effect or disability, longer survival, and prevention of death. Longer survival may occur in two ways: (1) the disease is totally eliminated by the treatment (eg, complete hysterectomy for carcinoma *in situ*); and (2) the length of time it takes for the disease to cause death is slowed down (eg, an individual may survive for 5 years with acquired immunodeficiency syndrome [AIDS] instead of 1 year).

A related issue is whether an efficacious procedure is effective. *Effectiveness* is the extent to which a procedure or intervention achieves its purpose when in general use. Effectiveness is determined by a variety of factors including the degree to which the procedure is accurately performed, the timing of administration, appropriate follow-up, and whether it is applied to the correct population. For example, a Papanicolaou test to screen for cervical cancer must be readily available, affordable, and accessible to the population of women at high risk for the condition, the women must avail themselves of the test on a regular basis beginning at the appropriate age when risk begins to increase, the Pap smear must be taken correctly by the clinician and processed and read correctly by the laboratory, and positive results must be followed up by appropriate diagnostic testing and treatment if cancer is present. A lack of any of these will impair program effectiveness, and cases will fail to be identified.

Case Definition

At this point, it should be apparent that the ability to determine who has a disease is an important aspect of studying and of treating a disease. Although diagnosing a disease may seem obvious, there can be multiple problems in identifying a person with a disease. A person who is identified as having a particular disease is called a *case*. Identification of a person as a case requires a set of identification criteria that allow the clinician or researcher to distinguish clearly between a case and a noncase. A case may be identified by a causative agent, a symptom complex, or laboratory, x-ray, or pathology findings. A combination of these may also be used. Cancer is diagnosed by malignant findings from a biopsy; a case of squamous cell carcinoma must be differentiated from a case of oat cell carcinoma. Diagnosis of carbon monoxide (CO) poisoning has traditionally been based on symptoms—headache, weakness, dizziness, and a carboxyhemoglobin of 35 g/100 ml (Waldbott, 1978). Diabetes has no clear-cut case criteria. Some clinicians require a single finding of a specific level of fasting plasma glucose or will accept a random elevated blood glucose or glucosuria to diagnose diabetes with or without symptoms. Some require this finding on more than one test, whereas others require a specific level of fasting plasma glucose and an abnormal glucose tolerance test (West, 1978). One published standard recommends confirming a diagnosis of diabetes with a fasting plasma glucose greater than 140 mg/dl on two or more occasions or a blood glucose greater than 200 mg/dl during a glucose tolerance test (Professional Guide to Diseases, 1989).

The clinical manifestations of a disease are the result of factors common to the body's reaction to any stressor and factors unique to the specific disease. The unique factors are often more useful than the nonspecific factors in identifying or diagnosing a disease. The headache, weakness, dizziness, and other neurological symptoms that are nonspecific characteristics of CO poisoning do not alone provide sufficient information for diagnosing CO poisoning. When these symptoms are present with the specific findings of a carboxyhemoglobin of 35 g/ml, a factor specific to this disease, then CO poisoning may be diagnosed.

Because multiple diseases may present similar symptom complexes, it is important to know the precise factor or factors that characterize the specific disease of interest. Although a nurse does not diagnose the disease, the nurse's plan of care requires knowledge of the natural history of the disease under treatment in the same way that a physician's plan of care depends on knowledge of natural history. For example, health care and prevention activities necessarily differ for the ketosis-prone diabetic and the ketosis-resistant diabetic (Kabadi & Kabadi, 1995). Although other criteria, such as presence or absence of an association with obesity, usual age at onset, and degree of abnormality of islands of Langerhans do vary for each, ketosis proneness or resistance is the critical criterion that differentiates them. Both, however, are labeled as diabetes. There is reason to believe that there may be several different types of diabetes with separate etiologies and natural histories (eg, diabetes induced by a beta-cell cytotoxic virus and diabetes induced by genetic defects associated with hyperinsulinemia and obesity) (West, 1978; DeFronzo, 1997). Because the same pathological endpoint may be produced in different ways, it is important that the clinician recognize different types or variants of a disease. Beta-cell destruction can be caused in any number of ways, all resulting in a disease called *diabetes*. The significance to the clinician is if different interventions are required or if the speed at which the disease develops in the different natural histories varies but each variant leads to a disease with the same name. In diabetes, weight control and modified diet may be used for an early stage of nonketosis-prone adult-onset diabetes. Oral hypoglycemic agents may be necessary in an individual with a later stage of nonketosis-prone adult-onset diabetes, and insulin therapy may be necessary in even later stages. A ketosis-prone juvenile-onset diabetic will most likely need insulin therapy at the point of detection.

Similarly, it is necessary to know with precision the natural history of specific types of cancer. Cancer of the breast and of the lung have different etiologies, different risk factors, and different patterns of progression even though both share the label of cancer. Even within a site-specific cancer, specification by cell type may be important in the natural history. For instance, oat cell carcinoma of the lung and squamous cell carcinoma of the lung may have different etiologies. They progress at different rates and they vary in their responsiveness to treatment.

THE STUDY OF DISEASE NATURAL HISTORY AS A PROCESS

The process of studying a disease is discussed to facilitate understanding of the current status of knowledge about the natural history of a disease. The phases (Table 12–1) are given for ease of discussion and to roughly parallel the order in which research on the natural history of a disease is conducted. For any specific disease, we commonly have more knowledge from the research or activities of the types listed in Phase I and less from Phase II-type activities. Epidemiological researchers, however, do not necessarily proceed in an orderly fashion through these phases.

Although the first case reports on a new disease may generate basic research on biochemical, metabolical, or other pathological processes that are responsible for the disease manifestation, the bulk of the research that follows usually will be epidemiological in nature. Epidemiological methods may be applied to determination of etiological factors, determination of the natural history of the disease, and determination of the efficacy of various screening, diagnostic, and treatment procedures. One epidemiological study may address one or more of these purposes at the same time.

Phase I: Identification of a New Disease

A new or previously unrecognized disease or syndrome has to be identified in some way. Legionnaire's disease was first recognized as a distinct disease after an outbreak of pneumonia among American Legion members attending a state convention

TABLE 12–1. EPIDEMIOLOGICAL PROCESS FOR STUDYING THE NATURAL HISTORY OF A DISEASE

Phase I
Clinician recognition of an undiagnosable and unusual complex of symptoms and clinical findings
Formulation of case definition for the first recognized cases
Case finding
Determination of incidence and prevalence rates and the duration or survival associated with the disease
Determination of factors associated with the disease
Formulation and testing of preliminary hypotheses

Phase II
Revision of case definition
Literature review
Hypothesis generation
Formulation of stage-specific case definitions
Determination of stage-specific incidence and prevalence rates
Determination of average duration in a stage
Confirmation of stages in the natural history
Determination of alternate pathways in the natural history
Determination of risk factors in the natural history
Experimentation

in Philadelphia (Centers for Disease Control, 1976). After the U.S. Centers for Disease Control (CDC) did an in-depth investigation of the Legionnaire's outbreak, a specific causative agent was found (Centers for Disease Control, 1977a). Subsequent to the identification of this organism, the CDC found that several pneumonia outbreaks before the 1977 Philadelphia American Legion's convention had been caused by the same organism (Centers for Disease Control, 1977a, b). Since that time, additional outbreaks of Legionaire's disease have been identified and studied to confirm and extend knowledge from the previous investigations. In other words, the disease had existed before its identification, or recognition, as a specific disease. In this case, recognition occurred because of the cluster of cases at the American Legion convention that were of unexplained etiology and because there was a high mortality rate associated with the problem.

A disease is new when clinicians are unable to label the problem (ie, there is no known specific diagnosis for the problem). Usually, recognition of new diseases requires awareness of several cases by one clinician or practice group. In addition to knowledge of several cases, recognition usually occurs because the cases have a severe or serious health outcome, such as paralysis, infertility, severe birth defects, or death. This means that most of the cases of the new disease are at the late clinical stage. Occasionally, an early clinical case may be encountered, but generally the first cases represent the worst clinical cases (ie, the late pathological stage).

A clinician who cannot locate any specific disease diagnosis that matches the complex of symptoms and clinical findings observed has several options: (1) to do nothing with the information; (2) to report the findings to a government agency such as CDC; or (3) to report on the case series in a publication. A published report on the cases may be the most common response, although there is no way of determining how many diseases have gone unrecognized for some time because of clinician inaction.

A published report on a case series will be descriptive in nature and for each case will describe age, sex, symptoms, significant history, clinical findings, treatment, and outcome. The clinician will report what he or she thinks is important or what he or she thinks may be risk factors for the disease. Presence of more than one case in the same family will be noted. If several cases have factors in common, such as excessive alcohol consumption, then that may be reported. An example of such a recent report is the case report of congenital permanent diabetes in two related male children of Arab origin. Both patients were negative for immunological markers of diabetes and for diabetes susceptibility alleles at the HLA locus. Insulin levels were undetectable, glucagon secretion, thiamine levels, and pancreatic ultrasound studies were normal. The authors suggested that their patients had a rare form of diabetes with isolated beta-cell defect and no additonal manifestations which differs from type I or type II diabetes and suggests autosomal recessive inheritance (Shehadeh et al, 1996).

Once there is awareness of a possible new disease or syndrome, additional case data will be accumulated and reported. These case series reports provide information similar to that given in the first report on a new disease, but they will also expand on the initial information. For example, if the original report described abnormal serum glutamic-oxaloacetic transaminase (SGOT) levels, secondary reports may include findings for a whole panel of liver function tests. Or if the original report described the failure of particular treatment regimens, the secondary reports may describe successful treatment regimens. Any potential causative factors described in the first report will usually be reported as present or absent in secondary reports. Factors not previously described that may be of importance in disease etiology will also be included in secondary reports. Once case reports begin to accumulate, epidemiologists usually begin to study the new disease.

Case Definition.   Before embarking on the study of a new disease, researchers must be reasonably certain that the syndrome in question really constitutes a unique new disease or syndrome. To be considered such, the disease must have a unique complex of characteristics that together result in a specific pathological condition. This represents the case definition. The *most* precise and specific case definition would be formulated from a number of cases after clinicians have identified *all* the findings associated with the disease or syndrome for each case including symptoms and the findings from hematology, blood chemistry, x-ray, nuclear magnetic resonance, histology, and pathology. Because such detailed and comprehensive information is seldom available for most of the initially reported cases, a case definition formulated at this point must be considered preliminary and should be revised as more information becomes available.

Once a preliminary case definition has been formulated, case finding, a concerted effort to find cases, must follow. Most often, case finding is done by clinicians and epidemiologists at major medical centers or state or federal government health agencies. Efforts are made through a variety of channels to request case referrals from the medical community.

State or federal agencies may publish preliminary information on the cases in state health publications or in the CDC's *Morbidity and Mortality Weekly Report (MMWR)*. Such reports will be largely descriptive, providing background information on the problem and the case definition. Incidence, prevalence, or attack rates or frequencies will be given. The outcomes or sequelae, such as permanent pathology and chronic illness or death, will be reported. Other syndromes found to be associated with the disease may be included, for example the report in the *MMWR* that Kaposi's sarcoma and pneumocystis pneumonia were likely to be associated with AIDS (Centers for Disease Control, 1981a, b). The initial report on AIDS was published early in 1981 (Centers for Disease Control, 1987). Periodic updated reviews of accumulating knowledge about the epidemiology of AIDS were published over the following years. An entire supplemental report summarizing all that was known at the time, was published in 1987 (Centers for Disease Control, 1987), followed by numerous updates since then. Periodic updates have been shown the increasing incidence and the spread of the disease in the heterosexual population.

Generating Causal Hypotheses.   At this point in Phase I, epidemiologists would investigate factors reported present in cases to determine which ones are associated with the disease and may play an etiological role for the disease. Hypotheses may be generated and tested for various risk factors suggested by primary and secondary case series reports. At this point in the research on AIDS, for example, it was determined that there was a strong association between AIDS and homosexuality (although it was not known if this was a reporting phenomenon) (Centers for Disease Control, 1981a, b). For Reyes syndrome, it was recognized that the cases were children in whom onset appeared to be associated temporally to a recent infection (Hattwick & Sayetta, 1979). Later research narrowed the infection to influenza B or varicella and showed associations with use of aspirin (Larsen, 1997). The hypothesis that aspirin could be causal seems to have been confirmed by the decline of cases in countries where public education campaigns were staged and aspirin products for children were withdrawn (Larsen, 1997). Such information may provide a basis on which to formulate etiological hypotheses. If there is no basis for a hypothesis, then research will generally be directed to various host, agent, or environmental factors including age, sex, race, smoking, alcohol, drug use, sexual preference, occupation, hobbies, infection history, general medical history, family medical history, and nutrition. This has been called a "fishing expedition," because the researcher is fishing and does not know what might be caught (in terms of causative agents). Such studies are necessary to look for leads on causation when no reasonable hypothesis exists.

Phase II: Refining the Case Definition

As further data become available, serious consideration must be given to refining the case definition for a disease because the preliminary case definition was based on a limited number of predominately late clinical cases and a limited amount of information about the cases. Publicity about the new disease may lead to earlier diagnosis of cases. Using the same methods relied on to formulate the preliminary definition, decisions based on more cases and more detailed information will be made to determine if revisions are needed. The most specific case definition would be based on *all* the findings associated with the disease or syndrome, including symptoms, hematology, blood chemistry, serology, immunology, x-ray, histology, and pathology. A complete set of such information should be collected for each organ or system of the body that may be affected by the disease. The same information and test results should be garnered for every individual who is believed to suffer from this disease. Testing procedures and test interpretation should be similar for all persons evaluated so that a standard definition of a case can be used to assemble cases for study. Lack of such comprehensive and consistent testing of the original or secondary cases frequently results in case definitions that are not as precise or specific as is desirable. Table 12–2 provides a list of minimum criteria needed for developing an adequate definition.

Testing Hypotheses.   The next step in refining a case definition is to decide which hypothesis of the natural history will be studied. A literature review of studies from laboratory and clinical disciplines may aid in choosing the most biologically plausible natural history hypothesis.

Epidemiological research on the hypothesized natural history of a disease may be seen as directed to answering a number of questions. These questions include: What are potentially causal factors? What are the identifiable stages of the natural history? What are the stage-specific incidence and prevalence rates? What are the average durations for each stage? In what ways, other than through progression to the next stage, might an individual leave a stage in the natural history? What risk factors are associated with each stage? What factors influence the stage-specific incidence rates? What factors are associated with how fast the natural history

TABLE 12–2. MINIMUM CRITERIA FOR THE MOST PRECISE AND SPECIFIC CASE DEFINITION[a]

Descriptive factors: age, sex, race, socioeconomic status, occupation
Significant medical/family history
Estimated date of onset
Estimated date of exposure, if relevant
Symptoms
Diagnostic test findings
    A standard comprehensive set should be used for all suspected cases. Similar methodology and interpretation should be used for each test
    Preferably these should be available for every organ or system that may be involved in the condition
Treatment
Outcome
Date of death or recovery

[a]This information must be uniformly available for a reasonable number of cases (usually 20 or more) to make it meaningful.

progresses? The whole array of epidemiological methods discussed in previous chapters is used in attempts to answer these questions. Confirmation of findings from cross-sectional and retrospective studies by prospective designs is often desirable.

Sometimes, however, ethical considerations make it impossible to do anything other than cross-sectional or retrospective research. For instance, a study of a factor that affects the rate at which those with carcinoma *in situ* develop invasive cervical cancer could not, ethically, be done prospectively. One would not purposely withhold treatment from women with *in situ* cervical cancer just to see how a factor influences their development of invasive cancer.

Risk factors must be considered separately for each stage of the disease. The important question is what factors influence the development of each stage or the movement between stages. For instance, are age, race, age at first pregnancy, and number of sexual partners risk factors for developing cervical dysplasia? Do they also influence progression? A risk factor may affect only one stage or may affect all stages, may affect an early stage but not a late stage, and a risk factor for a late stage may not be a risk factor for an early stage. To help sort out these relationships, it is useful to examine how the factor influenced the stage-specific incidence rate (negatively or positively, ie, does the rate increase or decrease and to what degree?). The next stage might develop more rapidly or more slowly because of a particular risk factor. Age seems to be a major factor in the rate at which the natural history progresses for many diseases and conditions. The question as to what factors are associated with staying in a stage versus moving to the next stage (or regressing back to an earlier stage) is also important to consider. Planning of intervention strategies for any one stage or level of prevention is greatly improved as a result of the findings associated with the stages and their risk factors.

Experimentation

The stages in the natural history and the factors affecting each stage can be conclusively determined only by evidence from experiments or randomized controlled trials. Such research is designed to determine whether control or minimization of a stage or a factor will eliminate the disease, reduce the disease, lessen the severity of the disease, or prolong the time in a stage. A study of whether immunization of those genetically susceptible to Coxsackie B_4 virus will reduce the incidence rate of IDDM is one example. Another example is to determine if reduction or elimination of exposure to a particular substance associated with a change from a latent stage to an active stage affects the natural history. For instance, if a substance or a factor is associated with cervical dysplasia changing to a carcinoma, a trial may be performed to determine the effect of eliminating or reducing the exposure. Computer simulations may assist in suggesting the most vulnerable, most effective factor or stage at which to intervene. Whenever feasible, intervention before clinical illness aimed at disease prevention is preferable.

USING INFORMATION ON NATURAL HISTORY IN CLINICAL PRACTICE

The epidemiological process for studying the natural history of a disease provides a basis for critical examination of the related literature as well as a mechanism for assessing the extent of available knowledge. To halt, reverse, or minimize the process of pathogenesis, the clinician requires a basic knowledge of disease progression and the factors that contribute to or cause the diseases of concern in their practice area, including the sequence of stages, stage-specific risk factors, factors associated with regression of a stage, efficacious intervention methods by stage, stage-specific incidence and prevalence rates, and average duration in each stage.

Prevention at any stage may not require a full understanding of the natural history of a disease. Banning asbestos or imposing stringent restrictions on asbestos exposure may eliminate mesotheliomas. Stopping smoking may drastically reduce risks of developing lung cancer and heart disease. Elimination of aspirin use in childhood infections may eliminate Reyes syndrome. In each example, primary prevention is possible based on information on risk factors that were identified by epidemiological methods. For each, very little is known about the natural history of the diseases, particularly the stage-specific risk factors. It is apparent that this lack of knowledge need not prevent the development of an effective intervention strategy. But what about all those individuals who never had any of the risk factors and still developed the disease? We all know of such people. Others who have all the risk factors never develop the disease. Only in understanding the entire natural history and the stage-specific risk factors will we be able to answer these questions.

On the other side of the coin are the diseases for which we not only know little or nothing about stage-specific risk factors but also have not identified risk factors that can be effectively eliminated. Age at menarche, age at menopause, late age at first pregnancy, and nulliparity are among the risk factors linked to breast cancer (Kelsey, 1993). Obesity, diet, alcohol intake, estrogen therapy, and environmental organochlorides have also been associated with increased risk (King & Shottenfeld, 1996). When one begins to menstruate or ceases menstruating is an acquired characteristic about which little is known. Having children is not always a choice (eg, never-married women and infertile women), and the association with number of children could be related to factors that also affect fertility. Although having children at a young age may reduce breast cancer risk, it is associated with an increased risk for cervical cancer and may be socially undesirable. Preventing obesity, per se, is unlikely to be an effective method of preventing breast cancer. Intervention on alcohol use and reducing environmental organochlorides might be possible, but these are thought to be relatively weak cofactors or to be causes of only small numbers of breast cancers. Thus, we do not know enough about the natural history and stage-specific risk factors of breast cancer to plan primary prevention strategies, although a low fat diet as primary prevention appears promising and is being tested in two trials, the Women's Health Initiative (WHI) and the Women's Intervention Nutrition study (WIN) (Greenwald et al, 1997). Secondary prevention through the use of mammography screening of women older than 50 years of age, however, is now common practice and national targets for percent of women over 50 screened are included in the Healthy People 2000 objectives (Institute of Medicine, 1990). In the past, radical mastectomy, although prolonging life, was a severe price to pay for the inadequate knowledge on the progression of the disease and the possibility that less radical treatment procedures may have been equally effective. Emerging knowledge has finally proved the safety of alternative treatment procedures at early stages (Gazet, 1996).

The inability to offer effective primary or secondary prevention alternatives means that tertiary prevention is the only choice for many diseases and conditions. Arthritis is a disease in this category. Primary and secondary prevention strategies are unavailable for many diseases because we know too little about their natural histories and the factors influencing them. Medical costs in dollars, in disability, and in deaths illustrate the tremendous burden of a health care system directed to tertiary prevention. We have no choice but to concentrate our efforts largely on tertiary prevention when we do not know enough about the natural history of diseases and the stage-specific risk factors associated with them.

The other aspect of prevention today is that most primary and secondary intervention methods are dependent on an individual choosing to reduce his or her risks through changes in unhealthy behaviors. When an individual chooses not to reduce risk, the person will frequently state "anything can kill you" or "Uncle Joe smoked and drank and was overweight and an obsessive worker and he was run over by a drunk driver at 90 years of age." If we could explain the chain of events (the stages) that lead to a disease outcome and the factors that influence the outcome of each stage to individuals who are nonbelievers, a greater willingness to change may occur. When we can tell someone what will happen, in what order, how and why and when it will happen or not happen at each stage, and the probability of it happening, it will have a much greater impact than telling someone they have a risk factor that may lead to a problem in 5, 10, 15, or 20 years. One of the keys to such information likely possessing sufficient motivational power to cause change is our ability to provide information that indicates a very high probability of disease. For instance, if we could tell someone that because of their characteristics they will have a 95% likelihood of dying from a given disease, it is far more likely that they will be motivated to change. There always will be individuals who will end up in the tertiary level of health care. For them, we must know the best intervention methods to halt, minimize, or reduce their pathological process. The clinical stages of the natural history and the factors that influence them then become crucial in planning effective tertiary care. Recognition of the role of estrogen and estrogen receptors in the clinical prognosis of breast cancer is an example of how such information may be valuable in planning treatment (Valavaara, 1997).

A list of the types of knowledge that are helpful to the clinician has been provided in Table 12–3. The clinician must consider which diseases, conditions, or syndromes are most prevalent in their practice area. For these conditions, the clinician should have up-to-date information on the natural history. If the clinician is unfamiliar with some of these, a reasonable way of updating knowledge is to prioritize study by the disease prevalence rate. That is, learn about the most prevalent conditions first.

TABLE 12-3. HELPFUL KNOWLEDGE FOR THE CLINICIAN ON THE NATURAL HISTORY OF A DISEASE

General information
    General description of disease
    Classifications and types of disease that may come under a general classification such as cancer or diabetes
    Basic pathology for the disease
    Methods of diagnosis: accuracy, sensitivity, and specificity of each
    Treatment for the disease
    Stages of the disease
    Risk factors associated with the disease

Tertiary prevention
    Clinical stages of the disease
    Description of characteristics of the disease at each clinical stage (ie, stage-specific case definitions)
    Treatment methods by stage
    Factors that influence prognosis
    Secondary conditions or disease that may be associated with the primary disease
    Factors that influence or are associated with the development of a secondary condition
    Side effects of treatment
    Factors associated with side effects
    Average duration of each clinical stage with and without treatment
    Outcome (eg, death, disability, sterility, paralysis)

Secondary prevention
    Prepathogenic or presymptomatic stages of the disease
    Description of the characteristics of each secondary stage (stage-specific case definitions)
    Intervention strategies and their efficacy
    Stage-specific risk factors for the secondary stages and the first tertiary stage
    Stage-specific incidence and prevalence rates (especially planners and administrators)
    Average durations by stage
    Alternate pathways and direction of change between stages
    Competing risks

Primary prevention
    Description of stages and sequence of stages, if more than one stage
    Factors associated with the stages or with likelihood of change to another stage
    Directions of change between stages
    Intervention methods and their efficacy
    Average time in a stage (ie, prepathogenic latency or induction period)

After gaining a basic, or general, knowledge about the relevant diseases and conditions, the clinician should consider the appropriate level of prevention for their practice area. Hospital staff see patients and diseases predominantly at the tertiary level of prevention, although they might identify risk factors among family members that require intervention and intervention with the patient and the family to increase smoking cessation might effect both primary and secondary intervention. Clinic and public health nurses see patients with problems that could be classified at all three levels of prevention. The type of clinic setting or specialty may affect where most patients are classified. Planned Parenthood clinics see patients at the primary level. A venereal disease clinic and a gynecological screening clinic see patients at the secondary and tertiary levels. The public health nurse may see patients predominately at the primary level whereas the visiting nurse may see them largely at the tertiary level.

Information about disease natural history may be sought by level of prevention or for the whole natural history. Although clinicians should be familiar with disease stages and risk factors, it is only in planning and implementing intervention strategies by level of prevention that it becomes necessary to have information about all details listed in Table 12–3.

Intervention and prevention strategies do vary by stage. Primary prevention strategies include such activities as health education, counseling, immunization, personal or environmental exposure control (eg, use of respirators or special ventilation when working with asbestos), isolation, restrictive laws (eg, drunk driving laws), and medication (eg, oral contraceptives). Secondary prevention strategies include screening, selective examinations, questionnaires to detect those at high risk followed by selective examinations, and abortion. Tertiary prevention is centered around medical treatment. The type of activities used at the primary level may also be used at the secondary and tertiary levels. For example, an obese woman with gallbladder disease should receive health education or counseling related to weight reduction. The clinician knowledgeable about risk factors for gallbladder disease will also know that estrogens and oral contraceptives are a risk factor. Documentation of estrogen use or contraceptive needs and use would therefore be important to this patient's care.

Tertiary Prevention

Tertiary prevention predominantly involves medical treatment. The epidemiological data most useful at this stage include knowledge of the types of classification systems used for the disease, the case definition for each type, the clinical stages of the disease, the clinical definitions for an individual in each stage, the intervention and treatment methods for each clinical stage, and any factors that influence the clinical stages or survival. Age almost always plays a role, as does general state of health. Attitude and psychological factors generally affect most diseases at the clinical level by influencing the pathological progression of diseases. Specific factors such as estrogen and estrogen receptors in breast cancer were already mentioned. Side effects of treatment may affect the health of the individual or attitude toward continuing care. The negative or undesirable effects of chemotherapeutic agents and radiation are examples where the health of the individual may be worse in the short term because of the treatment than because of the disease. Death from infections caused by chemotherapy-induced neutropenia is sometimes a problem in treatment of cancer patients.

In another aspect of tertiary prevention, a second disease or condition is caused by, or associated with, a primary condition or treatment for the primary condition. Knowledge of risk factors that may lead to a second disease is of particular importance. For instance, transplant patients tend to have cancer rates well above those of the general population. This is believed to be a consequence of immunosuppressive therapy rather than the primary condition that led to the need for the transplant

(Kinlen et al, 1979). Therefore, the clinician may counsel transplant patients about the importance of avoiding risks known to be associated with cancer. Risk factors such as smoking, heavy alcohol consumption, workplace exposure to carcinogens, and poor nutrition should all be avoided. A former burn patient with scarring is at increased risk for skin cancer and should be cautioned against tanning or unnecessary sun exposure.

The nurse, physician, or other health professional at the administrative level needs to be familiar with incidence and prevalence rates and the average durations of diseases in planning staff needs. Those responsible for planning prevention programs have to be knowledgeable about the entire natural history of the disease for which the programs are planned. Bed assignments in hospitals and nursing homes may need to be altered depending on the disease natural histories and the risk factors associated with their treatment. For instance, an infectious disease with a short period of communicability before diagnosis (ie, not diagnosable during its period of communicability) would not require isolation and therefore would not require a private room for the infected patient. The individual could be safely put in a ward but a person with an infectious disease with an extended period of communicability for example, tuberculosis, may require a private room to avoid exposing other patients. Development of policy and procedures for the protection of staff and patients is also a responsibility of the administrator that is dependent on knowledge of the risk factors and the natural history of a disease.

Secondary Prevention

Secondary prevention techniques are directed to the identification of individuals who are in the early pathogenic or very early clinical phases of a disease's natural history. Screening for early disease is the technique used most often. To screen for a disease, the clinician must know the stage-specific case definition for early pathogenic or early clinical cases. That is, the clinician must know the differences that characterize an individual who is clinically ill from one who is in an early pathological stage. The clinician must also know the difference between an individual who is in the susceptible or prepathological stages and one in the early pathogenic or early clinical stage. Men in their 30s or 40s who have a family history of heart disease, have high cholesterol levels, are overweight, smoke, lead sedentary lives, and have hypertension and abnormal exercise tolerance tests may be considered in the early pathological stages of heart disease. This could be a stage-specific case definition for early pathogenic heart disease. They may not be considered early clinical cases until angina is present on exertion. These stages could be differentiated from later clinical stages by the lack of any demonstrable artery disease or cardiac pathology. In this example, although the diagnosis is stage-dependent, there is no definitive way to differentiate the stages without doing a complete set of diagnostic tests. A man who reports never having had angina or heart disease may develop angina with the administration of an exercise tolerance test, part of the necessary workup for determining if a man is in a prepathological stage, an early pathogenesis stage, or in a early clinical stage. A history of heart disease may be denied, but resting electrocardiograms and the results of laboratory or other tests may suggest otherwise. Therefore, it is necessary to do a full set of tests whenever there is any doubt as to an individual's stage of disease.

The difference in treatment between the early pathogenic and the early clinical stages for the above example would be the utilization of sublingual nitroglycerin as needed for angina. Both groups would receive education and counseling on diet, smoking, alcohol, and weight reduction. And both groups would be encouraged to participate in or be provided with supervised exercise programs. Because of the abnormal exercise tolerance test, unsupervised exercise should be discouraged in men with early clinical disease. Both groups would also be treated with antihypertensive drugs. Periodic reassessment is necessary to determine if the individuals are still in these stages or if they have reverted to an earlier stage. Although some individuals always require antihypertensive agents and may continue to show abnormal exercise tolerance tests, others may no longer require drugs or have an abnormal exercise tolerance test.

The clinician uses information on the average duration of the early pathogenic and the early clinical stage in planning the aggressiveness and frequency of application of intervention methods. A short stage of early pathology or a short early clinical stage means that there is little time for treatment and that identification methods or screening tests must be performed more frequently.

Breast cancer may serve as an example to illustrate this point further. With breast cancer, it is likely that the same stages are present in all breast cancer cases but that in younger women the duration in a stage is greatly reduced. This would mean that the disease progresses more quickly through its natural history when younger women are affected. The previously discussed lack of efficacy for breast cancer screening with mammography among women younger than 50 years of age could be due to insufficient frequency of screening, rather than differences in the critical point.

Information on stage-specific incidence and prevalence rates assists the clinician in planning and evaluating screening and intervention programs and in educating and counseling the individual. The clinician may discuss with the patient how long they are likely to have the condition before it progresses, in the event changes are not made. At the same time, the individual may be told the probability with which certain actions are likely to result in reversal of the process, a slowing of the process, or halting of the process at its current stage. A clinician who is not knowledgeable about the natural history of the disease will not be in a position to provide such information and will be a less effective counselor or educator.

As in tertiary prevention, the health care administrator uses information on stage-specific incidence, prevalence, and duration in planning and evaluating secondary prevention programs. Surveillance programs may be necessary to detect drug side effects such as megaloblastic anemia in epileptic patients receiving anticonvulsants (several of the anticonvulsants are antifolate compounds). Monitoring oncology nurses for cytogenetic changes may be necessary if it is suspected that ventilation and personal protective devices provide inadequate protection when preparing chemotherapeutic agents and additional controls are not feasible under the current hospital administration. (Adequate ventilation and protective devices would be considered primary prevention.) Policy development, then, must also be considered for secondary prevention.

Primary Prevention

For most diseases and conditions, the bulk of the public may be in the stage of susceptibility. Exceptions include individuals who already have some later stage of the disease, those who are immune, or those who are no longer at risk because of removal of the involved organ. For example, women who have had a complete or radical hysterectomy are no longer at risk or susceptible to uterine or cervical cancer. Diseases confined to one sex, race, or ethnic background also limit the susceptible population.

Primary prevention can be aimed at the general population (eg, promoting a healthy diet or maintaining a safe water supply through clorination). Frequently, however, primary prevention targets a group at high risk of developing a disease because they have a set of risk factors that indicate a greater probability of developing the disease. Again, the clinician must be knowledgeable of the set of risk factors or criteria that make the individual at high risk or in the prepathological stage. Ordinarily, this classification of stage will be based entirely on risk factors and not on any laboratory, x-ray, or clinical evidence of a problem. By definition, these individuals are in a stage that precedes the presence of any such findings. For heart disease the definition might be a man between the ages of 25 to 70, who is overweight, sedentary, smokes, and has a family history of heart disease. Exercise tolerance tests, electrocardiograms, blood pressure, and other cardiac tests would all be normal. For breast cancer, the definition might be women between the ages of 35 to 70, who are slightly to greatly overweight, have a family history of breast cancer, a first child born after age 25 or having never given birth, and report an early first menses. Some clinicians would also include fibrocystic breast disease as part of a prepathological stage.

The type of primary prevention that is planned, then, requires a knowledge of the characteristics of individuals that would make them at high risk (ie, susceptible to the disease or health problem). It also requires a knowledge of the health problem or disease in the community. (See Chap. 15 for further discussion on community analysis.) Again, knowledge of the average duration and the stage-specific incidence and prevalence rates is necessary in understanding and planning intervention strategies and in providing education and counseling.

Many primary prevention activities are instigated by legislation or administrative decisions made at the community or institutional level. Clinicians are instrumental in assisting with such programs, including immunizations, health education, and occupational safety programs. Moreover, clinicians have numerous opportunities to engage in primary prevention as part of their daily practice. Knowledge of risk for various preventable diseases leads to identification of individuals who may be more susceptible to a particular condition. Once identified, health education aimed at reducing susceptibility of high-risk individuals can be initiated. A patient in the hospital for eye surgery needs education regarding how to maximize safety at home to prevent accidents. This same patient may have a family history of heart disease, a sedentary lifestyle, and a diet high in saturated fats. Education directed at changing exercise and diet habits to prevent heart disease is also appropriate primary prevention. Sometimes opportunities arise to engage in such primary prevention with a patient's family—the smoking son of an myocardial infarction patient, the overweight daughter of a diabetic patient. Knowledge of the natural history stages provides a framework for explaining risks to family members and steps that can be taken to reduce risks. Anticipatory guidance for new parents, counseling in preparation for retirement, or counseling the spouse of a terminally ill patient are all forms of primary prevention for which need may arise in daily practice.

Administrators also engage quite regularly in primary prevention activities based on knowledge of disease natural history. Development of policies and procedures to prevent the spread of communicable disease to other patients and staff—for example, covering care of equipment and linens of infectious patients, hand washing procedures, staff immunization requirements—builds on such knowledge. Needs may vary by unit. Awareness of potential hazards in the institutional setting is needed together with knowledge of probable effects of exposure. Musculoskeletal injuries, effects of exposure to radiation, anesthetic gases, ethylene oxide sterilizers, chemotherapeutic drugs, and infectious agents are among the hazards to be addressed through development of policies, procedures, and staff education programs.

REFERENCES

Centers for Disease Control. (1977a) Follow-up respiratory illness—Philadelphia. *Morbidity and Mortality Weekly Report, 26*(2), 9.

Centers for Disease Control. (1977b) Follow-up respiratory illness—Philadelphia. *Morbidity and Mortality Weekly Report, 26*(6), 43.

Centers for Disease Control. (1987) Human immunodeficiency virus infection in the United States: A review of current knowledge. *Morbidity and Mortality Weekly Report, 36* (suppl. no. S-6).

Centers for Disease Control. (1981b) Kaposi's sarcoma and pneumocystis pneumonia among homosexual men—New York City and California. *Morbidity and Mortality Weekly Report, 30*(25), 306.

Centers for Disease Control. (1981a) Pneumocystis pneumonia—Los Angeles. *Morbidity and Mortality Weekly Report, 30*(21), 250.

Centers for Disease Control. (1976) Respiratory infection—Pennsylvania. *Morbidity and Mortality Weekly Report, 25*(30), 244.

DeFronzo R. A. (1997) Pathogenesis of type 2 diabetes: Metabolic and molecular implications for identifying diabetes genes. *Diabetes Review, 5*(3),177–269.

Gazet J. C. (1996) Future prospects in limited surgery for early breast cancer. *Seminar on Surgical Oncology, 12*(1), 39–45.

Greenwald P., Sherwook K., McDonald S. S. (1997) Fat, caloric intake, and obesity: Lifestyle risk factors for breast cancer. *Journal of the American Dietary Association, 97*(7) (suppl.), S24–30.

Hattwick M. A. W., Sayetta, R. B. (1979) Time trends of Reyes syndrome based on national statistics. In J. F. S. Cocker (Ed.). *Reyes syndrome II.* New York: Grune & Stratton.

Institute of Medicine. (1990) *Healthy people 2000. Citizens chart the course.* M. A. Stoto, R. Behrens, C. Rosemont (Eds.). Washington, D.C.: National Academy Press.

Kabadi U. M., Kabadi M. M. (1995) Combinations sulfonylurea and insulin therapy in diabetes mellitus. *Comprehensive Therapy, 21*(12), 731–736.

Kelsey J. L., Gammon M. D., John E. M. (1993) Reproductive factors and breast cancer. *Epidemiologic Reviews, 15*(1), 36–47.

King S. E., Shottenfeld D. (1996) The "epidemic" of breast cancer in the U.S.—Determining the factors. *Oncology (Huntingt) 20*(4), 453–462.

Kinlen L. J., Sheil A. G. R., Peto J., Doll R. (1979) A collaborative UK-Australian study of cancer patients treated with immunosuppressive drugs. *British Medical Journal, 2,* 1461.

Larsen S. U. (1997) Reyes syndrome. *Medicine, Science and Law, 37*(3), 235–241.

Mettlin C., Smart C. R. (1994) Breast cancer detection guidelines for women aged 40 to 49 years: Rationale for the American Cancer Society reaffirmation of recommendations. *CA: Cancer Journal for Clinicians, 44*(4), 248–255.

National Institutes of Health. (1997) *Report of the Concensus Development Panel on Breast Cancer Screening for Woman Ages 40–49,* Bethesda, Md.

Nelson J. H. Jr., Averette H. E., Richart R. M. (1989) Cervical intraepithelial neoplasia (dysplasia and carcinoma in situ) and early invasive cervical carcinoma. *CA: Cancer Journal for Clinicians, 39*(3), 157–178.

Nerup J. (1981) Etiology and pathogenesis of insulin-dependent diabetes mellitus: Present views and future developments. In J. M. Martin, R. M. Ehrlich, F. J. Holland (Eds.). *Etiology and pathogenesis of insulin-dependent diabetes mellitus.* New York: Raven Press.

Professional Guide to Diseases. (1989) *Diabetes mellitus.* Springhouse, Pa.: Springhouse Corporation, pp 816–819.

Pitot H. C. (1981) *Fundamentals of oncology.* (2nd ed.). New York: Marcel Dekker, Inc.

Shehadeh N., Gershoni-Baruch R., Mandel H., Nutenko I., Etzioni A. (1996) Congenital permanent diabetes: A different type of diabetes? *Acta Paediatrics, 85*(12), 1415–1417.

Shapiro S. (1977) Evidence on screening for breast cancer from a randomized trial. *Cancer, 39,* 2772–2782.

Valavaara R. (1997) Reliability of estrogen receptors in predicting response to antiestrogens. *Oncology (Huntingt), 11*(5) (suppl. 4), 14–18.

Waldbott G. L. (1978) *Health effects of environmental pollutants. (2nd ed.).* St. Louis: C.V. Mosby Co.

West K. M. (1978) *Epidemiology of diabetes and its vascular lesions.* New York: Elsevier.

Disease Control
and Surveillance

lthough health care encompasses the health of individuals, families, and communities, the major focus of education and practice has traditionally been the individual. Health of the family has probably gained the most attention in community nursing practice and family practice medicine. This focus on the individual is somewhat ironic because the general health of a community may have impact on the health of individuals within that community. Certainly, monitoring health events in a community is crucial to early detection of disease outbreaks so that prompt intervention with control measures can prevent the spread and limit the incidence of disease. The greatest impact on the health of individuals may be made through control activities directed at high-risk groups that have been identified through surveillance or research. If one's objective is to improve the health of the individual, therefore, at least a portion of one's attention must be focused on the community. This chapter addresses the operational definition of surveillance and the planning, implementation, and evaluation of surveillance systems in the context of community monitoring and its role in controlling disease and maintaining the health of the population. Such monitoring clearly has an important role in managed care.

SURVEILLANCE SYSTEMS

Definition

Surveillance may be defined as ongoing monitoring, generally using methods distinguished by their practicality, uniformity, and timeliness, rather than by complete accuracy. The main purpose of surveillance is to detect changes in trend or distribution in order to initiate investigative or control measures. A flowchart of the surveillance/intervention process is shown in Figure 13–1. The surveillance of a particular disease or health problem encompasses all aspects of the natural history of disease occurrence and spread pertinent to effective control. A surveillance system may also be a reporting system wherein reports are made for a specific purpose, for example, a *registry* to which all cases of a particular disease or other health-relevant condition in a defined population are reported. Use of a defined population relates the cases to a population base, allowing calculation of incidence rates. Some authors, myself included, differentiate between a reporting system and a registry by including in the latter the regular following of cases to determine case status (ie, deceased, in

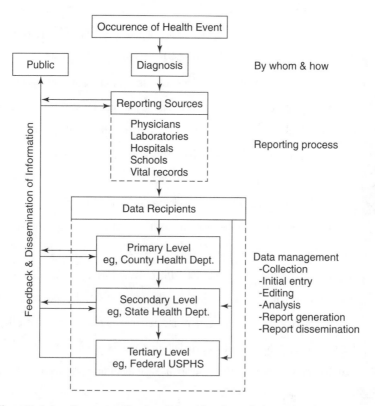

Figure 13–1. Surveillance system flowchart. (*Adapted from Centers for Disease Control. Guidelines for evaluating surveillance systems.* Morbidity and Mortality Weekly Report, 1988; 37 [suppl. S-5.].)

remission, and so on). Date of diagnosis and case status may then be used to determine prevalence and survival rates and to evaluate effectiveness of changes in screening and diagnostic or clinical treatment interventions applied to the population. By these definitions, the pattern of cancer in the community may be monitored by a reporting system (first diagnosis only) or by a registry (includes stage at diagnosis, treatment, and ongoing reports of status). Birth defects are usually under surveillance through initial reporting only, although high-risk infants may be followed on a registry. Cancer surveillance, in contrast, is usually ongoing.

Purposes of Surveillance Systems

Surveillance of a disease or health problem may be carried out for several purposes. The primary purpose is to detect new or developing problems quickly and bring them under control. Problems can be as varied as an increase in the incidence of a disease, untoward effects of medical procedures, or changes in population behaviors, for example, the increasing use of herbal preparations, which potentially can interact with medical drugs prescribed by a clinician. A secondary purpose is to evaluate the effectiveness of control measures. Yet another purpose is to monitor quality of care. Recently, surveillance systems such as the Health Plan Employer Data and Information Set (HEDIS) have been put in place to provide data that allow purchasers and consumers to reliably compare the performance of managed health care plans in eight performance domains for which measures were or are being developed. These include effectiveness of care; access/availability of care; satisfaction with the experience of care; cost of care; stability of the health plan; informed health care choices; use of services; and plan descriptors. Measures meet criteria of relevance, scientific soundness, and feasibility (for collection) and the same measures are collected for all health plans (National Committee for Quality Assurance, 1997). The process of collecting the data provides a tool for the health plans to monitor their own performance. For all purposes, the ultimate goal is to provide optimal care and reduce or eliminate unnecessary suffering and disease. Table 13–1 lists a variety of outcomes that illustrate the value of surveillance systems.

Surveillance allows clinicians and administrators to quickly become aware of a potential problem (in terms of who, what, when, where, and how much). Investigation

TABLE 13–1. VALUE OF SURVEILLANCE

- Defines problem
- Permits quick awareness of potential problem
- Permits quick investigation and control
- Reduces lost work time, worker's compensation, and insurance costs
- Affords legal protection
- Supports later research
- Allows evaluation of control measures
- Stimulates thought and increases awareness
- Reduces cost of *ad hoc* morbidity and mortality studies

of the potential problem is the next step, for there is little or no value in awareness if no reason is determined as to why a sudden change in frequency of disease (a potential epidemic) has occurred. The investigation can both determine whether a problem really exists, and if so, describe it more fully and identify a probable cause of the problem. Once a probable cause is identified, control efforts can be developed and applied. An example of immediate application of control measures might be the hospital infection control nurse identifying an outbreak of an infection among patients on a medical unit and finding that all patients infected were hospitalized for renal dialysis. The nurse has the dialysis machines cultured and discovers that one dialysis machine is positive for the organism causing the infection. Immediate action is then taken to sterilize the machine and all component parts, even before the source from which the agent was transmitted to the machine is identified. In other instances, investigation and delineation of a possible cause may lead to more in-depth research to document the cause. One such recent example was in regard to injuries and deaths associated with use of snowmobiles in Maine. When surveillance activities by the Department of Inland Fisheries and Wildlife (DIFW) and the Maine Office of the Chief Medical Examiner noted an increase in the number of deaths annually associated with snowmobile use, they reviewed data routinely collected by DIFW wardens and other law enforcement officers and death certificate data from the Bureau of Human Services for time of occurrence, weather conditions, terrain, alcohol use, helmet use, and cause and circumstances of the accident. Other data examined included age, sex, place of residence, education, marital status, and blood or vitreous alcohol levels and cause of death for those who died. Findings indicated associations of excessive speed, careless operation of the vehicle, alcohol use, and darkness with snowmobile accidents. Findings are being incorporated into a statewide strategic plan to improve snowmobile safety (Centers for Disease Control, 1997a).

ESTABLISHED SURVEILLANCE SYSTEMS

Many surveillance systems exist today. Sources of surveillance data include systems established for other purposes, such as birth or death certificate systems. Many sources of routinely collected health-related data are useful for surveillance purposes. These sources of data were discussed in Chapter 4. Other systems are specially designed for surveillance of a particular condition. The U.S. Centers for Disease Control (CDC) have monitored some infectious diseases for years. Many states, as well as the World Health Organization (WHO), have surveillance programs with mandatory reporting of communicable diseases. The American Hospital Association sets requirements for surveillance of infectious diseases in hospitals. Health professionals need to familiarize themselves with local, state, and federal reporting requirements in order to comply. Information may usually be obtained from local public health agencies.

For practical reasons, the American Public Health Association divides reportable communicable diseases into five classifications. The first class of case reports, *universally mandatory reportable diseases,* requires quarantine and includes plague, cholera, yellow fever, and smallpox. Louse-borne typhus fever and relapsing fever, paralytic poliomyelitis, malaria, and viral influenza are also reportable under WHO requirements. These illnesses are usually reportable first by telephone or FAX followed by a full written report. Rapidity of report is vital to containment of a widespread outbreak. The second classification of *regularly reportable diseases* has two subclasses: (1) those diseases requiring rapid reporting (eg, typhoid fever and diphtheria) to the local health authority followed by weekly reports mailed to the next superior agency (eg, state health department); and (2) routine weekly reports to local health agency of diseases such as brucellosis or leprosy. The third major classification is *selectively reportable diseases* in endemic areas. This class has been subdivided into three categories based on speed of reporting needed (the telephone being the most practical means; and weekly collective report by mail). Examples of selectively reportable diseases include tularemia, coccidioidomycosis, and clonorchiasis. Food poisoning, infectious keratoconjunctivitis, and others come under the fourth major class, *obligatory report of epidemic—no case report required.* Outbreaks of such problems should be rapidly reported (telephone) to the local health department. Class five, *official report not ordinarily justifiable,* includes diseases that are usually sporadic and uncommon or where the report is of informational value but of no practical value. *Control of Communicable Diseases in Man* (Benenson, 1990) is a handy and practical guide to the likelihood of reporting being mandatory. Because local and state laws vary, it is best to consult this guide or your local health department to be sure that compliance is maintained. Table 6–5 provided a list of nationally reportable infectious diseases in the United States.

The CDC and other federal agencies maintain a variety of surveillance systems in addition to those for infectious diseases. These surveillance systems include surveillance for reproductive health, chronic fatigue syndrome, behavioral risk factors, respiratory disease, injuries, and birth defects (Centers for Disease Control, 1997b). Some state health departments have sudden infant death syndrome (SIDS) surveillance systems. Cancer surveillance systems or registries exist in several states including Connecticut, Iowa, Wisconsin, and New Mexico. The American College of Surgeons sets requirements for hospital tumor registries. Surveillance systems exist in some states for farm accidents, acute pesticide poisonings, birth defects, occupational accidents, and others. Death certificates are frequently used as surveillance tools for maternal and infant mortality, cancer, heart disease, diabetes, accidents, suicide, and other purposes. Worker's compensation data are used for surveillance of occupational accidents and diseases by many states. State health departments can provide information on these reporting systems in their state.

PLANNING A SURVEILLANCE SYSTEM

The Concept of Community

A surveillance system is generally designed to monitor events for a particular community. A community need not be conceptualized as a large geopolitically defined area such as a neighborhood, city, or county. For health professionals working in an institution such as a hospital, the community that affects individual health can be conceptualized as a "micro"-community composed of the hospital patient and staff populations. The health status of this community can be assessed and monitored for occurrence of unusual health events using the same methods applied to the geopolitical community. Within this setting, implementation of control measures aimed at the identified causes of unusual events can contribute to maintaining the health of individuals within this hospital community.

The appropriate target group or community thus depends on the practice setting and the types of health care problems that are encountered. To a public health nurse, the community or population of interest may be infants born in a particular county. Neonatal death rates may have been observed through a review of death certificates to be much higher in a city within the county than in its surrounding areas. The clinician may wish to determine whether this difference results from differences in prenatal care, delivery practices, or other factors that vary between the city and the rest of the county. Such an investigation may lead to recognition that in the city there is an increase in live (as opposed to stillborn) deliveries of infants weighing less than 500 g. Because infants weighing less than 500 g do not generally survive, these live deliveries lead to an increase in the reported neonatal mortality. This increase requires no control activities as it results from medical care changes and reporting practices, and there is presently no control activity known that could save these infants.

Hospital supervisors will be interested in the inpatient population of their hospital. A hospital patient surveillance system may have suggested a sudden increase in hepatitis A cases, and the supervisor wishes to quickly determine if the cases are predominantly in one unit (eg, dialysis), one diagnostic group (eg, leukemics), or in particular types of units (eg, surgical). It may be determined that a new nurse had hepatitis when hired and spread the disease to all units where she worked as a float nurse. Control measures would include assuring that this nurse does not work again until treatment is instituted and the nurse is no longer contagious, that all identified cases are isolated and treated, that all immediate contacts are treated with immunoglobulin or gammaglobulin, and that hygiene practices are reviewed with the nurse.

An outpatient care coordinator working in the medical office of a managed care organization is responsible for managing the flow of patient care services provided to health plan members who use that facility. Sudden increases in demand for services require staffing changes or other responses to ensure that adequate care is available. Analysis of patterns of utilization can illuminate annual patterns, such as the increased incidence of influenza-related visits in the early fall, and lead to implementation of proactive prevention efforts, such as a flu immunization program in the early fall or staffing adjustments to meet such periods of unusual demand. If the clinic appointment system was designed to provide data for monitoring usage of services, then regular analysis of the aggregate data collected through the system for characteristics of users, proportional distribution of diseases seen at visits, and so forth can illuminate patterns that allow the coordinator to better meet demand for services. As illustrated in these examples, groups or populations to which surveillance and control methods are applied may be defined according to the interests of the clinician or administrator.

Steps in Developing a Surveillance System

Development and use of a surveillance and control system, whether for hospital infections (eg, *Staphylococcus aureus*), community infectious diseases (eg, measles), chronic diseases (eg, cervical cancer), untoward effects of drugs (eg, nausea, birth defects), or untoward effects of medical procedures (eg, pain, bladder infections) can be broken down into several steps.

1. Defining the purpose and goals
2. Collecting the data
3. Analyzing the data
4. Interpreting the data
5. Investigation (when indicated)
6. Control (when required)
7. Evaluation

A successful surveillance system will deal with health problems of importance to public health and have a well-defined and specific statement of purpose. Additional factors that contribute to the success of a surveillance system are simplicity, flexibility, timeliness, representativeness, acceptability to the individuals and organizations that participate in the system, sensitivity to detecting epidemics, and accuracy of case reporting (Centers for Disease Control, 1988).

Planning of the surveillance system may be viewed as a series of questions (Table 13–2) that need to be answered before a system can be implemented. Before addressing these questions, however, review of any previously developed surveillance systems with similar purposes can be helpful in the design of the new system. Such a review should include an examination of purposes of the system, reporting forms used in each system, source of the reports, frequency of reporting, and adequacy (effectiveness) of the system.

Defining the Purpose and Goals

The purpose and goals of a surveillance system need to be stated clearly and in operational terms. For example, if the purpose of a system is to monitor and control the incidence of hospital-acquired staphylococcal infection, then goals would

TABLE 13–2. SUMMARY OF BASIC QUESTIONS IN SURVEILLANCE

- How is a case to be defined and what is to be reported?
- Where is the information to come from?
- Who reports it?
- Who is responsible for it?
- How frequently is it to be reported/analyzed?
- What is to be done with the raw data once it is in hand?
- How is it to be evaluated?
- Who needs the information?
- Who will evaluate the generated information?

specify the steps needed to achieve this purpose. Goals might thus reflect the process of monitoring and intervention to: (1) define a case of hospital-acquired staphylococcal infection; (2) establish the background (endemic) rates; (3) track rates over time and identify when rates exceed the endemic level; (4) investigate and identify practices, procedures, or patient risk factors associated with the outbreak; and (5) implement appropriate prevention and control measures.

Data Collection

Deciding what data to collect is crucial to success or failure of the system. Is one looking for all infectious diseases regardless of level of confirmation or severity? If one is interested in community surveillance of herpes, should reports be made of any recurrent genital lesion not diagnosed as syphilis, gonorrhea, or venereal warts, or is laboratory verification of herpes necessary? If oral or ophthalmological herpetic lesions are suspected, should both children and adults be reported? Should a sexual partner of a genital herpes case be reported if this partner does not have a lesion and reports never having had a lesion but is the only potential source of infection for the *index case* (the first case in a family or other defined group to come to the attention of the investigator)? Are all potential contacts to be reported? It can be seen from these questions that instituting a herpes surveillance system is not quite as simple as saying all herpes cases must be reported. Rather, a specific definition of what constitutes a case for reporting purposes must be delineated. The following items are often components of a case definition.

1. Specific name of disease or health problem (eg, not kidney disease but glomerular nephritis), using existing coding systems, such as International Classification of Disease (ICD) codes, where available
2. Any laboratory tests or confirmation requested or required to be reported as a case (eg, positive breast biopsy required for a report of breast cancer; a radiological finding only would not be acceptable)
3. Date of onset
4. Precipitating factor (eg, verification of drug utilization may be necessary to define a case associated with side effects of drugs)
5. Date or dates of likely contact or exposure to a precipitating factor (eg, in infectious disease, environmentally or occupationally induced disease)
6. Symptoms or symptom complex (which may be used to define a case)
7. Time period (duration) of symptoms, if relevant
8. Age of case if age criteria are required to define a case (eg, a case of menstrual toxic shock was defined as being in women older than 12 years of age)

These items delineate how broadly or narrowly a case is to be defined and assist clinicians in determining when an individual should be reported as a case. Figure 13–2 shows use of the case definition for the chronic fatigue syndrome surveillance system. This definition uses both inclusion and exclusion criteria.

The next decision relates to what other information to collect about each case. In making the final determination of which pieces of raw data are to be collected, it

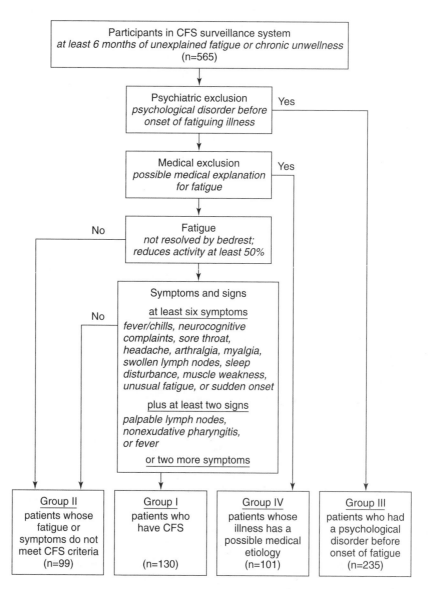

Figure 13–2. Use of the 1988 case definition for chronic fatigue syndrome (CFS) to classify participants in the CFS surveillance system, by diagnostic category—Atlanta, Wichita, Reno, and Grand Rapids, September 1989–August 1993. (*Adapted from Centers for Disease Control. Surveillance for chronic fatigue syndrome—four U.S. cities, September 1989 through August 1993. Morbidity and Mortality Weekly Reports, 1997; 46[No. SS-2], 6, Fig. 1.*)

must be recognized that the success of the system will be, in part, dependent on collecting the minimum amount of information necessary, yet sufficient for analysis, interpretation, and determination of whether an investigation will be needed. Completeness of reports, compliance with reporting schedules, and cooperation of personnel are often a function of how much data are to be collected. As a result, the value of the entire reporting system may be dependent on the length and ease of completing the report forms.

The following items relevant to the natural history may be of interest.

- Demographic data
- Site of problem (eg, vagina, eye, bladder, skin, postoperative wound)
- Date of onset
- Date of probable contact (infectious)
- Potential contacts (infectious)
- Laboratory or other tests performed
- Date of tests
- Types of symptoms
- Symptom duration and severity
- Treatment
- Current status
- Sequence of events (accidents, infections)
- Source of report and date of report
- Instruments or procedures possibly or probably contributing to or causing this problem
- Where condition was acquired
- Agent or likely agent
- Protective measures used or not used
- Alcohol or drug use (accidents, birth defects, etc.)

A decision on which of these items to include in the report can be facilitated by considering the issues discussed in the following paragraphs.

Sources of Data.   An important issue to address is *where the information is to be obtained?* Table 13–3 lists some sources of information that may be used in a surveillance system. An occupational health surveillance system may use several sources, for example, employee health records, workman's compensation data. In a hospital infection surveillance system, all units in the hospital may be asked to report; a state cancer surveillance system may use the medical records department of each hospital in the state as the sole source of information. In making a decision about which source or sources of data to use, the planner should consider likely compliance with the request to report, whether reports will be reliable and on time, completeness of information available at a given source, comparability between sources (if several sources are used), and cost factors.

Accountability for Reporting.   The next question is, *who will complete the written report?* If more than one individual must provide information, *in what order should the information be completed?* The patient, the unit clerk, the physician, the nurse, the medical records department librarian, the hospital administrator, the local health offi-

TABLE 13–3. SOURCES OF INFORMATION FOR SURVEILLANCE

- Medical records
- Preemployment physicals
- Patient or employee (questionnaires, interviews)
- Spouse
- Absentee reports
- Hospital records
- Medical insurance
- Life insurance
- Worker's compensation records
- Other clinical records (in-house)
- Local clinic, emergency room, or other hospital records
- Discharge physical (from company)
- Union records
- Personnel records

cer, the pharmacist, the school nurse, the insurance company clerk, the clinic nurse, or the pathologist may all provide relevant information. In making a decision about who should report, consideration must be given to the level of accuracy needed, the likely completeness of the report (ie, who provides more complete information), the timeliness required (time may be vital), and the likelihood that a report would be submitted. Switching from a physician-based cancer reporting system to one in which the hospital medical records librarian reports generally increases both completeness of reports and improves timeliness; the librarian deals with records as part of the job and building into the daily routine a process for completing a report is fairly easy.

If there are several tiers in the reporting chain, it is important to identify the individuals who are responsible at each level. For example, a case of salmonellosis may be reported by a physician to the local health officer (at the local health department), who then reports to the regional or state health department epidemiologist, who then reports it to the CDC. The person responsible (eg, secretary, unit clerk, nurse, physician, pharmacist, medical records librarian, pathologist) should be specified at each level of the reporting system. At the administrative level of the surveillance system, one individual should be ultimately responsible for seeing that reports are made.

It is often helpful to have people who will participate in the reporting system help with the design of the system. If they are part of designing the system it is more likely to be successful because the system is more likely to meet their needs, both by making the reporting process feasible for the reporting sites and by identifying what they would like to learn from the data collected through the system. Such planning will contribute ideas, clarification, and identification of problems. For example, physicians reporting cancer cases may report more completely and accurately if representative doctors participate in determining what type of information may be of help in planning treatment and followup frequency for their cases. The physicians may wish to compare survival rates for their hospital with other similar types of hospitals in the state in order to see if their rates are lower or higher. If they learn their survival rates are lower, they will likely want data that will enable them to determine what is different about their cases, treatment, or frequency of followup visits in order to consider interventions. Going through all the steps in designing the system jointly with the principal system designer will help those doing the reporting to understand the decisions that are made and lead to a personal interest in the quality of the system. At the same time, the principal designer will obtain a more complete and accurate system.

Timeframe. The next two questions to address in designing a surveillance system are: *How frequently are data to be reported?* and *How frequently are data to be analyzed?* A case may be reported as soon as it occurs, or cases may be reported daily, weekly, monthly, or yearly. The frequency of reporting depends on the nature of the disease or health problem, the specific purposes of the surveillance system and urgency of intervention. Thus, carbon monoxide poisoning should be reported immediately while cancer may be reported monthly.

Analysis is often completed with the same frequency as reporting, so that if daily reports are required, analysis would also occur daily. Exceptions do occur. It may be necessary to report cases of acquired immunodeficiency syndrome (AIDS) immediately so that sexual contacts can be located and further contacts eliminated or reduced, but analysis of frequency data to describe trends in AIDS occurrence may only be needed monthly or quarterly. In the case of birth defects, reporting may be monthly, but annual analysis may be sufficiently frequent. Another reason for more frequent reporting than analysis is that infrequent reporting may cause those who report to forget to report because of the time interval. For instance, a nurse is more likely to report a drug side effect if he or she has to complete a report form at the time the effect occurs rather than completing the reports once a month. Frequency is also dependent on time and staff resources. There is little value in frequent reporting and analyses if the system staff do not have the time to monitor and investigate the data that are produced from frequent monitoring.

Data Analysis and Interpretation. Additional questions to address in planning a surveillance system are: *What are you going to do with the raw data once you have it?* and *Who needs the information provided by the system?* As indicated previously, both the items on the report that are to be analyzed and the analytic procedures should be selected during planning of the surveillance system. Then, at the time analysis is carried out, data necessary for analytic procedures such as case counts, incidence or prevalence rate calculations, graph preparation, and other descriptive procedures to be used will be in place. Statistical tests of differences or of trends may also have been selected. Such statistical tests usually test the current situation against some previous situation. For example, an infection control nurse might wish to determine if there is a statistically significant increase in the hepatitis case rate for one month (or week) when compared with the previous month (or week). With some health problems, such changes are obvious from descriptive data and tests of significance are unnecessary.

In general, the information generated by a surveillance system should result in regular and periodic summary reports distributed to the providers of the data and to others who need or wish to have the information. Summary reports may provide comparative data, for example, how a local hospital's treatment and survival patterns compare with other hospitals in the registry or reports of investigations completed and interventions initiated as a result of the generated information. For example, the CDC routinely report such investigations based on their surveillance data in the *Morbidity and Mortality Weekly Report.* Such a CDC report may describe an investigation of a giardiasis outbreak in a rural Colorado town or an investigation of health complaints associated with a particular baby food.

At the minimum, general frequency counts and rates are generated. These may also be examined within categories of place, time, and age. In producing these data the analyst seeks to determine if the incidence or prevalence rate is unusual (suggesting an epidemic) or if there is a trend that would indicate that a problem may be developing. In the context of monitoring health care quality, the analysis would be designed to identify progress toward specified goals (eg, 80% of infants under age 2 years having had all recommended immunizations) or, in the case of critical events, such as medication errors that indicate a problem, to identify where system problems may be developing.

The decision as to whether both frequency counts and rates will be generated must be based on whether the counts are of sufficient size to make rates meaningful in view of the size of the population denominator to be used. In general, rates are preferable. Extremely rare diseases, however, are usually reported in surveillance system reports as frequency counts because the number of events in the numerator is too small relative to the denominator to reliably detect changes in rates.

Analyzing the surveillance data within subcategories of place, time, and age may identify unusual changes or trends. If an incidence rate is unusual within a particular part of the hospital, a particular school, a particular community, a particular age group, or in a particular period of time, it can provide useful clues as to what may be contributing to an increase or trend. Another reason for such analyses is that sometimes a change in rates may not be apparent at the general population level but becomes readily apparent with more detailed analyses (a dilution-type effect). The following hypothetical example may make this clearer. Analysis of hospital infections determines that 14 cases of staff needle punctures per month is the usual number for the hospital. The latest analysis has determined that there are 15 cases during the current month. Fifteen cases are no more than would be within the expected range for the hospital. If the hospital has a staff of 1,000, the needle puncture rate would be 15 in 1,000 or 1.5 per 100 staff. One staff member suggests that it is possible that the needle sticks are much more frequent than 1.5 per 100 staff in her unit. A more detailed analysis is then performed by determining the rate of needle sticks for each unit. Table 13–4 presents the findings. It is apparent that unit 6 has a much higher rate than that which is generally the case for the other hospital units. General analysis would have missed this finding. Investigation is now required to determine why this unit has such a high rate of staff needle punctures.

Assuring That the Data are Useful.   As previously stated, to determine if the data show a potential problem that requires investigation, some analysis of the information generated (the frequency counts and rates) must be performed. Issues of staff availability, time, and cost can play a vital role in the type of interpretation that is made of data or whether any interpretation is made. For example, in a hospital with several

TABLE 13–4. HYPOTHETICAL DATA ON NEEDLE PUNCTURES BY HOSPITAL UNIT

UNIT	FREQUENCY	STAFF SIZE	RATE (PER 100 STAFF)
1	1	65	1.54
2	1	55	1.82
3	1	50	2.00
4	2	200	1.00
5	1	110	0.91
6	5	80	6.25
7	0	100	N/A
8	1	90	1.11
9	1	50	2.00
10	2	200	1.00
Total	15	1,000	1.50

nurse epidemiologists, a borderline increase in rates will likely be detected as a suspect epidemic and investigated. With only one nurse epidemiologist on the staff, such a borderline increase may be overlooked or ignored, particularly if the epidemiologist is already busy with investigating a previously identified problem. One investigator often has time to investigate what appears to be a potential epidemic, but if the surveillance system simultaneously suggests potential epidemics of pneumonia, staphylococcal infection, and *Salmonella,* the increase in *Salmonella* cases may be ignored. At the same time, a stimulus such as a press report of a small nonepidemic increase of some problem (eg, infants born with ductus arteriosus) may lead administrators to divert resources to investigate this problem.

Where computer resources are unavailable, hand tabulation and review are required. In such situations, an informal evaluation where someone merely looks at the information generated (without additional analysis) for possible epidemics or serious upward trends might be used. For example, the nurse epidemiologist may look at the data in the needle puncture example and decide to investigate the cause of the excess in unit 6. Or, in a larger data series, a statistical test may routinely be performed to determine if the current rate is significantly different from that for some previous period of time. Although the statistical test to be used depends on the characteristics of the data, the chi-square test of differences is used most frequently. Statistical tests of differences or of trends may also compare one group with another (eg, one surgical unit compared with another one or one county compared with another county). Comparison of groups, however, as in the latter case, is usually completed only after initial analysis and interpretation rather than as a routine procedure. The intent of all such analysis is the determination of whether an epidemic exists.

The scarce staff resources available in an agency for review of data can often be used most efficiently if the data system is computerized. The increasingly routine use of computer analysis may contribute to routine use of statistical tests. Although the latter should not entirely replace the informal procedure, it does have the advantage of extremely rapid evaluation of large amounts of information. This would mean that the reviewers would have to spend time considering only likely problems, not all the data, reducing the work load. It also avoids the problem of tired, overworked individuals missing important information because they have had too large a volume of data to review. The thalidomide tragedy is one classic example where the increase in severe birth defects should have been readily recognizable but simply was not recognized until a large number of children had been affected (Taussig, 1962). The ultimate purpose of a surveillance system is to detect new or developing problems quickly before needless suffering occurs. To accomplish this, data must be effectively reviewed and evaluated.

Recognizing an Epidemic

An epidemic is "the occurrence in a defined population of cases of a particular illness, a specific health-related behavior, or other health-related event, clearly in excess of normal expectancy." To determine if this definition is met, it is necessary to know what is normally expected. Normal expectations can most easily be obtained from a previous period of time or from a similar comparison population. With a surveillance system, previous data from a comparable time period are generally available and can be used. The definition of an epidemic also includes the phrase "clearly in excess." When a hospital unit that normally only has two *nosocomial* (arising while patient is in a hospital or as a result of being in a hospital) staphylococcal infections in a month experiences ten cases in one week, it has a clear excess and thus an epidemic. With many diseases and health problems, such a clear excess is not always present. When the difference in frequency is a statistically significant difference (ie, not likely caused by chance), it is considered in clear excess.

In doing such comparisons, the time periods being compared must be equivalent, for example the case rate for the current week must be compared with the case rate for one previous week. Some epidemics may not be recognized as epidemics because an inappropriate comparison time period is used. Ideally, if seasonal variations in rates normally exist, then comparisons should be made between similar seasons. If reporting quality or completeness has changed substantially over time, presence of an epidemic could be masked or, conversely, appear to be present when it is not. There is little value in doing tests of differences if quality or completeness has changed substantially.

Trends over a prolonged period of time are frequently documented by surveillance systems. Unfortunately, little has been done to investigate such trends within the context of routine surveillance system investigations. In addition to looking for sudden significant changes, analysis for trends must also be routine. In the past, if work was completed to study such trends, it was more often performed by outside parties who became interested in the phenomena. Surveillance systems have thus been criticized as insensitive methods of recognizing or becoming aware of potential problems. If the time from the first exposure to a causative factor until onset of an epidemic is short, a problem may be recognized relatively easily. Conversely, a long latent period accompanied by a slow increase in the rate of exposure to a causative agent may make it impossible to label an apparent problem as an epidemic. This would be true, for example, in the case of a carcinogen such as asbestos, which has a 20- to 40-year latency period from exposure to onset of disease symptoms leading to diagnosis of mesothelioma. Diagnosed cases resulting from a single site of occupational exposure to asbestos (eg, one shipyard) may be scattered throughout many years and geographical locations and therefore not be identifiable as related to the prior common exposure. Similarly, new drugs or medical procedures are often introduced slowly over a period of time; even with a short latency period between exposure and onset of the associated disease, new cases may be scattered in time and place and thus be difficult to relate to the common exposure (the drug or the medical procedure). Oral contraceptives are a classic case in point. It was several years after use of the birth control pill began before anyone recognized the association between the pill and strokes, myocardial infarction, and thromboembolisms in women older than 35 years (Ory et al, 1980). Unless drug companies establish surveillance systems when a new drug is marketed, such associations will continue to go unrecognized, since side-effect testing during drug development is relatively short term.

Interactions of the disease, population at risk, and medical practice dynamics may also mask presence of an epidemic. For example, the frequency with which hysterectomy was performed for conditions other than cancer of the uterine cervix (eg, fibroids, endometriosis, and uterine prolapse) varied over time, by geographic region, and age of the woman (Centers for Disease Control, 1997c). Thus, the number of women at risk of developing cancer of the uterine cervix varies according to the number of women in the population who have a uterus and a cervix. During the same time period that changes in hysterectomy practices were occurring, so were patterns of sexual behavior, a risk factor for cervical cancer.

Interpretation of the data, thus, is basically focused on the question of whether there is evidence that an epidemic exists or that a problem is developing. Remember, a surveillance system is not designed to give answers to causal questions; it is meant to alert clinicians, administrators, or public health officials to potential problems so that an intervention can be initiated. If an investigation is not completed and, as a result, an existent problem is not identified, the system has not fulfilled its purpose. Such a circumstance puts both the health professional and the organization in the rather precarious legal position of having ignored what was known to be a possible problem.

Investigation

The goal of the investigation is to confirm whether a problem exists (an epidemic or upward trend over time) and to delineate potential causes so that control measures can be implemented. While ability to identify causal agents is helpful, control efforts may be applied even though causative factors have not been verified. For example, in the early 1980s, AIDS was, through its epidemiological features, highly suspected to be related to male homosexual activity with multiple partners. Even though the specific causative agent was unknown, control efforts could be directed at reducing homosexual contacts. Utilization of the Pap smear for nearly 50 years to reduce cervical cancer mortality through early detection is another example of control efforts in the absence of a known cause for the disease. Only in the last 10 years has the human papillomavirus (HPV) been convincingly implicated in an etiologic role (Nelson et al, 1989).

Preliminary Investigation.   Investigation may be divided into two phases, preliminary and active followup. During the preliminary phase additional information is collected, eg, that from a literature review related to previously identified epidemiological features such as natural history, latency period, susceptible age groups, time trends, and suspected or known etiological agents. Regardless of whether a literature review is needed, the investigator should first consider the simplest explanations for the apparent problem. A new, young, and aggressive physician who reports religiously may have a drastic impact on the number of cases reported. Introduction of a new diagnostic technique may mean that previously unrecognized cases are reported. Changes in reporting as a result of staff changes or new diagnostic tools are the most likely simple explanations for what may appear to be a problem. If such explanations are eliminated, the second phase is entered.

Active Followup.   The second phase of the investigation encompasses review of case definition with modifications of definition as necessary, verification of case status for all reported cases (ie, meets case definition), delineation of an appropriate comparison group, additional case ascertainment (previously unreported), collection of any new data identified as needed, analysis of new data, interpretation, and statement of conclusions. The investigator must make sure that the information gathered for both case and comparison groups are subject to the same data collection procedures and depth of ascertainment. Failure to do so may result in faulty interpretation and conclusions.

During the course of an investigation it may become apparent that more assistance or knowledge is needed. Assistance may be sought from the local health department, which may request help from the state health agency, which may in turn request assistance from the CDC. Although it is usually recommended to pursue a request for assistance through the hierarchy: local agency first, district or state second, then the CDC, in some cases it may be necessary to go directly to the CDC in order to stimulate state or local interest. Staff at the CDC are often personally acquainted with state epidemiologists and know how best to approach these individuals.

IMPLEMETATION OF MEASURES TO CONTROL DISEASES AND OTHER HEALTH PROBLEMS

Control measures are those activities that will reduce or eliminate the epidemic or problem that has been identified. Control measures may include:

- Quarantine
- Immunizations

- Preventive therapy (eg, administration of gammaglobulin to an individual who has been exposed to hepatitis)
- Eradication or reduction of host vector (eg, rats or mosquitoes)
- Medical treatment of individuals who may spread the disease (eg, syphilis)
- Early diagnosis (eg, cervical cancer or contacts of venereal disease cases)
- Reduction or removal from exposure (eg, environmental or occupational exposure to asbestos)
- Market ban or selective restriction of an agent (eg, pesticides or drugs not to be given during pregnancy)
- Nutritional supplements (eg, iron or folate for anemia)
- Other medical treatment or product modifications (eg, childproof safety caps)

Which control measure or measures are used depends on the problem identified, what caused the problem, and the likelihood for success of a given measure. The simplest, most effective, most practical, and least resource-consumptive method or methods represent the best choice. The reader should refer to Chapter 6 for a discussion of control measures related to infectious diseases and Chapter 7 for discussion of control measures related to diseases of noninfectious etiology.

During the development of a control plan, the administrator or clinician must consider several aspects of the situation. What is the appropriate target population at whom to direct the control measures? The best approach may be to apply control efforts selectively to a certain segment of the population. This strategy was used for the international control of smallpox; immediate contacts of known cases were isolated and vaccinated first, then entire population groups were vaccinated. The physical location for control efforts must also be considered. For example, will only a single unit in the hospital or in a particular school be the target or does adequate control necessitate measures to be applied in the whole hospital, in all classes at one school, or in all schools in the community? The final factors to consider are the period of time during which control efforts will be required and the planned startup and completion dates for the control effort.

Data collection must continue during and after control efforts so that the effectiveness of control measures can be evaluated. Implementation of control measures may have little or no effect if the wrong or inadequate measures are taken or if they are implemented after the epidemic has already peaked. Inability or failure to effectively implement control efforts eliminates the value of a surveillance system.

Evaluating the Surveillance System

It cannot be emphasized enough that evaluation ought to be a routine component of surveillance and disease control programs, with system revisions made as necessary. A surveillance system that has never been evaluated may be a totally worthless system. Both process and outcomes should be part of the evaluation.

Administrative or process-related questions that might be addressed in a system evaluation are quality of reporting, timeliness of reporting (late reports are of little value if they are so late that the epidemic is over before it is even recognized), adequacy of the reporting frequency (relative to the system requested frequency), completeness of reporting (ie, what proportion of all cases are actually reported), timeliness of summary reports, and how well needs of report providers are being met. Such process review should occur periodically during the regular operation of the surveillance system. This periodic review should consider the process-related items already discussed (ie, quality of reporting, timeliness of reporting, completeness of reporting, and adequacy of the reporting frequency). During the first phase after implementation of a surveillance system, consideration should also be directed to the appropriateness of the data sources selected and the individuals responsible for reporting. The periodic review of the data collection process is intended to determine if the data collection process is working. Regular review and elimination of problems should avoid a late realization that the purpose of the surveillance system was not met because of problems in the data collection process.

Part of the development of the surveillance system should have been identifying desired outcomes. These should be expressed as measurable goals, so they provide a framework for evaluating the system. The evaluation plan should address questions that ultimately answer *whether the purpose of the system was met?* For instance, were there any investigations carried out? Did these investigations identify a problem that was subsequently controlled or eliminated? What proportion of investigations led to control or elimination? What were the effects of the resulting interventions on disease incidence or prevalence? Other system evaluation questions might include whether a problem was identified earlier than it would have been without the system. How much earlier? Did the reduction in time to recognition have an impact on the rate of suffering? Table 13–5 summarizes system evaluation questions.

In the interest of controlling costs of health care, the need for surveillance systems must be clearly delineated and goals established. Evaluation of the system can then focus on how well goals are met. Assuming that the original goals were well conceived to meet community health needs, such review will provide a reasonable basis for evaluating the costs and benefits of the surveillance system. If goals are not being met, the surveillance system can be redesigned to better meet the goals or eliminated and funds diverted to better use.

TABLE 13–5. SYSTEM EVALUATION QUESTIONS

Questions Related to System Goals
Was the purpose of the system met?
    Were there any investigations carried out?
    Did these investigations lead to identification of a problem that was subsequently controlled or eliminated?
    What proportion of investigations led to control or elimination?
Was a problem identified earlier than it would have been without a system? How much earlier?

Administrative and Process Questions
How high is the quality of the reporting?
How timely are the reports?
Is the reporting frequency adequate?
How complete is the reporting?

REFERENCES

Benenson A. S. (Ed.). (1990) *Control of communicable disease in man* (15th ed.). Washington, D.C.: American Public Health Association.

Centers for Disease Control. (1998) Guidelines for evaluating surveillance systems. *Morbidity and Mortality Weekly Report, 37* (suppl. S-5).

Centers for Disease Control. (1997c) Hysterectomy surveillance—United States, 1980–1993. *Morbidity and Mortality Weekly Report, 46*(SS-4), 1–15.

Centers for Disease Control. (1997a) Injuries and deaths associated with use of snowmobiles—Maine, 1991–1996. *Morbidity and Mortality Weekly Report, 46*(1), 1–4.

Centers for Disease Control. (1997b) Reports published in CDC surveillance summaries since January 1, 1985. *Morbidity and Mortality Weekly Report, 46*(SS-3), i–iii.

National Committee for Quality Assurrance. (1997) *HEDIS 3.0: Narrative—What's in it and what we need to know.* Washington, D.C.: National Committee for Quality Assurance.

Nelson J. H., Averett H. E., Richart R. M. (1989) Cervical intraepithelial neoplasia (dysplasia and carcinoma in situ) and early invasive cervical carcinoma. *CA: Cancer Journal for Clinicians, 39*(3), 157–178.

Ory H. W., Rosenfeld A., Landman L. C. (1980) The pill at 20: An assessment. *Family Planning Perspectives, 12*(6), 178.

Taussig H. B. (1962) A study of the German outbreak of phocomelia. *Journal of the American Medical Association, 180*(13), 80.

Screening

n this chapter, screening is discussed as a strategy for secondary prevention of disease in populations. Both mass screening and case-finding uses of screening are considered. Screening is defined and contrasted with diagnostic tests. Characteristics of effective screening tests and screening programs, including operational measures of test accuracy such as reliability, validity, sensitivity, and specificity are presented. Issues of effectiveness versus efficacy are discussed. Finally, generally agreed upon screening recommendations are presented.

DEFINITION AND TYPES OF SCREENING

A major strategy for secondary prevention of disease is screening. *Screening* is defined as the presumptive identification of unrecognized disease or defect by the application of tests, examinations, or other procedures that can be applied rapidly and inexpensively to populations. Its purpose is to distinguish among apparently well persons, those who probably have a disease from those who probably do not. Screening is not intended to be diagnostic; persons with positive results on a screening test require additional diagnostic tests and examinations to establish a definitive diagnosis. Screening procedures may include cytological tests, blood tests, x-rays, urinalysis, amniocentesis, examination for scoliosis, and a variety of other procedures.

Screening tests may be applied unselectively to an entire population (eg, blood pressure screening of all persons attending a health fair) or may be applied selectively to certain groups of persons known to have a high risk for a disease. Examples of selective application to high-risk population groups are screening workers exposed to bladder carcinogens by cytological analysis of urine for bladder cancer, using mammograms to screen women with a family history of breast cancer, or doing tuberculin tests on children in inner-city schools. Such applications of screening tests, whether unselectively to entire populations or selectively to high-risk groups, are examples of *mass screenings.*

Screening may also be used as part of periodic health examinations in a private physician's office or a health maintenance clinic. Pap smears, for example, are often included as a part of the routine examination for women, and electrocardiograms are standard for middle-aged men. Regular height, weight, hearing, and vision measures of children are taken in pediatricians' offices, well-child clinics, or on home visits by nurses to detect early lags in growth and development or early impairment of hearing and vision. This type of screening, where clinicians use screening tests to search for disease among their own patients who have come in for a general checkup or for consultation regarding unrelated symptoms, is called *case finding.* With case finding, the clinician has an explicit responsibility to follow up any abnormal results. In mass screening, followup is usually limited to referring those individuals who test positive to their private physician or to a facility with followup capability.

Multiphasic screening, the use of a variety of screening tests on the same occasion, is another application of screening. Recent advances in technology have led to automated, sophisticated test techniques that permit many tests to be run on a single blood sample. These procedures have been used for a variety of purposes including: (1) establishing baseline data and classifying persons entering care at a particular health care facility; (2) periodic surveillance of persons with established disease; (3) hospital preadmission and preoperative examinations; (4) health evaluations for employment and life insurance; (5) as adjuncts to sickness consultations or periodic health examinations; and (6) risk-factor appraisal.

Questions have been raised about such uses of multiphasic screening. Part of the concern arises from the fact that the basic definition of normal versus abnormal is based on the customary normal curve, a statistical concept, rather than a clinical one. Abnormalities are defined as laboratory values that lie outside some specified range, usually two standard deviations from the mean. On this curve there will always be normal persons who are defined as abnormal. In any general population resembling the normal population from which the laboratory derived its normal range, one could expect one person in 20 to have an abnormality. In the case of multiphasic screening where many tests are performed simultaneously, the probability of a falsely abnormal result is considerably increased, yet a clinician feels obligated to follow up abnormal results because failure to do so could be legally risky. Because abnormal values on many of the clinical laboratory tests could be a sign of any of a variety of disease conditions, the patient may be thrown into what Schneiderman (1981) has called the *subspeciality loop* in an attempt to rule out systematically each of the conditions that potentially explain the elevated value.

As a way of minimizing this problem, Elvebach (1972) proposed using age- and sex-specific percentiles rather than standard deviations to define abnormality. This approach overcomes dependence on the normal curve, which is inappropriate in any case for the many biochemical values that are not normally distributed, and deals with the problem that a value normal for one group (eg, older women) may be highly abnormal for another group (eg, young men), and recognizes that health and disease represent a continuum on which separation of one from the other by a simple cutoff is quite arbitrary.

Mass screening, case finding, and multiphasic screening are all examples of prescriptive screening—screening performed for the purpose of better controlling disease through early detection in presumptively healthy individuals. Screening is also used by epidemiologists for research purposes. Screening of a population may be performed to estimate prevalence of disease. Furthermore, these screened populations may be followed over time, using periodic screens to identify new cases of the disease to determine incidence rates.

CHARACTERISTICS OF SCREENING TESTS

Screening Tests Versus Diagnostic Tests

How do screening tests differ from diagnostic tests? A major difference is the stage in the disease process at which the test detects the condition. Screening tests detect the disease before symptoms appear. Diagnostic tests are generally used on patients who have come to a treatment center seeking an explanation for symptoms they are experiencing. Diagnostic tests are ordered by a physician, often require specialized equipment or expertise to administer, are generally expensive, often time consuming, and may incur a degree of discomfort, pain, or risk for the patient. Results of diagnostic tests are usually of sufficient accuracy to establish a definitive diagnosis; they can thus be used as a basis for initiating treatment.

In contrast to diagnostic tests, screening tests are generally offered to apparently healthy populations as a way of determining whether it is probable that they have a disease; it is presumed that identifying probable disease before symptoms appear permits early initiation of treatment and, therefore, will affect the prognosis for the patient. The scientific basis for establishing the validity of this presumption was discussed in Chapter 12. The accuracy of screening tests is insufficient as a basis for initiating treatment; followup diagnostic testing of individuals with abnormal results on the screening test must be performed. For example, an individual who tests positive on a tuberculin test would need to have a complete history taken and, at a minimum, have a chest x-ray and a sputum test that can be cultured for the tubercule bacillus. Although the initial cost of doing a screening test may be low because these tests are generally inexpensive and can be administered by an individual with minimal training, the economic cost of the followup testing of those screened as abnormal can be considerable. If the yield of confirmed cases of disease is high among those screening abnormal and the test can identify most diseased persons in the screened population, then the cost of screening and followup can be justified. If the yield of confirmed cases is low relative to the number of positives on the screening test who are confirmed healthy, then screening becomes harder to justify.

The particular characteristics of screening tests that need to be considered are shown in Table 14–1 and are compared for screening and diagnostic tests. As

TABLE 14–1. CHARACTERISTICS OF SCREENING AND DIAGNOSTIC TESTS

CHARACTERISTIC	RATING OF SCREENING TEST	RATING OF DIAGNOSTIC TEST
Accuracy	Low–moderate	High
Simplicity	High	Moderate–low
Cost	Low	Moderate–high
Safety	High	High–low
Acceptability	High	Moderate–low

mentioned previously, screening tests are generally simpler, less accurate, less expensive, less risky, and more acceptable to a presumably well population than are diagnostic tests. These characteristics make mass screening programs feasible. To induce participation, an ideal screening test should take only a few minutes to perform, require minimal preparation by the patient, and require no special appointments. Tests requiring special diets (eg, fasting blood sugar) are not feasible for mass screening. Neither are tests that involve special appointments, discomfort, or risk (eg, proctoscopy carries risk of bowel perforation). Tuberculin testing as a screening procedure is feasible only if the screening population is "captive" (eg, children in a school), because a followup reading is required. Quick and simple examinations such as blood pressure determinations or the Snellen eye chart for vision screening are ideal screening tests from the standpoint of acceptability.

Test Accuracy

The cost of the test is a function of both the cost of the procedure itself and of the cost of subsequent evaluations performed on patients with positive test results. The need for followup testing is a function of the accuracy of the test. Accuracy is dependent on two characteristics, the validity and the reliability of the test.

Reliability involves the repeatability or replicability of the results—the ability of a test to give consistent results in repeated applications. Reliability is dependent both on the precision of the test—how much variation is present in the test itself—and on variation introduced by different persons applying the test. Variability in the result of a test procedure administered at two different times to the same sample by the same tester (eg, a split sample of blood) could be a function of variability in how the procedure was performed or interpreted by the tester (intra- and interindividual variability), or a function of variability in the test conditions (eg, the effects of change in room temperature on the chemical reagent used or the age and storage conditions of the reagent). Variability inherent in the test is called *test–retest reliability* and is obtained by doing the test two or more times on the same sample and calculating the statistical correlation of results across these samples. The measure of variability introduced by different persons applying the test is usually tested by examining the correlation of the results when two or more persons administer the test separately to the same individual or sample. This correlation is known as *interrater reliability*. Another correlative measure, *intrarater reliability*, assesses the consistency of a single individual at performing the test and interpreting the results.

Validity indicates how well a test result represents reality. In the case of screening tests, validity is assessed by the frequency with which the result of the test is confirmed by more vigorous diagnostic procedures. Validity is measured by the sensitivity, specificity, and predictive values of the test. *Sensitivity* is the frequency with which persons who have the disease test positive (ie, the probability of the test correctly identifying a case). *Specificity* is the frequency with which persons who do not have the disease test negative (ie, the probability of correctly identifying noncases). These measures are illustrated in Table 14–2. The distribution of a population with respect to disease status and screening test results, which are used as the basis for these measures, is shown in Table 14–3. Those persons with the disease (reading down in Table 14–3) can have two test results, true-positives or false-negatives. Sensitivity then is the percentage of all those with the disease (true-positives plus false-negatives) who test positive. Thus, the formula for sensitivity, as shown in Table 14–2, is

$$\text{Sensitivity} = \frac{\text{True-positives}}{\text{True-positives} + \text{False-negatives}} \times 100$$

Persons without the disease may have false-positive results on the screening test or true-negative results (see Table 14–3). Specificity is based on the percentage of these two test results that are true-negatives (see Table 14–2).

Sensitivity and specificity for a new test are determined by applying the test to a population for which disease status is known. These values are independent of disease prevalence. They are reciprocal to some degree, however, in that increasing sensitivity inevitably causes some decrease in specificity. Conversely, increasing

TABLE 14–2. MEASURE OF RELIABILITY AND VALIDITY OF SCREENING TESTS

CHARACTERISTIC	MEASURES	HOW CALCULATED
Validity	Sensitivity	$\dfrac{\text{True-positives}}{(\text{True-positives} + \text{False-negatives})} \times 100$
	Specificity	$\dfrac{\text{True-positives}}{(\text{True-negatives} + \text{False-positives})} \times 100$
	Predictive value positive test	$\dfrac{\text{True-positives}}{(\text{True-positives} + \text{False-positives})} \times 100$
	Predictive value negative test	$\dfrac{\text{True-negatives}}{(\text{True-negatives} + \text{False-negatives})} \times 100$
Reliability	Test-retest reliability	Correlation of results on two tests on same samples
	Interrater reliability	Correlation of results on same samples completed by two or more evaluators
	Intrarater reliability	Correlation of results on same samples performed several times by a single evaluator

TABLE 14–3. DISTRIBUTION OF DISEASE STATUS AND SCREENING TEST RESULTS IN A POPULATION

SCREENING TEST RESULT	TRUE DIAGNOSIS		
	Diseased	Not Diseased	Total
Positive	True-positives	False-positives	True-positives + False-positives
Negative	False-negatives	True-negatives	False-negatives + True-negatives
Total	True-positives + False-negatives	False-positives + True-negatives	True-positives + False-positives + False-negatives + True-negatives

specificity decreases sensitivity. This is particularly true for tests based on a continuous distribution of test values. A level called the *screening level,* must be chosen somewhat arbitrarily to represent abnormality. Because there is an overlap in the distribution of test values for individuals with and without the disease at any cutoff level defining abnormality, some individuals will be misclassified. In blood pressure measurement, for example, 140 mm Hg and 90 mm Hg, respectively, are frequently used as cutoffs for systolic and diastolic pressures for declaring a person positive for hypertension in a screening program. A significant number of persons testing positive on the screen may be false-positives whose pressure was temporarily elevated because of anxiety over having their pressure taken or because of some stressful event on the way to the screening site (eg, a near accident in the parking lot). This cutoff, although likely to correctly classify as probable hypertensives all those who truly have hypertension, will also misclassify as probable hypertensives many who are not. Sensitivity is excellent, but specificity is low. Using a cutoff of 160 mm Hg and 100 mm Hg may misclassify some true hypertensives as normal but is less likely to misclassify individuals without hypertension as abnormal; at this level, sensitivity is lower, but specificity is higher than in the previous example.

Consider the following example: Phenylketonuria (PKU) is an inborn metabolic defect affecting metabolism of protein. This condition can be detected by a blood test for phenylalanine levels. Approximately three fifths of the 50 states require or recommend testing newborn infants for this condition before hospital discharge (Sprinkle et al, 1994). Retesting is recommended for those tested before 24 hours of age (Sinai et al, 1995; Hanley et al, 1997). In a population without PKU, blood levels of phenylalanine may vary from 0 to 12 mg%. In a population with the disease, phenylalanine levels may range from 6 to more than 50 mg%. Levels in an individual may vary from time to time depending on factors such as recency of ingesting protein-containing foods, which metabolize to produce phenylalanine, and the amount of such foods ingested. Levels also vary by age. Thus, the distribution of phenylalanine values in infants with and without PKU may resemble that shown in Figure 14–1. Between 6 and 12 mg% there is overlap in the distribution,

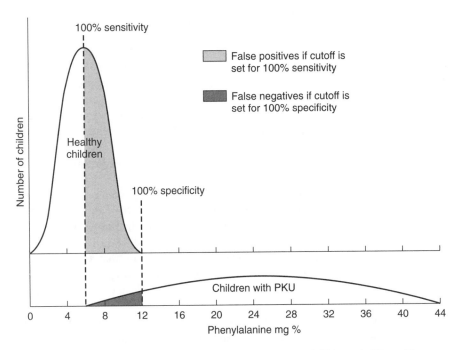

Figure 14–1. Illustrative distribution of phenylalanine values in normal children and children with phenylketonuria (PKU).

with many healthy children and some children with PKU. Some value must be chosen to serve as the cutoff level for declaring normal versus abnormal. In the diagram shown, declaring 6 mg% as the cutoff (screening level) would represent 100% sensitivity—all diseased children would be correctly screened as positive; there would be no false-negatives. This, however, would produce a large number of false-positives (Fig. 14–1). Using 12 mg% as the cutoff for declaring normal versus abnormal would produce a test that is 100% specific; this, however, would produce a substantial number of false-negatives. Therefore, to maximize sensitivity and specificity of the test, an intermediate value such as 9 to 10 mg% represents an acceptable compromise, maintaining reasonably high sensitivity and reasonable specificity.

Predictive values of a screening test, unlike sensitivity and specificity, are measures dependent on the prevalence of disease in the population to which the test is applied. Predictive values describe the frequency with which test results represent correct identification of disease status among those screened. The predictive value of a positive test is the proportion of those testing positive who have the disease. The predictive value of a negative test is the proportion of those testing negative who do not have the disease. These are usually expressed as percentage of positives or percentage of negatives who were correctly identified (see Table 14–2).

Using Predictive Values for Decision Making

Because predictive values vary with the prevalence of disease in the screened population, they are useful in deciding whether to use a particular test in a given population. For a test with a fixed sensitivity and specificity, increasing the prevalence rate of the disease in the population to be screened increases the predictive value of a positive test. Because groups at high risk of developing a disease are likely to have a higher prevalence of that disease than a general population, screening of high-risk populations can improve the predictive value to a positive test. This means fewer false-positives relative to true-positives to be followed up for diagnostic testing (Table 14–4).

Returning to the previous example of PKU, let us examine the effects of disease prevalence on predictive values in two hypothetical population distributions of disease and phenylalanine levels. In a general population, the prevalence of PKU was determined to be 9.6 in 100,000 among white births and 4.6 in 100,000 among nonwhite births (National Research Council, 1975). Suppose that sensitivity and specificity of the test have been determined to be 94% and 90%, respectively. Applying these approximate values in a screen of 100,000 white newborns would produce the values shown in Table 14–5(A). Nine of the ten infants with PKU would be correctly diagnosed, and one would have a false-negative test. Among the 99,990 infants without PKU, 4,999 would have false-positive test results and require a diagnostic workup to determine that they do not have PKU. The predictive value of the positive test is a dismal 0.180%; 555.4 subjects with false-positive tests must be given a diagnostic workup for every case detected (4,999 divided by 9). Predictive value of a negative test is excellent at 99.999%.

Unfortunately, to date no high-risk group for PKU has been identified. Let us suppose, however, for illustrative purposes, that some high-risk group was identifiable. Further, let us assume that the likely prevalence of disease among this high-risk population is 10 in 1,000. Using the same screening test with the same sensitivity and specificity to screen 100,000 high-risk persons produces the results shown in Table 14–5(B). Nine hundred cases of PKU are detected. Predictive value of a

TABLE 14–4. PREDICTIVE VALUE OF A POSITIVE TEST AS A FUNCTION OF DISEASE PREVALENCE FOR A LABORATORY TEST WITH 95% SENSITIVITY AND 95% SPECIFICITY

PREVALENCE OF DISEASE IN SCREENED POPULATION (%)	PREDICTIVE VALUE OF POSITIVE TEST (%)
1	16.1
5	50.0
10	67.9
20	82.6
50	95.0

TABLE 14–5. RESULTS OF HYPOTHETICAL SCREENING FOR PHENYLKETONURIA (PKU)

A. TEST RESULT	PKU PRESENT	PKU ABSENT	TOTAL
Positive test	9	4,999[a]	5,008
Negative test	1	94,991	94,992
Total	10	99,990	100,000

Prevalence = 10/100,000
Sensitivity = 90%
Specificity = 95%

$$\text{Predictive value positive test} = \frac{9}{5008} = 0.180\%$$

$$\text{Predictive value negative test} = \frac{94,991}{94,992} = 99.999\%$$

B. TEST RESULT	PKU PRESENT	PKU ABSENT	TOTAL
Positive test	900	4,950	5,850
Negative test	100	94,050	94,150
Total	1,000	99,000	100,000

Prevalence = 10/1,000
Sensitivity = 90%
Specificity = 95%

$$\text{Predictive value positive test} = \frac{900}{94,150} = 15.385\%$$

$$\text{Predictive value negative test} = \frac{4,050}{94,150} = 99.894\%$$

[a]Numbers have all been rounded to the nearest whole number because persons do not exist as fractions.

positive test has increased to 15.385%; only about 6.5 subjects with false-positive results must be followed for every case detected. Predictive value of the negative test shows only a negligible change.

CRITERIA FOR SCREENING PROGRAMS

The criteria that should be met by a good screening program are listed in Table 14–6. These criteria address the scientific, social, and ethical issues relevant to screening. They imply careful selection of tests based on accuracy, good epidemiological description of the natural history of the disease, evidence of the efficacy of earlier treatment (see discussion of lead time bias, Chap. 12), and a positive cost–benefit to society. The criteria for screening programs also imply careful selection of the population to be screened and inclusion of plans for program evaluation.

TABLE 14–6. CRITERIA FOR A SCREENING PROGRAM

1. Test has high sensitivity and specificity.
2. Test meets acceptable standards of simplicity, cost, safety, and patient acceptability.
3. Disease that is focus of screening should be sufficiently serious in terms of incidence, mortality, disability, discomfort, and financial cost.
4. Evidence suggests that the test procedure detects the disease at a significantly earlier stage in its natural history than it would present with symptoms.
5. A generally accepted treatment that is easier or more effective than treatment administered at the usual time of symptom presentation must be available.
6. The available treatment is acceptable to patients as established by studies on compliance with treatment.
7. Prevalence of the target disease should be high in the population to be screened.
8. Followup diagnostic and treatment service must be available and accompanied by an adequate notification and referral service for those positive on screening.

The Individual's Risks Versus Benefits

Because screening procedures are applied to well persons and because of the potential economic and psychological costs incurred by misclassification of disease status, a benefit should accrue to the individual screenees as a result of the program in addition to the cost–benefit to society accruing from earlier detection and treatment of the disease.

Consider the four possible outcomes of a screening test: (1) true-positive, (2) true-negative, (3) false-positive, and (4) false-negative. Individuals with accurate results, the true-positives and true-negatives, can benefit from screening. Individuals with true-negative results benefit from the peace of mind that comes from knowing they are disease-free. Those screenees with true-positive results, however, will benefit from the detection of their disease only if three conditions are met: (1) the screening test has detected their condition at an earlier stage of disease than would have the presence of symptoms; (2) earlier detection can lead to improving their prognosis because an effective treatment is available; and (3) the available treatment is acceptable to the patient and the physician. If these conditions are not met, then there is no benefit to individuals with true-positive results. For example, screening for sickle cell anemia has been criticized in the past on the grounds that no benefit accrued to the diseased individual because no effective treatment was available to change the prognosis; the patient merely lives longer with anxiety about having sickle cell disease. However, more recently, research delineating the mechanisms by which sickle cell produces its clinical manifestations has led to more effective treatments that supplement the supportive therapies of the past with treatments directed to the disease's unique pathophysiology (Rodgers, 1997). If the three conditions are met, then the economic cost of treating the condition is likely to be lower than it would be without screening, both because of less complicated initial treatment and because of the decreased probability of disability.

Screened individuals with false-positive results are likely to be somewhat unhappy with the screening program. First, they experience a period of time when they must worry about whether they have the disease. Second, they must undergo a series of diagnostic tests that, at the very least, take time away from work, home, and friends; these tests may be uncomfortable or painful and involve unpleasant side effects or some degree of risk. Finally, someone must pay for these tests; if health insurance pays, such costs eventually will be reflected in higher premiums. Individuals who do not have health insurance must pay the costs out of their own pockets. Although individuals will be relieved to learn that they do not have the disease, they are likely to resent the unnecessary economic and psychological costs. Followup testing also imposes a burden on the health care system. If the positive predictive value of a screening test is low, then large numbers of false-positives must be processed through diagnostic procedures. Time, facilities, and personnel must be available, and a good referral program must be in place.

Finally, there is the individual with the false-negative test. This individual also may be harmed as a result of the screening program. Although it could be argued that this individual is no worse off than if they had not been screened, such is not always the case. Major harm would arise if, when symptoms appear, the individual recognizes them as early signs of the disease for which they were recently screened negative and ignores them rather than seeking medical attention. As a result, the cost of treating the condition may be higher than otherwise would be the case, and the patient's prognosis may be negatively affected. Legal action could ensue. As a precaution, some health education about signs and symptoms and the possibility that these could develop in the future despite negative screening results might be useful to include in the screening program.

PROGRAM PLANNING AND EVALUATION

The principles of planning and evaluation described in Chapter 16 are readily applicable to screening programs. Program planning and evaluation relies on epidemiological data (see discussion of secondary prevention in the section of Chap. 12 entitled "Using Information on Natural History in Clinical Practice"). The following facts about each disease must be sought:

1. Incidence, prevalence, and mortality from the disease, preferably age- and sex-specific
2. Progression of the disease with and without treatment at various stages, to include morbidity, mortality, and length of the early asymptomatic period (latency)
3. Risk factors associated with development of the disease
4. Availability of screening tests, their safety, sensitivity, and specificity in the early stages of the disease, and their unit cost
5. Demonstrated efficacy of the screening tests in changing disease outcomes

Decisions about which screening tests should be used in mass screening programs in a particular community need to consider disease frequency as well as the demonstrated ability of the test to identify the disease at a stage of the natural history when intervention can change the prognosis. Availability of followup services and resources in the community are also considerations.

General measures of community health, such as changes in morbidity or mortality related to the disease, specific demographic and followup data on screenees to evaluate rates of diagnostic followup, and the predictive values of positive and negative results should all be included in evaluation protocols. An example of the importance of such monitoring is a program in the inner-city area of an eastern U.S. city that screened for cervical cancer using the Pap test. This is a test with demonstrated efficacy, reasonable sensitivity, and specificity. The inner-city was targeted for the screening program because residents were considered high risk in terms of the high prevalence of behaviors that increased their risk for cervical cancer. Although substantial numbers of women were screened, the predictive value of the positive test was low; very few cases of cervical cancer were detected. Review of the intake records revealed that most participants were middle-income married women rather than the lower-income single women at high risk of developing cervical cancer who were targeted by the screening program. Thus, disease prevalence among those screened was low. This example demonstrates that a screening program that uses an efficacious test may not be effective. *Efficacy* is tested under ideal conditions, usually a randomized clinical trial. *Effectiveness* refers to how well a program performs under field conditions, ie, when introduced into service settings where the oversight and controls imposed by a research protocol are lacking. While a research screening program may demonstrate high predictive value, results are often dissimilar when programs are implemented in communities because there is not the strict control on whether the populations screened were those targeted, laboratory readings may be less closely monitored, as well as other factors. Thus, monitoring and evaluating of programs after implementation is essential. Such monitoring permits early identification of problems and implementation of corrective strategies that may increase the effectiveness and cost–benefit of the program.

Efficacy and Survival Estimates

The question of whether a particular screening procedure actually minimizes or prevents damage is an important one requiring knowledge about the natural history of the disease. Minimizing or preventing damage means that the natural history will be changed or altered in some way by the intervention after diagnosis of the disease. Changes or alterations considered beneficial are elimination of the disease, minimization of effect or disability, longer survival, and prevention of death. Longer survival may occur in two ways. In the first, the disease is totally eliminated by the treatment (eg, complete hysterectomy for carcinoma *in situ*). The second way is to slow down the length of time it takes for the disease to cause death. For example, an individual may survive for 30 years with diabetes instead of 5 years.

Screening efficacy is the extent to which the screening test produces a beneficial result under ideal conditions. Ideally, the determination of efficacy is based on the results of a randomized controlled trial. But much of the available literature reporting on the efficacy of various screening tests does not have data from randomized clinical trials. Rather, they compare screen-detected cases with nonscreened cases and compare survival. In evaluating the efficacy of a screening method, the researcher who conducts the study and the clinician who reads research results must determine that appropriate analysis is used to evaluate survival. Two major issues should be considered: lead time and length bias. *Lead time* is the time gained in treating or controlling a disease because of earlier diagnosis (ie, the interval from detection to the time at which diagnosis would have been made without screening). Lead time is desirable if it permits early treatment and changes the disease prognosis. But evaluation of screening time must address lead bias—a systematic overestimation of survival time that can result if lead time has not been accounted for. Figure 14–2 illustrates lead time. Suppose that two women of the same age, Mary and Susan, develop a breast cancer that became pathogenic at the same point in time for each of them (point *a* in Fig. 14–2), and each dies at age 35 years from breast cancer (point *b*). Suppose Mary, at age 30 years, detected a lump in her breast, went to her physician, and after a biopsy was diagnosed and treated for breast cancer (point *K*). Susan, however, read about a local center that was screening for breast cancer using mammography. At the age of 25 years (point *L*), she had a mammogram that detected a lesion, was followed up by biopsy, and was diagnosed and treated for breast cancer. Mary survives until she is 35 years old, 5 years since her diagnosis. Susan also survives until she is 35 years old, which is 10 years after her diagnosis. Can it be concluded that screening improved survival? In the past, most studies evaluating the effects of screening programs calculated survival for screened patients beginning

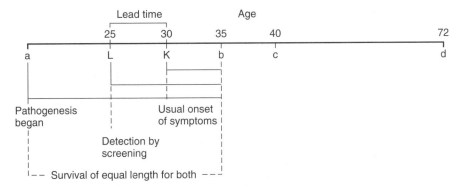

Figure 14–2. Comparison of breast cancer detection and survival for two women. (If two women develop a breast cancer at the same point in time [point *a*] and both die of breast cancer at age 35 years [point *b*], then they have an equal survival. If survival is measured from point of diagnosis, point *L* for the woman whose lesion was discovered in screening and point *K* for the woman whose lesion was discovered at the usual onset of symptoms, then the survival of the two women would appear to be different, point *L* to point *b* for one woman [10 years] and point *K* to point *b* for the other woman [5 years]. The interval between *L* and *K* is considered lead time and only reflects a difference in when awareness of the presence of disease existed. If the woman detected at point *L* had lived to be 40, then there would have been a true difference in survival, point *b* to point *c*, a true difference of 5 years.)

with the time of diagnosis by screening and ending with their death. Patients diagnosed after seeking care for symptoms were used as the comparison group. Their survival time was measured from diagnosis (symptom onset) to death. If screening detects disease during early pathogenesis before symptoms are present, say point L rather than point K (see Fig. 14–2), *lead time* is gained. Lead time is the extra time during which there is an awareness of the presence of disease, extra in the sense that it was recognized before symptoms were present. The lead time in this example is 5 years, the period in Figure 14–2 between points L and K. In the case of Mary and Susan, the 5 extra years for Susan merely reflects the lead time in detecting her disease. Presumably by detecting a disease earlier, treatment will be more effective and the disease can be prevented from progressing. This is only true, however, if the screening method can detect the pathological change before the critical point. A false conclusion of increased survival may be made if comparisons of survival for patients detected by screening are made with the survival of those diagnosed because symptoms are present, unless lead time is subtracted out. Lack of control for this effect in such survival comparisons is called *lead time bias*. To be valid, survival comparisons must take account of lead times.

The other methodological issue of concern in evaluating studies of screening efficacy is length bias, also called *length-biased sampling* and *prognostic selection*. *Length bias* is defined as a systematic error in estimation of survival time after screening because of a propensity for a screening test to identify cases destined to have a relatively benign course. The issue to be considered in evaluating a study of screening efficacy is whether the screening test selectively identifies the slow-growing as opposed to the fast-growing cases. If it does, this alone could create the impression that the test is efficacious; outcomes for the screened group will be better than for the unscreened group simply because fast-growing cancers generally have worse outcomes than slow-growing cancers. Unless the study can address the extent to which length bias is operating and estimate its effect on the differences in outcome, it must be interpreted conservatively. (For more extensive discussion of lead time and length bias, refer to Morrison, 1985.) Because lead time and length bias have been inadequately addressed in most screening studies reported in the literature and because for many screening tests there are no randomized controlled efficacy trials, there may be controversy over whether use of a particular test should be recommended. The current controversy regarding screening for prostate cancer with the Prostate Specific Antigen (PSA) test is an example.

PRACTICE GUIDELINES

Although a variety of published protocols provide primary health care practitioners with guidelines for use of screening procedures in preventive health practice, there is far from unanimous agreement on screening protocols. For example, there is disagreement between the American Cancer Society and the National Cancer Institute on the appropriateness of annual screening of women aged 40 to 49 with mammography (Leitch et al, 1997; Report of the Consensus Development Panel, 1997).

Also, as new studies are completed it is frequently necessary to reevaluate recommendations about a specific screening protocol. The American Cancer Society in 1980 changed its position regarding the use of chest x-rays for lung cancer screening based on reevaluation of the evidence (Mettlin & Dodd, 1991). Fecal occult blood (hemoccult) screening for colorectal cancer was controversial until a series of efficacy trials were recently completed. After reviewing the results from these trials, the American Gastroenterological Association published guidelines for colorectal cancer screening that included annual fecal occult blood testing (Winawer et al, 1997). The updated American Cancer Society recommendations also include mass screening of the population over age 50, with colonoscopy followup of positive tests (Byers et al, 1997).

Each clinician must evaluate the proposed screening program in terms of the criteria in Table 14–7 and in terms of the actual dollar cost relative to the health benefits to individuals and society. There is an extensive literature quantifying cost–benefit, but this is beyond the scope of this chapter. Administrators will need to attach dollar figures to various programs and relate this cost to benefit for purposes of obtaining funding; they will need to demonstrate the benefit of their preferred program relative to others competing for the same source of funds and to present convincing scientific arguments for their recommendations. Clinicians must be able to evaluate the cost of case finding to their practice and their patients, weighing the harm versus benefit of using a particular test, the impact of using the test on cost of health services and use of resources within their own practice setting, the burden of suffering associated with the condition both for individuals (patient and family) and for society, and the risk status of the particular patient. The clinician is in a position to collect the information necessary to establish likely risk—a thorough health and behavioral history is invaluable. If the clinician is familiar with the epidemiological evidence regarding risk factors, they are in a position to identify patients at high risk for specific diseases. Use of screening tests selectively on high-risk patients rather than on all patients in a broad category is likely to be most effective. For example, a cytological analysis of urine for a patient occupationally exposed to bladder carcinogens who is also a heavy smoker makes some sense, but routine cytological analysis on all adults does not. Electrocardiographic testing of an overweight, hypertensive middle-aged man who smokes and has a family history of heart disease may be useful, but to routinely screen all middle-aged men is probably of little use.

With these issues in mind, the U.S. Preventive Services Task Force recommended screening tests and procedures for inclusion in clinical encounters (1989). These recommendations were included in Chapters 8 through 11. Similarly, the Canadian Task Force on the Periodic Health Examination (Canadian Task Force, 1979) developed a set of recommendations for periodic health examinations that includes appropriate screening tests and screening examinations. Table 14–7 lists the screening tests and examinations recommended by the Canadian Task Force. The procedures included in these table received a rating of A or B from the Task Force to use with the specified population. A recommendation of A means that there is good evidence to support the use of a periodic health examination; a recommendation of

TABLE 14–7. RECOMMENDED SCREENING TESTS FOR EARLY DETECTION BY MASS SCREENING OR SCREENING OF HIGH-RISK GROUPS[a]

TEST FOR GENERAL POPULATION AND HIGH-RISK GROUPS	DISEASE	APPLICABLE POPULATION
Serological testing	Syphilis	Pregnant women before 16th week
Thyroxine testing	Neonatal hypothyroidism	All neonates
Microbiological inhibition and fluoro-metric tests	Phenylketonuria	All neonates
Maternal serum alpha-feto protein testing	Neural tube defects	Pregnant women
Visual acuity testing	Refractive vision defects	School children
Blood pressure measurement	Hypertension	General population
Mammography	Breast cancer	Women older than 45 years[b]
Papanicolaou smear	Cancer of the cervix	All sexually active women
Blood group and antibody tests	Blood group incompatability in pregnancy	Pregnant women
Microbiological examination of urine	Bacteriuria in pregnancy	Pregnant women
Cervical and urethral smears	Gonorrhea	Pregnant women
Iontophoresis sweat test	Cystic fibrosis	Siblings of cystic fibrosis patients
Serum creatinine phosphokinase determination	Duchenne's muscular dystrophy (DMD)	Female relative of DMD patients
Resistance of serum hexosamine to heat inactivation	Tay-Sachs' disease	Ashkenazi Jews and other high-risk groups
Amniocentesis	Down's syndrome	Parents with translocation of chromosome 21 or family history of Down's; pregnant women older than 35 years of age
Serological testing for *Toxoplasma gondi*	Toxoplasmosis	Nonimmune pregnant women who keep a cat or who eat raw meat
Cervical and urethral smears	Gonorrhea	Women with history of multiple sexual partners
Blood tests	Syphilis	Persons with history of multiple sexual partners
Blood hemoglobin concentration	Iron deficiency anemia	Premature babies; babies of multiple pregnancy or an iron-deficient woman; persons of low socioeconomic circumstances
Stool test for occult blood	Cancer of colon and rectum	Persons with history of colitis, familial polyporis or villous adenomas, or family history of cancer of the colon; persons over age 50 years
Cytological analysis of urine[c]	Cancer of the bladder	Workers occupationally exposed to bladder carcinogens; smokers
Urine testing for glucose	Diabetes mellitus	Family history of diabetes; abnormalities associated with pregnancy; physical abnormalities such as circulatory dysfunction and hand vascular impairment
Tuberculin test	Tuberculosis	Family of tuberculosis patients; children living in high prevalence areas (generally lower socioeconomic conditions); elderly in high prevalence areas

[a]Recommendations based on Canadian Task Force. Periodic health examination. *Canadian Medical Association Journal,* 1979; *121,* 1193–1254.

[b]Canadian Task Force recommends women aged 50 to 59 years; American Cancer Society recommends women older than 40 years. Frame and Carlson recommend it only for women older than 50 years with large fatty breasts (Frame P., Carlson S. A review of periodic health screening using specific criteria. *Journal of Family Practice,* 1975; *2,* 29–36).

[c]American Gastroenterological Association and American Cancer Society Recommendation.

B is supported by fair evidence. Procedures with ratings of C through E, reflecting poor evidence to support their use, were not included in the table. The reader is referred to this report and to a four-part review of screening tests by Frame and Carlson (1975), which is mostly consistent with the Canadian recommendations. The Frame and Carlson articles are particularly helpful in detailing the rationale behind each recommendation. Since this report was issued the evidence regarding colorectal cancer supported screening, so this has been added to the table.

The reader will note that some tests that are widely used or frequently proposed for use are not included, for example, mass screening with prostate-specific antigen (PSA) tests for prostate cancer, self-testicle examination, and breast self-examination (BSE). We shall consider the issue of BSE as an example of how to think through the screening issues.

It has been suggested that BSE be taught to high school girls as a form of screening for breast cancer. Similar issues are relevant to proposals to teach testicular examination to high school boys. It is hypothesized that habits established at an early age, in this case monthly practice of BSE, are more likely to become routine behaviors and if all women were to develop the habit of monthly BSE, early detection of breast cancer would lead to early treatment and substantial reductions in mortality. In fact, self-examination by the patient is the way in which 90% of breast malignancies in one study were detected (Thiessen, 1981), whether or not the patient had been instructed in systematic periodic breast examination. In a study of women receiving annual physician examinations, 38% of all breast tumors were discovered by the patients between physician examination (Venet et al, 1971). Because women seem to be so successful at finding tumors and because BSE is inexpensive and can be performed frequently without much investment of health care resources, this recommendation seems more than reasonable at first glance, particularly since establishing the habit early should overcome the patient compliance problem. Since these early studies, several longitudinal studies have tried to assess the efficacy of BSE for preventing mortality. Results are inconclusive; two studies found no significant reduction in breast cancer mortality associated with BSE-detected tumors (Auvinen et al, 1996; Holmberg et al, 1997), while a third did find a reduction for tumors detected by BSE, when mammography was used for diagnosis (Gastrin et al, 1994). Some additional problems that have not been considered in this recommendation follow:

1. Studies have documented time lags ranging from 6 to 18 months between the time women detect a lump and the first physician contact.
2. It has been demonstrated that it is difficult for women with large, pendulous, or fatty breasts to detect lumps (Thiessen, 1981). These same women may have a higher risk of developing breast cancer.
3. No increase in survival has been demonstrated among women younger than 50 who are screened by a combination of mammography plus palpation (Consensus Development Conference Panel, 1997), let alone by BSE. Although there is little question that treatment of stage I breast cancer is associated with dramatically longer survival than either untreated stage I cancer

or cancer diagnosed at later stages, it has never been demonstrated that BSE more frequently detects stage I cancer.

4. Although breast cancer is the leading cause of death due to cancer in women, its incidence is age-related. The disease is rare before age 30. The U.S. incidence data from the Surveillance, Epidemiology, End Results Program (SEER), 1987 to 1991, shows the annual incidence per 100,000 women to be 1.0 between ages 20 and 24, 7.8 from ages 25 to 29, 25.6 from ages 30 to 34, and 63.6 between ages 35 and 39. By age 65 to 69, incidence is 412.1 in 100,000 and by 80 to 84, it is 477.1 in 100,000 (Ries et al, 1994). The likelihood that any one woman younger than 40 will have breast cancer is minute; from high school age to age 25, it is nearly nonexistent.

5. Of breast lump biopsies performed at all ages, somewhere between 10% and 40% (1 in 2.5 and 1 in 10.0) are malignant (Bassett et al, 1997). In younger age groups the ratio will be closer to 1 in 10 because of the low incidence of breast cancer. If all young women were to do BSE, it would become even lower because nearly all lumps found would be benign and, therefore, false-positives. Many lumps are never biopsied; an examining physician, particularly a breast specialist, is often expert at determining when a presumed lump is part of normal breast structure and at ruling out malignancy by palpation. Thus, the specificity of BSE is very low. Many lumps found will require a physician's visit followed by referral to a breast specialist. Even if biopsy is not required, these women undergo enormous psychological stress. For those requiring a biopsy to rule out malignancy, the psychological and physical pain are substantial, as is the economic cost. Bassett and coworkers (1997, p. 173) stated it well—"Excessive biopsies for benign lesions have adverse effects on society and on the women who undergo them because they increase the costs of screening, cause morbidity and anxiety, and add to the barriers that keep women from using a potentially lifesaving procedure."

Clinicians and administrators must continually make decisions about sponsoring public screening programs and whether to use various screening tests in their own practice. Medical supply companies are continually developing new technologies for screening that are marketed to clinicians, administrators, and with increasing frequency, the general public for use at home. Home screening raises not only concerns about the burdens of following up false-positives but also major issues regarding false-negatives primarily because there is no control over whether the test procedure is correctly performed. Studies of home pregnancy testing kits found false-negative rates as high as 50% in consumer use when they were first available (Baker et al, 1976); improved kits still yielded false-negative rates as high as 33% (Valanis & Perlman, 1982). Issues that arose included concern that false-negative rates might be more frequent among high-risk pregnancies (ie, teenagers and those of lower socioeconomic status) as a result of poorer compliance to test procedure among these groups. Such negative results might lead these groups to delay seeking prenatal care even longer than usual or those wishing to have an abortion to seek care too late for a simple first trimester abortion. The news media frequently pick up on such issues, and those in clinical practice must be informed about the relevant epidemiological data to speak out on these issues, as they are so often asked to do.

The National Human Genome Project in the United States, designed to identify and map all human genes, is likely to lead to availability of tests to detect individuals with genes that make them high risk for one or more diseases. One case in point illustrates some of the issues and concerns that arise with such testing. Recently, a test for the BRCA1 gene for breast cancer became available. This test has raised additional issues in regard to screening, since we are screening not for an early stage of the disease, but for a gene that indicates higher risk of developing the disease. However, while those with the gene are at higher risk of developing breast cancer, having the gene does not mean they will get the disease. Further, the cause of breast cancer has not yet been determined, so we know little about how to prevent the disease. Low fat diet has been suggested as a possible cause; its causal role is only now being tested in a randomized clinical trial, the Women's Health Initiative (Matthews et al, 1997; Rossouw et al, 1995). Chemoprevention of breast cancer for high-risk women through use of tamoxiphen has been suggested, but results from the clinical trial testing its efficacy have not yet been published (Nayfield, 1995). Some surgeons have recommended prophylactic oophorectomy or bilateral prophylactic mastectomy for high-risk women, but the value of these procedures has never been demonstrated in a randomized trial and many women find this approach unacceptable. Early detection through regular screening is the only definitive option available to women testing positive for the gene and they could obtain routine mammograms without knowing they have the gene. To date, the only action available to women screened positive is to avoid reproduction so the gene is not passed on to a daughter. Thus, being screened for gene positivity does little to assist the woman or her physician in preventing breast cancer and the cost of the test is high. Mass screening would definitely not make sense. More controversial is whether to use the test in a clinical setting to screen individual women with a family history of breast cancer or other factors making them at high risk for this disease.

In this era of limited fiscal resources for health, screening programs must be objectively based. Because few testing programs are systematically evaluated by clinical trial before widespread use, available data related to the criteria for screening programs must be reviewed. As new information on disease natural history and changes in treatment becomes available, reevaluation of existing recommendations may be necessary. Clearly, screening procedures are best used in conjunction with a longitudinal program of periodic health assessment, rather than sporadic, one-shot screening programs.

REFERENCES

Auvinen A., Elovainio L., Hakama M. (1996) Breast self-examination and survival from breast cancer: A prospective follow-up study. *Breast Cancer Research and Treatment, 38*(2), 161–168.

Baker L. D., West L. W., Chase M. D., et al. (1976) Evaluation of home pregnancy tests. *American Journal of Public Health, 66,* 130–132.

Bassett L., Winchester D. P., Caplan R. B., Dershaw D. D., Dowlatshahi K., Evans W. P. III., et al. (1997) Stereotactic core-needle biopsy of the breast: A report of the Joint Task Force of the American College of Radiology, American College of Surgeons, and College of American Pathologists. *CA: Cancer Journal for Clinicians, 47*(3), 171–190.

Byers T., Levin B., Rothenberger D., Dodd G. D., Smith R. A. (1997) American Cancer Society guidelines for screening and surveillance for early detection of colorectal polyps and cancer: Update 1997. *CA: Cancer Journal for Clinicians, 47*(3), 154–160.

Canadian Task Force. (1979) Periodic health examination. *Canadian Medical Association Journal, 121,* 1193–1254.

Elvebach L. R. (1972) How high is high? A proposed alternative to the normal range. *Mayo Clinic Proceedings, 47,* 93.

Frame P., Carlson S. (1975) A critical review of periodic health screening using specific criteria. *Journal of Family Practice, 2,* 29–36; 123–129; 189–194; 283–288.

Gastrin G., Miller A. B., To T., Aronson K. J., Wall C., Hakama M., Louhivuori K., Pukkala E. (1994) Incidence and mortality from breast cancer in the Mama Program for Breast Screening in Finland, 1973–1986. *Cancer, 73*(8), 2168–2174.

Hanley W. B., Demshar H., Preston M. A., Borczyk A., Schoonheyt W. E., Clarke J. T., Feigenbaum A. (1997) Newborn phenylketonuria (PKU) Guthrie (BIA) screening and early hospital discharge. *Early Human Development, 47*(1), 87–96.

Holmberg L., Edbom A., Calle E., Mokdad A., Byers T. (1997) Breast cancer mortality in relation to self-reported use of breast self-examination. A cohort study of 450,000 women. *Breast Cancer Research and Treatment, 43*(2), 137–140.

Leitch A. M., Dodd G. K., Constanza M., Linver M., Pressman P., McGinnis L. M., Smith R. A. (1997) American Cancer Society guidelines for the early detection of breast cancer: Update 1997. *CA: Cancer Journal for Clinicians, 47*(3), 150–153.

Matthews K. A., Shumaker S. A., Bowen D. J., Langer R. D., Hunt J. R., Kaplan R. M., Klesges R. C., Ritenbaugh C. (1997) Women's Health Initiative. Why now? What is it? What's new? *American Psychologist, 52*(2), 101–106.

Mettlin C., Dodd G. D. (1991) The American Cancer Society Guidelines for the cancer-related checkup: An update. *CA: A Cancer Journal for Clinicians, 41*(5), 279–282.

Morrison, A. S. (1985) Screening in chronic disease. In *Monographs in epidemiology and biostatistics.* Vol. 7. New York: Oxford University Press.

National Research Council. (1975) *Genetic screening programs, principles and research.* Committee for the Study of Inborn Errors of Metabolism, Division of Medical Science. Washington, D.C.: National Academy of Sciences.

Nayfield S. G. (1995) Tamoxifen's role in chemoprevention of breast cancer: An update. *Journal of Cellular Biochemistry, 22*(suppl.), 42–50.

Ries L. A. G., Miller B. A., Hankey B. F., Kosary C. L., Harras A., Edwards B. K. (Eds). (1994) *SEER Cancer Statistics Review, 1973–1991: Tables & Graphs.* (NIH Publication No. 94-2789). National Cancer Institute, Bethesda, Md.

Rodgers G. P. (1997) Overview of pathophysiology and rationale for treatment of sickle cell anemia. *Seminars in Hematology, 34* (3 suppl.), 2–7.

Rossouw J. E., Finnegan L. P., Harlan W. R., Pinn V. W., Clifford C., McGowan J. A. (1995) The evolution of the Women's Health Initiative: Perspectives from the NIH. *Journal of the American Medical Women's Association, 50*(2), 50–52.

Schneiderman L. (1981) *The practice of preventive health care.* Menlo Park, Calif.: Addison-Wesley.

Sinai L. N., Kim S. C., Casey R., Pinto-Martin J. A. (1995) Phenylketonuria screening: Effect of early newborn discharge. *Pediatrics, 96*(4) (Pt. 1), 605–608.

Sprinkle R. H., Hynes D. M., Konrad T. R. (1994) Is universal neonatal hemoglobinopathy screening cost-effective? *Archives of Pediatric–Adolescent Medicine, 148*(5), 461–469.

Thiessen, E. V. (1989) Breast self-examination in proper perspective. *Cancer, 28,* 1537–1545.

U.S. Preventive Services Task Force. *Guide to clinical preventive services: An assessment of the effectiveness of 169 interventions.* Baltimore: Wilkins & Wilkins.

Valanis B., Perlman C. (1982) Home pregnancy testing kits: Prevalence of use, false-negative rates and compliance with instructions. *American Journal of Public Health, 72,* 1034–1036.

Venet L., Strax P., Venet W., Shapiro S. (1971) Adequacies and inadequacies of breast examinations by physicians in mass screening. *Cancer, 28,* 1546–1551.

Winawer S. J., Fletcher R. H., Miller L., Godlee F., Solar M. H., et al. (1997) Colorectal cancer screening: Clinical guidelines and rationale. *Gastroenterology, 112*(2), 594–642.

15

Clinical Decision Making

he process of caring for patients requires systematic assessment, diagnosis, intervention, and reassessment. Many clinical decisions about an individual patient are based on information about the probability of certain events occurring, and on the collective experience of multiple clinicians with groups of similar patients. Expert clinicians have often relied on intuition based on experience rather than an analytical process for making decisions. But the current rate of change, the barrage of new information, and the emphasis on outcomes and cost-effectiveness make it more important than ever that systematic analysis plays a role in clinical decisions. The rapid development of new procedures and tests for patient assessment and diagnosis, new treatments, advanced communication technologies, and complexities of social and cultural changes require incorporating new elements into the process of making these clinical decisions. The clinical issues addressed in this chapter include: (1) normality versus abnormality, which involves questions relevant to diagnosis and risk assessment; (2) selection of treatment; and (3) prognosis. Questions of cause and decisions about screening, although clinically relevant, are discussed in other chapters because, except for case finding, they relate to groups of persons; this chapter focuses on decisions regarding individual patients. Clinical issues regarding prevention were discussed in Chapters 8 through 11 relative to life cycle stage. The role of formal decision–analysis and of practice guidelines based on an analytical synthesis of information as tools to assist clinicians in their decision-making process are presented. Finally, questions to ask when reading the clinical literature are discussed.

CLINICAL EPIDEMIOLOGY

On a daily basis, clinicians make decisions with respect to individual patient care. These decisions include which tests or assessments should be performed to aid in diagnosis, whether or not to treat, and which treatments are likely to be most effective. The ability to deal with these issues by making rational decisions that will lead to optimum therapeutic outcomes is a signal characteristic of an outstanding clinician. How are these clinical decisions reached? Scientific method, insofar as it consists of observation, classification of phenomena, measurement, hypothesis, and reasoning, has been a part of clinical disciplines largely in the laboratory, where experiments test physiological and biochemical hypotheses about how specific organ systems work. In actual clinical practice, where intervention by the clinician involves procedures to clarify diagnosis or to maintain or improve the patient's well-being, the scientific method is much less often used. Unlike laboratory investigators who must both specify and justify their decisions, clinicians making decisions about individual patient care often make choices on the basis of a hunch, intuition, or a nebulously defined clinical experience. Perhaps this is one reason that clinical professions like nursing, medicine, and physical therapy are considered at least as much art as they are science. Research has, in fact, demonstrated that expert clinicians are more likely than novices to perceive situations holistically, solve complex problems faster and more accurately, and rely on unspecifiable knowledge (Benner & Tanner, 1987; Antrobus, 1997). However, even expert clinicians are finding it more difficult to function without systematic analysis in the present health care environment where they are barraged with new technology and information.

Many clinicians view as alien the idea that any or every action of intervention undertaken in the course of individual patient management should be exposed to the rigors of scientific method. They do not consider the need to collect evidence that will allow others as well as themselves to judge whether that action was justified. When a new intervention becomes available, how often do clinicians review the evidence on efficacy before adopting it for use with their own patients? How does a clinician decide whether a patient is at high risk for developing a condition and should therefore be screened, or whether a particular intervention will make a difference? On what basis is a judgment made as to what will likely happen to the patient without intervention? These are all questions considered by the science of *clinical epidemiology*—the application of epidemiological principles and methods to the day-to-day care of patients. Such scientifically oriented health practice uses a systematic, data-based problem-solving process to determine if a patient has a problem requiring professional intervention, what kind of intervention is needed, and if

TABLE 15–1. CLINICAL ISSUES AND QUESTIONS IN THE CARE OF PATIENTS

ISSUES	QUESTIONS
Normality/Abnormality	Is a person sick or well?
	What precipitating event led the patient to seek health care?
Risk	What factors are associated with an increased likelihood of disease? With likelihood of a specific disease?
	Will altering the factor change the probability of developing disease?
Diagnosis	What are the objective signs, physical findings, or laboratory data?
	How accurate are diagnostic tests or strategies used to find a disease?
	What are the costs and risks of diagnostic tests?
	Which of several possible diagnoses is more likely, based on disease frequency distributions?
Treatment	What are the ultimate objectives of treatment?
	What treatment options are available?
	How does each change the future course of a disease?
	What are the advantages and risks of treatment compared with no treatment?
Prognosis	When should treatment be altered or stopped?
	What is the probable clinical course of this disease?
	What are the consequences of having the disease?

the intervention has been effective. The realization that this systematic approach is required to make sense of available clinical data arose from the recognition that clinical observations are made on patients who are free to do as they please—they are not laboratory rats under control of the investigator; clinicians have variable skills and prejudices, so observations may be influenced by a variety of systematic errors that can distort the true nature of events and therefore be misleading; and chance plays a role in determining outcomes.

Clinical epidemiology deals both with the systematic collection and interpretation of clinical data and with the application of findings from these studies in daily clinical decision making. Prior chapters of this book have addressed the acquisition of epidemiological data and considerations in evaluating such data. This chapter focuses on uses of available epidemiological data in clinical practice, specifically on how epidemiology is used to make decisions regarding care of individual patients. The clinical issues most relevant to clinical practice addressed in this chapter are listed in Table 15–1 along with illustrative questions relating to each issue.

NORMALITY VERSUS ABNORMALITY

It is rare that patients present with something so grossly different from the usual that it can immediately be recognized as abnormal and categorized by diagnosis. More often, when a patient presents with a complaint, the clinician is immediately faced with the need to determine whether this symptom represents a normal, expected event or a physiological abnormality. If it is abnormal, is it a transient everyday complaint not worth pursuing aggressively or is it a subtle manifestation of disease?

For example, is the sore throat a garden-variety pharyngitis or a dangerous streptococcal infection? Does the patient with abdominal pain have self-limited gastroenteritis or a more serious intestinal disorder such as peptic ulcer, colitis, or a tumor? Is a 5-foot, 6-inch tall woman weighing 160 lbs obese? Does her weight pose a risk to her health? What are the risks? Is weight alone sufficient justification for a program to reduce her weight? If so, how much should she lose and how fast is it safe to lose the weight? What risks are attached to the use of medication as an aid to lose weight? This first decision as to whether an observation reflects illness serves as a precursor to action. If the observation has clinical significance in terms of representing either a risk factor for future illness or probable illness in the present, then intervention is initiated. If it is decided that the observation does not represent illness or abnormality, then no action is taken. The observation is useful in either instance as a yardstick for judging improvement or deterioration. Decisions about normality may also be used as the basis for social and legal decisions (eg, whether compensation is due or whether someone is mentally competent).

Very few separations of normal from abnormal are based on a clear-cut, dichotomous, yes-or-no measure yielding discrete data. Exceptions are conditions such as cleft lip or cleft palate. Other exceptions are infectious conditions for which there is a laboratory procedure that can grow an organism from the cultured sample only if it is present. A positive culture indicates presence of disease, a negative culture indicates absence of the disease, assuming complete reliability of completing a valid culture procedure. In these instances, decisions about normality are somewhat straightforward.

More often, however, the measures that must be used in assessment are continuous in nature, for example, blood pressure. The likelihood of hypertensive symptoms increases as blood pressure increases. So does the predictive value of blood pressure for occurrence of other conditions such as myocardial infarction or stroke. But the question faced by clinicians is, "When is blood pressure abnormal? When does it require me to do something?" In the case of a blood pressure of 150/90 in a 35-year-old man, for example, the clinical significance can be inferred only from knowledge of the extent to which it is present or absent in other members of the general population, both well and ill, and from measures of the strength of the association between various levels of blood pressure and independent pathological or clinical confirmation of the presence of illness. The objective is to determine where on the continuum of health to illness this particular patient fits. The natural history of a disease represents this health–illness continuum (see Chap. 3 and Chap. 11). Such information on the natural history of each disease is available in the epidemiological literature. Most medical and nursing schools include these data in the content of didactic or clinical courses.

Natural History and Abnormality

During the prepathogenic phase of the natural history of any disease, the host is healthy. Once a susceptible host becomes exposed to a pathogenic agent, physiological changes begin. Some of these factors represent signs of elevated risk for developing a disease but can also be steps in the development of the disease, although not all individuals go on to develop the illness. At some stages along the health–illness continuum, the only detectable signs of abnormality are subclinical changes that can be detected by laboratory tests. Later, one or several symptoms may appear. As the number or intensity of symptoms increases, the patient will recognize that something is wrong and go to a health care center for diagnosis and treatment. The task of the clinician is to identify where on the natural history continuum the patient currently falls (Table 15–2). This decision serves as the basis for action; appropriate treatment is usually a function of stage of disease progression.

Depending on the particular point along the natural history continuum where the patient's illness lies at the time he or she presents at the health care center, different signs and symptoms will be observed. A physician working in a specialized hypertension clinic will have a very different impression of signs and symptoms associated with hypertension than will a nurse who manages a full caseload in a health maintenance clinic. The physician in the specialty clinic sees many patients who were referred because there was something so unusual about their presentation that general practitioners or internists were either unable to decide on hypertension as a diagnosis, the patient's hypertension did not respond to usual treatment, or the patient has a complex of chronic diseases requiring a specialist's evaluation of the safest way to treat the newly detected hypertension. Furthermore, once this physician has arrived at a diagnosis and instituted treatment, the patient is usually sent back to the referring source for follow up. The specialty physician can never really evaluate effectiveness of the treatment. He or she may never see a patient again unless treatment failed, and perhaps not even then. Some patients may not comply with the prescribed treatment; some will do well and some will do poorly, but in neither case will they be a part of the physician's professional frame of reference.

The nurse who manages patients in the health maintenance clinic will see a more representative range of signs and symptoms associated with elevations in blood pressure. He or she will observe patients with a normal range of blood pressures, temporary, stress-related elevations, gradual increases in pressure that may indicate some underlying disease process, patients whose pressure is on the high side but who have been assessed and declared not to require treatment, and patients who may have a sudden increase in blood pressure caused by an underlying disease process. This nurse will observe a wide variety of symptoms associated with hypertension among patients in the clinic. There will be more opportunity to observe

TABLE 15–2. POSSIBLE DECISIONS ABOUT THE NATURAL HISTORY STAGE OF A PATIENT

1. Essentially normal (no risk, no illness)
2. At risk
3. Disease agent present
4. Signs of disease present
5. Symptoms of disease present
6. Disability from disease present
7. Risk of death

long-term compliance with the hypertension treatment regimen and to see both suc-cessful and unsuccessful outcomes of treatment. However, even though the nurse's experience is more representative than that of the speciality physician, it is limited by little, if any, experience with the unusual or difficult-to-manage patient. Further-more, the nurse does not see those persons living in the community who are not re-ceiving regular health care monitoring and follow up. Thus, the nurse, too, needs the epidemiological database to give a complete picture of the disease natural his-tory and frequency of signs and symptoms and how they are distributed in relation to time of disease onset, severity of disease, and response to therapy.

Because health care is often fragmented or specialized, many clinicians deal with a very limited spectrum of the natural history/health–illness continuum, limit-ing experience. Clinicians are therefore dependent on information derived from epi-demiological studies to provide a complete picture of the disease natural history in-cluding disease frequency, distributions of signs and symptoms, and how they are distributed in relation to time of disease onset, severity of disease, and response to therapy. In addition, data from epidemiological studies are needed to answer ques-tions about relative effectiveness of patient treatment or management.

Epidemiological Criteria for Abnormality

Abnormality can thus be defined through epidemiological data on frequency and on the natural history of the condition. For practical purposes, abnormality is usually defined on the basis of three criteria: (1) it is statistically unusual; (2) it is regularly associated with disease, disability, or death; and (3) treatment leads to a better outcome.

Clinicians generally define normal as whatever occurs often and abnormal as what occurs infrequently. This statistical definition is most often based on fre-quency of the characteristic in a general population. Often, an arbitrary cutoff point of two standard deviations from the mean is used to separate normal from abnor-mal, with all values beyond two standard deviations considered to be abnormal. An alternative approach suggested by Elvebach (1972) is the use of percentiles, particu-larly age- and sex-specific percentiles. This approach has some advantages over the standard deviation approach because it does not assume a normal distribution of values, which is characteristic of few biological measures. Using age- and sex-specific populations as the basis for defining normality increases precision. How-ever, neither of these statistical approaches to normality is adequate in all situations. Fletcher and associates in their book, *Clinical Epidemiology* (1988), listed four ways in which the statistical definitions might be ambiguous or misleading:

1. If all values beyond a certain limit (eg, the 95th percentile) are considered abnormal, then the prevalence of all diseases would be the same (5%). This is, of course, contrary to our usual way of thinking about disease—few dis-eases have the same prevalence.
2. There is no general relationship between the statistical definition of how un-usual the value or symptom is and clinical disease in terms of prognosis for getting worse, developing some other symptom or disease condition, or

dying. For some diseases, only extreme values are clinically significant, and values at the 95th or 98th percentile would mean nothing. Further, although some extreme values are unusual, they may be preferable to more usual ones. A systolic blood pressure of 100 is more unusual than one of 160, but is definitely preferable.

3. Patients may be clearly diseased even though values for laboratory tests diagnostic of their disease are in the usual range for healthy people. For example, some individuals have intraocular pressures within normal range but clearly show retinal damage typical of glaucoma.

4. For many laboratory values, the entire range of values from low to high are associated with risk of disease. For serum cholesterol, for example, risk of coronary heart disease increases throughout the normal range; there is nearly a 3-fold increase in risk from "low normal" values to those in the "high normal" range.

For these reasons, statistical definitions of normality must be considered simultaneously with the other two criteria. First, it is necessary to know which values are regularly associated with disease, disability, or death. Deciding what level of risk is worth preventing is a judgment call based on the data. With blood pressure, for example, 150/90 is used by the National Center for Health Statistics as representing a clinically useful level of risk to begin treatment. Many physicians, however, would institute treatment at 140/90 in a younger person (Fletcher & Bulpitt, 1992). Others do not feel that treatment is justified unless one or both of the values are higher. When some current clinical trials are completed, there may be sufficient evidence to resolve this issue once and for all. It cannot be resolved without systematic collection of data.

The third criterion—what is defined as abnormal should be treatable—is a pragmatic one. Labeling something as abnormal makes little sense if it cannot be treated; the labeling merely causes anxiety for the patient. It is often necessary to reevaluate what is treatable as new data accumulate. The definition of treatable hypertension has changed over time as new evidence from clinical trials accumulated (Fletcher & Bulpitt, 1992).

DIAGNOSIS

Clinical diagnosis is a process, not a single action. The process is initiated with data collection (eg, medical history) and analysis, from which an initial diagnostic hypothesis is derived, tested, and refined. Once a diagnostic decision is reached, planning and implementation of appropriate interventions follow. The process ends with evaluation of a patient's responses to the interventions.

A medical diagnosis is a judgment about what disease process explains the complaints or abnormalites presented to the clinician by the patient. This judgment then drives a plan for treatment. Nurses hold primary accountability for making clinical judgments regarding the status of the patient and their family's daily life as it affects or is affected by the patient's health. Treatment plans are aimed at helping the individual and the family to manage effectively within the constraints imposed by the medical diagnosis and treatment, presenting circumstances, health-related activities, and demands of daily life. In many settings such as industry, home care, private practice, and nurse-managed clinics, nurses hold delegated responsibility for making accurate, appropriate clinical judgments about a patient's pathophysiological health status. On the basis of these judgments, nurses must decide whether to recommend that a patient continue in self-care, continue under nursing management, perhaps seeking consultation from the physician about altering the medical treatment regimen, be referred to a physician for medical diagnosis and treatment, or be retained under the existing medical regimen. Therefore, the following discussion includes illustrations relating both to biomedical and nursing diagnoses.

Deciding whether a laboratory test value or observed symptom represents health or illness is clearly a first step in the process of reaching a diagnosis. The second step is differentiating among the alternative conclusions that can potentially be reached about a patient's condition. This step involves three substeps: (1) reviewing patient characteristics in relation to possible explanatory data, (2) choosing the appropriate clinical measurements for obtaining further information, and (3) reviewing and synthesizing the evidence to determine what diagnostic classification or label best fits the evidence. Once this process is complete, the stage of disease progression can be determined and a treatment can be selected.

Clinical Interpretation of Observations

Suppose a laboratory value, a symptom, or a cluster of symptoms has been identified as abnormal. What is to be done? Clearly, until the clinical meaning of these observations is established, no action can be taken. Just as epidemiological thinking is useful in deciding initial issues of normality versus abnormality, so it is used in narrowing down the diagnostic options. Epidemiological questions to be considered are:

1. What diseases are prevalent in the community at this time? If, for example, there was a local influenza epidemic at the time a patient presents with fever, headache, weakness, cough, and myalgia and these symptoms were of recent origin, a clinician would be likely to attribute the symptoms to influenza and make recommendations accordingly. At other times, if there was no influenza outbreak, the clinician might be more inclined to consider laboratory tests to rule out other explanations.

2. What diseases characterized by these symptoms would fit the characteristics of this patient? As part of the clinical history, information about patient characteristics such as age, race, sex, occupation, habits, and geographical area of residence is gathered. If a middle-aged woman presents with a nonspecific lung lesion, has no history of smoking or hazardous occupational exposure but lives in the Mississippi Valley, histoplasmosis might be immediately expected. If this same woman lived in Arizona and presented with these same symptoms, other diagnoses would need to be explored. No tests

may be required when a 38-year-old nonsmoking mother who uses little alcohol and has been generally healthy in the past now presents with recent weight loss, fatigue, faintness, forgetfulness, and upset stomach if the screening clinician is aware that this woman was widowed 3 months before. These are symptoms frequently associated with the stress of unresolved grief. Thus, many diagnostic decisions can be tentatively reached before examining the patient or doing diagnostic tests, simply by collecting appropriate information and "thinking epidemiologically." In general practice settings (primary care practice), the probability of finding a serious underlying disease associated with symptoms is much less than in referral settings. Very often, the action taken will be to treat the symptom without additional diagnostic tests. Where there is suspicion of underlying disease, however, additional tests may be required.

Choosing a Diagnostic Procedure

With advances in medical technology come a wide array of new diagnostic procedures and techniques. When a patient presents with several symptoms, the physician, nurse clinician, or other clinical personnel must choose from among the available tests those that are most likely to provide useful, valid information in order to arrive at a diagnostic classification of the problem that can be used to plan treatment. Cost of the tests and risks to the patient must also be considered. In the best of all possible worlds, information on the relative efficacy of each test or combination of tests, based on prospective studies, would be available relative to each disease of interest. This, however, is rarely available in practice. More is known about tests that have been in common use for some time than about many of the newer, less used tests.

The same criteria discussed in relation to screening tests in Chapter 14 are important in choosing diagnostic tests: reliability; validity as measured by sensitivity, specificity, and predictive values; cost; safety; and acceptability. The most accurate tests—the gold standards—are often relatively elaborate, expensive, and risky (eg, cardiac catheterization, other radiological contrast procedures, and tissue biopsies). Usually, in the initial stages of a diagnostic workup, simpler, less accurate tests are used. Clearly, when the suspected disease is life-threatening but treatable, high sensitivity of the test is essential (eg, childhood leukemia). Sensitive tests are also useful when the patient's symptoms represent many possible disease conditions and the objective is to rule out diseases and reduce the number of viable possibilities that must be considered. For example, tuberculin skin tests, which are highly sensitive but not highly specific, can rule out tuberculosis as an explanation for lung infiltrates; a negative test would direct the diagnostician to look for alternative explanations. Sensitive tests, in these latter instances, are thus most helpful when the result is negative.

Because highly specific tests are rarely positive in the absence of disease, such tests are useful for implicating or confirming diagnoses suggested by other tests. Such tests are necessary before instituting treatment. Thus, one strategy in the use of diagnostic tests is to begin with tests of high sensitivity but reasonable cost and risk. As the number of diagnoses being considered is decreased, then more specific tests are used. Tests with high specificity are also, more often than not, more expensive and pose greater risk to patients (eg, cardiac catheterization). Such tests are also highly sensitive.

Another strategy for maximizing the effectiveness of any diagnostic procedure is to maximize the likely prevalence of the disease by selectively applying the test to those patients at highest risk by history and symptoms for developing the disease. This strategy maximizes the predictive value of the positive test just as screening high-risk populations increases the predictive value of a screening test.

Yet another strategy is to use multiple tests for the same disease. Because many diagnostic tests have less than 100% sensitivity and specificity, use of a single test frequently results in an intermediate probability of disease (eg, 40% or 60%). Because treatment cannot be instituted on the basis of a 60% certainty that the disease exists (eg, pancreatic cancer), more information or certainty is needed. Multiple tests can be used in parallel (at the same time) or serially (consecutively). With multiple tests, a high degree of certainty is achieved when all tests are positive or negative. Serial testing can be used when rapid assessment is not required (eg, when the suspected disease progresses slowly, is not life-threatening, and the patient can be easily followed up, as in an office or ambulatory care clinic). It is also used when some tests are risky or expensive; these risky or expensive tests are used only after the simpler tests are positive. With serial testing, testing is stopped when a negative result is obtained. Serial testing maximizes specificity and positive predictive value but lowers sensitivity and negative predictive value. This approach is useful when no individual test is highly specific. The most specific test should be used first to minimize the number of persons who must be followed up (Fig. 15–1). The possibility of a false-negative result must be considered if no alternative diagnostic explanation is confirmed or if additional symptoms that are consistent with the diagnosis develop (Fletcher & Bulpitt, 1992). It is often the nurse who may be engaged in followup care of such patients and who will be in a position to observe these symptoms and initiate referral to a physician for further testing.

Parallel tests are used when rapid assessment is required—when the suspected disease has a rapid course with high case fatality rates, when patients are hospitalized, or in cases of emergency. They may also be considered for ambulatory patients who may have difficulty returning for additional visits. This approach increases the sensitivity and negative predictive value of results over those obtained by any individual test. Specificity and positive predictive value are, however, lowered. Although disease is less likely to be missed than with serial testing, a higher rate of false-positives requiring additional testing or unnecessary treatment results.

Nurses and Biomedical Diagnoses

In an increasing number of settings, nurses are functioning in roles that involve not just nursing diagnoses, but medical diagnoses, usually based on protocols under the supervision of a physician. Nurses are faced with such decisions when they work as triage nurses in an emergency room, in nurse-run clinics, and in the telephone

Population of 1000 individuals
Disease Prevalence = 20%
(200 individuals with disease; 800 without disease)

Administer Test A	Administer Test B
(sensitivity = 0.80 specificity = 0.90)	(sensitivity = 0.90 specificity = 0.80)

Positive Test	Negative Test	Positive Test	Negative Test
160 with disease	40 with disease	180 with disease	20 with disease
80 without disease	720 without disease	160 without disease	640 without disease
240	760	340	660

Retest with Test B	Retest with Test A
(sensitivity = 0.90 specificity = 0.80)	(sensitivity = 0.80 specificity = 0.90)

Positive Test	Negative Test	Positive Test	Negative Test
144 with disease	16 with disease	144 with disease	46 with disease
16 without disease	64 without disease	16 without disease	144 without disease
160	80	160	180

Figure 15–1. Effect of test order on followup and outcome in serial testing. (*Adapted from Fletcher R., Fletcher S., Wagner E. Clinical epidemiology—The essentials. Baltimore: Williams & Wilkins, 1992, Table 3.5, p 68.*)

advice role. A nurse faced with the need to make a biomedical diagnosis must do so without access to a sophisticated array of laboratory tests, although in some settings he or she may be able to order or carry out some basic ones, such as a complete blood cell count (CBC), Pap smear, stool culture, or hemocult test. The nurse's diagnostic task is not to affix a precise diagnostic label but to infer and classify the status of the patient on the basis of present or readily available data. The nurse must determine whether the presenting symptoms represent a mild or self-limiting condition that can be alleviated through nursing intervention or a more serious disease that requires medical diagnosis and treatment.

Suppose that a patient presents with a complaint of watery diarrhea and abdominal cramping. Such symptoms may be acute symptoms of either an infectious process or of exposure to a toxin, or, if chronic, may be a manifestation of a serious disorder. Based on the patient's description of altered fecal output and other history factors such as age, sex, race, occupation, dietary patterns, recent travel experiences, recent stressful incidents, and drug intake—and in some settings results of a physical examination—the nurse can reach some conclusions about the probable cause of the symptoms. Acute onset with no history of psychological, occupational, or pharmaceutical causes suggests an infectious etiology. Epidemiological evidence suggests that viral infections generally have a short duration of 1 or 2 days and few distinguishing characteristics. Symptoms produced by bacterial organisms that cause diarrhea through production of a toxin rather than infection of the bowel (eg, staphylococcal food poisoning), while producing severe cramps and diarrhea, are characterized by the suddenness of onset, lack of fever, and self-limited course. Other bacterial and protozoal infections are not apt to be self-limiting, will become more severe with time, and require referral for differential diagnoses to distinguish these inflammatory states from other causes so that appropriate medical treatment can be instituted.

Parameters for assessing diarrhea lasting longer than 3 days include: (1) frequency and urgency, which can provide clues to the site of the lesion, (2) amount and character of stools, (3) relationship of abdominal pain to defecation and eating, (4) presence or absence of blood in stools, unrelated to dietary intake, (5) presence or absence of mucus, and (6) weight loss. Diagnostic tests that might be ordered by the physician include stool testing for occult blood; microscopic examination for pus, ova, or parasites; a stool culture; other laboratory analyses of the stool; protoscopy or sigmoidoscopy, or both; x-rays; serum carotene levels (for steatorrhea); and tests for electrolyte losses.

Nursing Diagnoses

One type of diagnostic challenge facing the nurse clinician is the diagnosis of abnormal health status resulting from a prescribed medical treatment regimen. Epidemiological studies provide data on likely complications of various treatments. Awareness of common complications or side effects enables the nurse to diagnose such problems promptly. An epidemiologically oriented nurse caring for a patient on high-dose, short-term steriod therapy would be alert to the potential for alteration in glucose metabolism. Because this patient is at higher risk for such outcomes, the nurse would routinely monitor the patient's urine for glucose and acetone, monitor results of serum glucose tests, and observe the patient for signs and symptoms of steroid-induced diabetes, such as polydypsia, polyuria, and polyphagia. Positive results on these measures would likely lead the nurse to a diagnosis of steroid-induced alteration in glucose metabolism. This diagnosis then offers several alternatives for intervention, including teaching the patient to limit their intake of high carbohydrate foods and alerting the physician who may wish to alter the steriod therapy or institute additional treatment for diabetes. In this same patient, if the nurse detects a temperature elevation accompanied by cough, skin lesions, dysuria, redness, swelling, heat, or pain in eyes, ears, throat, abdomen, joints, or genital or rectal areas, flushed appearance, or malaise, lethargy, or myalgia, an infection will most likely be diagnosed and the physician alerted.

Risk Assessment for Health Promotion Intervention

Risk assessment is a way of estimating personal risk for developing a disease. It provides a basis for offering practical advice on how to reduce that risk by changing lifestyle. The media publicity given to many epidemiological studies has generated public interest in disease risk and how to lower it. Risk is the probability that an untoward event will occur (eg, the probability of becoming ill or dying within a stated period of time or by a specific age). The term *risk factor* is variously used by epidemiological authors to mean any of the following (Last, 1988):

1. An attribute or exposure associated with an increased probability of a specified outcome, such as occurrence of a disease. Also called a *risk marker*, it need not be a causal agent
2. An attribute or exposure that increases the probability of occurrence of a disease or specified outcome (ie, a determinant)
3. A determinant that can be modified by intervention, thereby reducing the probability of occurrence of a disease or other specified outcomes. May be referred to as a *modifiable risk factor*

As used in the following discussion, risk factor refers to modifiable risk factors as in definition 3.

Many lifestyle factors are known risk factors for specific diseases. Examples were discussed in Chapters 8 through 11 in relation to stages of the life cycle. In Chapter 12, risk factors were discussed in relation to onset and progression of disease. Identification of individuals at risk of specific diseases was discussed in relation to disease prevention and control in Chapters 2, 6, 7, and 13. The following brief discussion centers on a currently popular approach to health risk appraisal in clinical practice.

Based on their natural history, specific precursor risk factors can be identified for many of the diseases that are major causes of morbidity and death. For example, risk of heart attack caused by atherosclerotic heart disease is associated with age, sedentary lifestyle, smoking, being overweight, hypertension, diabetes, and triglyceride levels. These risk factors can be combined to give a composite risk using either a mathematical formula or probability tables based on *relative risk* data from epidemiological research, usually cohort studies. Such quantified risk assessment became popular in the 1980s and was known as a *health risk appraisal function* (D'Agostino et al, 1995). Some patients are motivated by such numerical feedback. Health risk appraisal continues to be widely used, despite equivocal evidence for its effectiveness; adding individually tailored behavior change information appears to improve the likelihood that patients will change at least one behavior (Kreuter & Strecher, 1996).

Risk appraisals continue to be used often in occupational settings to identify candidates for worksite intervention programs (Anderson & Staufacker, 1996; Wilson et al, 1996). Interest is growing in developing health risk appraisals for the elderly, particularly for identifying high-risk individuals in a managed care setting. Health risk appraisals with the elderly are being tested to identify their effect on functional decline (Breslow et al, 1997) and to test the benefits of selected preventive services on health behaviors (Elder et al, 1995).

It is, of course, not necessary to quantify risk precisely. A major advantage of quantification is that it seems to express risk in terms that are easy for both the clinician and the patient to understand, provides a baseline against which progress can be measured subsequent to lifestyle changes, and provides a database with both baseline and followup data that could be used to study the effects of lifestyle changes as long as adequate information is recorded about these behavioral changes.

Without quantification, as long as clinicians are well informed about the natural history of these conditions they can still identify for individual patients the risk factors for the specific major causes of death. Monitoring of biological and behavioral risk factors can be used to assess whether changes in health behaviors and/or treatment to reduce biological risk factors have produced concurrent changes in the biological risk factors. Using the example of atherosclerotic heart disease, cholesterol, triglycerides, blood pressure, and weight could be monitored concurrently with patient reports of changes in smoking, exercise, and so on. If drugs are given to lower cholesterol or blood pressure, effects of these on the relevant biological risk factor can be monitored.

Another aspect of risk assessment concerns the identification of factors that place patients at higher risk of particular complications from medical interventions. These are discussed further in the following sections of this chapter on "Prognosis" and "Choosing a Treatment."

PROGNOSIS

The disease prognosis represents the expected clinical course and outcome for the patient (ie, the relative probabilities that a patient will develop each of the alternative outcomes of the natural history of the disease). In the absence of intervention, prognosis is a function of the general progressive nature of the disease itself, the pathogenicity and virility of the disease agent, and characteristics of the host. Influenza, for example, is usually an acute, self-limiting condition, producing unpleasant symptoms in the host, but not threatening life. Certain variants of the influenza virus may be more virulent than others. These occasional virulent strains may be characterized by a much higher attack rate and by higher case fatality than for the more common less virulent strains. Certain subgroups of the population— the elderly, the very young, and the poor—may be more susceptible to infection and more likely to have clinically apparent disease with complications that may lead to death.

Thus, knowledge of prognosis guides decisions about the need for intervention. What we tell the patient about their illness is based on knowing the prognosis. Should we reassure the patient that the illness is trivial or prepare them for major changes in health status or even death in the future? Is there anything the patient can do to alter the prognosis, for example, changes in lifestyle after myocardial infarction? Prognosis also influences what we do for the patient, whether we merely follow for observation or initiate treatment.

Medical intervention in the form of treatment is intended to change the disease prognosis and lead to a more favorable outcome for the patient. Each time a physician prescribes a medicine or performs an operation, they must weigh the potential for benefit against the potential for harm. Similarly, nursing interventions are intended to change patient outcome and must be weighed in terms of potential for benefit versus harm. Many therapeutic interventions offer potential for harm as well as benefit. Drugs have undesirable side effects; even the ubiquitous aspirin tablet presents a risk to certain individuals, eg, hemophiliacs. Surgical procedures carry risk of infection, organ failure, and death. Extended bed rest may be as undesirable as excessive exertion. Bladder catheterization of a postoperative patient with a severely distended bladder may be helpful in preventing refluxing of urine to the kidneys, rupture of the bladder, or other complications but also poses the threat of introducing infectious organisms into a patient whose resistance may be low. Although this risk may be low in the average patient, in an immunosuppressed patient this risk must be weighed against the risks to the patient of waiting too long to void.

CHOOSING A TREATMENT

Choosing between two or more possible treatments requires that each be clearly identified and that a method be available to assess the overall value of their outcome. Data from epidemiological and clinical studies provide information as to the probable effects of a treatment on the prognosis for the disease, both generally and for particular subgroups of patients. Even where adequate data are available, two additional elements influence the decision-making process: (1) uncertainty about the future outcome and (2) the value or worth assigned to the various possible outcomes. These conditions apply to physicians who must decide, for example, whether to prescribe or not to prescribe a particular drug or whether or not to perform surgery. They also face such decisions in regard to whether or not to prescribe drug treatment for prevention of disease. An example of the latter is whether to put postmenopausal women on estrogen to prevent osteoporosis and heart disease. Evidence that long-term estrogen therapy can prevent osteoporosis is strong and includes data from clinical trials (Rizzoli & Bonjour, 1997). The evidence for prevention of cardiovascular disease looks good, but awaits the outcome of the Women's Health Initiative. However, the extent to which long-term estrogen therapy may increase breast cancer is controversial at present (Smith et al, 1996). Thus, there is uncertainty about possible outcomes. What might be viewed as positive on a population basis is less clear-cut for a clinician dealing with an individual woman patient. Given adequate evidence, a public health administrator would likely decide to support routine administration of hormone replacement therapy (HRT) to women in order to produce a large decrease in the number of annual cardiovascular deaths among women, despite some small increase in the number of breast cancer deaths. For the clinician making a decision with a patient on whether to begin long-term HRT, personal risks and benefits are crucial considerations. Further, side effects, such as bleeding, breast tenderness, headaches, fluid retention, or irritability, particularly when the combined estrogen–progestin regimens are given to prevent endometrial hyperplasia, may interfere with quality of life (Scharbo-Dehaan, 1996) and be important considerations for the patient. The value assigned to these various outcomes and side effects may vary by physician and by patient.

Nurses also must make decisions about treatments. For example, a hospital nurse must decide whether to administer morphine to a postoperative patient complaining of pain, but who appears to be suffering signs of respiratory distress. Busy physicians will often delegate to nurses the responsiblity for walking patients through the options and risks available to them, eg, for decisions about taking long-term HRT versus alternative approaches to prevention of osteoporosis and heart disease through diet, weight-bearing excercise, smoking cessation, calcium supplementation, and so forth.

Today, patients are faced with treatment decisions in many situations; they are required to give informed consent for medical procedures such as surgery. In other instances, they may need to decide among alternative treatments; for example, a woman may have one physician recommend a modified mastectomy for treatment of breast cancer whereas another physician may have recommended a lumpectomy with subsequent radium implant. The issue of long-term estrogen therapy for prevention of osteoporosis or coronary heart disease is another example of how patients need to participate in the decision or whether to accept a treatment or not. Male patients may be faced with a choice as to whether to have a biopsy after a positive prostate-specific antigen (PSA) test for prostate cancer or to pursue "watchful waiting."

Sound clinical judgments in any of the above situations require a command of a sufficient body of facts and the skill to combine facts appropriately. Such skills are rarely taught; rather it is assumed that with acquisition of sufficient experience, the clinician will somehow acquire clinical judgment. But the essence of clinical judgment resides in the ability to weigh advantages and disadvantages of a diagnostic or therapeutic procedure and to choose a course of action for a particular patient based on estimates of costs and benefits.

Sackett and coworkers (1991) identified three principal decisions inherent in determining the rational treatment of any patient:

1. Deciding the ultimate objective of treatment, whether cure, palliation, symptomatic relief, limitation of structural or functional deterioration, preventing later complication or recurrence
2. Selecting the most efficacious specific treatment
3. Specifying an identifiable (measurable) treatment target as a guide for when to stop or alter treatment. Poor progress toward the target suggests a need to change the intensity or form of treatment

Making and recording these decisions provides a basis for coherent patient management, even by a treatment team. Without such decisions, chaos can ensue. For example, unless a decision to provide only palliative care and to maintain comfort and dignity for a terminally ill patient is recorded, personnel covering when the primary physician is off duty might order x-rays, blood counts, and antibiotics if the patient spikes a temperature.

Treatment decisions must be based on the best available evidence on risks and benefits of treatment. Ideally, evidence is available from studies on patients with characteristics similar to the one being treated. Critical assessment of the validity and applicability of the evidence is essential. The other elements to be considered are the patient's social, psychological, and economic circumstances.

Clinical decisions about treatment should be made only after a patient's need is determined. The issue becomes one of choosing from among several potential interventions the one that will have the highest probability of achieving the most valued or desirable outcome. The four components to be considered are: (1) a set of possible actions, (2) potential outcomes associated with those actions, (3) the probability that a particular outcome will occur if a given action is taken, and (4) the value of the outcome to the decision maker. It is assumed that the patient's values are an element in determining relative values of particular outcomes to the decision maker. Certainly the value of an outcome to a patient will affect his or her compliance with the treatment. In general, clinical decision making takes place in an open system (ie, complete knowledge of factors affecting the outcomes is usually unknown). These unknowns lessen the complete rationality of the decision-making process. Even so, nursing and medical decisions can be made more objective and systematic if outcomes are consciously and deliberately narrowed to a limited number that are then ordered by their values and if the relative potential of available actions to achieve these outcomes is weighed. Practical strategies for such decisions are found in decision analysis.

Decision Analysis

The necessity of making treatment decisions in the face of uncertainty about outcome is an integral part of the life of a clinician. Confronting uncertainty is never easy. Uncertainty is minimized, however, when all available information enters into the process of decision making in a logical manner. Imagine a family practice physician encountering a 59-year-old woman who is concerned about osteoporosis because her mother experienced a hip fracture, but a bone scan shows she has not suffered any substantial bone loss. The woman has no family history of heart disease, but does have a family history of breast cancer and a personal history of fibrocystic breast disease. She no longer is experiencing any hot flashes or other perimenopausal symptoms and never took estrogen replacement therapy for symptom management. She is concerned about the findings of excess risk of breast cancer associated with taking long-term HRT. She has a relatively inactive lifestyle and is a smoker. Options for intervention include putting her on HRT, calcium/vitamin D, or the newly approved specific estrogen receptor modulator, Rolaxifene, which has no long-term safety findings and little side effects data. (Because of limited available data, their uncommon use by those in mainstream medicine, and for simplicity's sake, we are ignoring herbal preparations and phyto-estrogens in this example.) In theory, increasing excercise and calcium in the diet are also options, but in most clinical situations would probably be used as adjuncts to one of the drug treatments. The HRT is associated with a variety of unacceptable side effects for many women and must be taken long-term to sustain bone integrity. Calcium and vitamin D may be associated with gastrointestinal upset and possibly increased risk of renal stones. Rolaxifene is an unknown quantity, since it was just approved by the Food and Drug Administration for prevention of osteoporosis in December 1997. The final decision must be the patient's; therefore, the physician's recommendation will probably include a discussion of the pros and cons of all of the alternatives. But, as the expert, the physician must choose and support the option that is likely to have the best outcome.

The example given above is vexing, but if one alternative is chosen and presents compliance or side effect problems, the other options are still available. For some other decisions, such as whether to use a medical treatment or surgery for a patient with severe angina that interferes with functional status, who has occlusion of several arteries, and who has chronic emphysema, the clinician faces more difficult challenges, since function and risks associated with surgery introduce additional dimensions that need to be considered. In the face of such decisions, many clinicians are turning to formal decision analysis as a way of arriving at the best possible logical decision.

Decision analysis involves application of analytical and mathematical tools to assist in making the "best" choice. Decision analysis assumes that (1) decision makers wish to maximize some measure of value for outcomes of the decision and (2) people are generally limited in the amount of information they can process at any one time about complex decisions. Thus, the goal of decision analysis is to break complex decisions into smaller, more easily assimilated pieces that human decision makers can handle well, and then to use mathematical techniques to put all the pieces together to solve the larger, more complex decision. This process is operationalized through the decision tree, a diagram showing the interrelationships of three pieces of the problem: (1) possible actions, (2) possible outcomes associated with each possible action, and (3) probability of each outcome occurring if a given action is taken. The values of the outcome to the decision maker and to the patient also need to be considered and may be included in the decision tree.

Figure 15–2 shows relationships between possible actions and outcomes in a simple decision tree format. The root of the tree is the initial available decision alternatives. Branches of the tree move away from the root showing these alternatives. The point of branching is called a *decision node*. Each alternative leads to several potential, mutually exclusive outcomes, one of which must occur. These represent additional branches coming out from the appropriate initial branch. The ordering of branches from the root represents information in the order in which it becomes available to the decision maker and, therefore, the order in which the decisions must be made. For example, in Figure 15–2 if treatment A is done first, the three possible outcomes are a successful outcome (the patient recovers), an equivocal outcome (the patient is improved, but not recovered), and a negative outcome (no improvement or condition worsens). Consider a decision about how to treat a patient with unstable angina who also suffers from emphysema. Twenty years ago, medical treatment might have been an easy choice. However, now percutaneous transluminal coronary angioplasty (PTCA) and coronary artery bypass grafting (CABG) are commonly used with these patients. Imagine that treatment A is drug

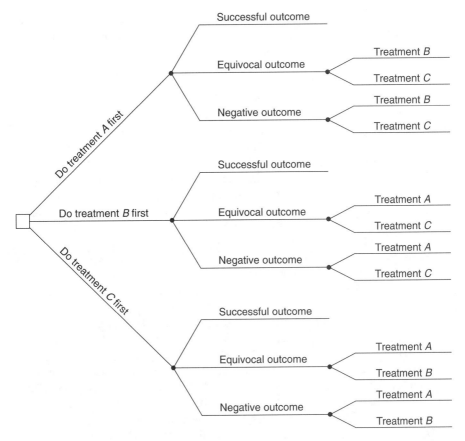

Figure 15–2. Hypothetical decision tree where three potential treatments are available.

treatment, that treatment B is PTCA, and that treatment C is double bypass surgery. If the surgeon considers CABG, he or she knows that there is some probability of a negative outcome associated with the surgery (eg, death, stroke, or other surgical complication), particularly due to the patient's emphysema. Clinical trials have shown similar risks of these outcomes for PTCA and CABG; 4.6% and 4.4% of patients undergoing these procedures died within the next 2 to 7 years and the combined rate of cardiac death and nonfatal myocardial infarction was 9.9% and 9.3%, respectively (Corr, 1996). On the other hand, the probability of prolonging life is excellent. Patients undergoing PTCA in the clinical trials were more likely to require a subsequent procedure in the first year after the first procedure and were less likely to be totally free of angina than those having CABG, but they were also likely to recover more quickly than patients having CABG. The failure rate of CABG graphs rises sharply after 5 to 8 years and a second surgery carries higher risks than the first one, while a second PTCA is no more hazardous than the primary procedure and 80% of patients were successfully managed by PTCA.

If the clinician were to choose one of the surgical treatments as first choice, in the event of the negative outcomes, except death, medical options could be tried, but any damage cannot be corrected. Before making a decision, the surgeon would assess probabilities for various outcomes if treatment A or C were tried first. To assign values to the various outcomes, the physician needs to consider how each outcome would affect the patient's ability to support the family, maintain self-esteem, or whatever else might be important for that patient. Numerical values to represent these patient values can be assigned to each outcome if the surgeon wishes to do a mathematical analysis of the decision tree. These numerical values, called *utilities,* would be multiplied by the probabilities of the occurrence for each alternative decision. Scores for the alternatives can then be compared. Alternatively, the physician could choose to restrict the analysis to a qualitative analysis. (For more detailed discussion of quantitative decision analysis, including legal issues, see Birkmeyer & Welch, 1997; Lawler, 1995; Detsky et al, 1997; Krahn et al, 1997; Ursu, 1992; Simpson, 1994; Hagen, 1992, among others.)

The decision tree does not indicate a single best decision, only options and possible consequences. The best decision is based on a variety of factors that can be assigned to one of two categories: (1) probabilities of the various outcomes (obtainable from epidemiological data combined with judgment of the clinician) and (2) values of the various outcomes to the patient and the decision maker. Both the probabilities and the values of particular outcomes are a function of the condition or circumstances of the patient in question. For example, potential options and outcomes remain the same for virtually all patients for whom arteriography is considered, but probabilities of particular prognostic outcomes and the associated values differ from patient to patient; the decision is influenced accordingly. The probabilities and assigned values of a particular outcome can be added to the branches of the decision tree and either a formal, quantitive analysis or a qualitative analysis of the tree can be performed. To simplify either analysis, probabilities and the values of various outcomes can be used to "prune" the tree. Pruning involves removing branches that are relatively unimportant (eg, of low probability for this particular patient) and consolidating others to reduce the problem to manageable proportions.

Informal Decision Making

In many clinical situations, a thought process similar to constructing and pruning a decision tree occurs instinctively and informally without the clinician describing or being able to describe the process. Such behavior would be expected of the experienced clinician whose knowledge and experiential base of probabilities and knowledge of probable utilities of potential outcomes lead to an instinctive best decision. For the younger, less experienced clinician, however, conscious use of a decision tree can develop the sound patterns of decision making that will eventually lead to such intuitive decisions in the future.

Probabilities are derived from empirical and clinical studies. Many of these probabilities are part of the knowledge base acquired by clinicians during their professional education and may be a subconscious factor used in making clinical decisions. Grier, in a study of nurses' decision-making methods about patient care, demonstrated that when nurses were asked to rank alternative actions, the preferred actions were generally consistent with the nurses' knowledge of the probabilities of the various outcomes and with the nurses' values for the outcomes. Values of the outcomes varied by whether the nurses worked in an inpatient or community setting (Grier, 1976). This variation in values assigned to outcomes probably results because judgments about the value or utility of an outcome are necessarily more subjective than are probabilities of an outcome occurring. Assessment of probabilities is exclusively the responsibility of the clinician and requires up-to-date knowledge of the most recent research. Because different individuals assess the value of outcomes differently, assessment of values must be completed in cooperation with the patient and the family. For example, a 45-year-old patient with hypertension may prefer to take antihypertensive medications for an indefinite period rather than to face the risks and discomforts involved in a diagnostic evaluation and surgical correction of hypertension of probable renovascular origin. Another patient of similar age, cardiovascular status, and other characteristics may prefer the risks of the diagnostic and surgical maneuvers to the prolonged need of drug therapy.

In a more nursing- or social work-oriented example, a 78-year-old widowed blind woman with diabetes may prefer the option of sharing her home with a stranger in need of a place to live who would help with shopping, cooking, and her insulin injections to the option of moving in with a relative. Another woman experiencing similar circumstances may prefer giving up the independence of her own home and living with relatives or moving to an assisted-living setting rather than trusting a stranger living in her home.

Let us consider the following example of how a decision tree approach can be used by a nurse. The visiting nurse visits the home of the Jacksons, an elderly couple in their mid-70s. Mr. Jackson, the patient, is recovering from a stroke and is paralyzed on his right side. His wife, who has been caring for him since his return home from the hospital appears to have an upper respiratory infection. She is slightly flushed and appears tired, which is unusual. Although she claims to have a slight cold that does not amount to anything, she continues to carry out her busy schedule of caring for her husband, keeping their home clean and neat, baking treats for her husband, and making dolls for a church bazaar. Her oral temperature is 101.2°F and other vital signs are somewhat elevated. Her throat is red, she has considerable nasal congestion, and some shortness of breath. The nurse must decide what activity recommendation would be best for Mrs. Jackson—continue ambulating, sitting, or staying in bed. Outcomes that need to be considered are effects on (1) circulation/ventilation, (2) fatigue/overexertion, (3) gastrointestinal/urinary elimination, (4) image of self, (5) muscle/joint mobility, (6) sensory stimulation, (7) skin integrity, and (8) resistance to infection. Figure 15–3 shows a decision tree for decisions in relation to effects on fatigue/overexertion and resistance to infection along with probabilities quantifying the probability of each outcome. The tree has been pruned to show resistance to infection outcomes for only those mobility outcomes that favor maintaining present mobility. The probability of each outcome is

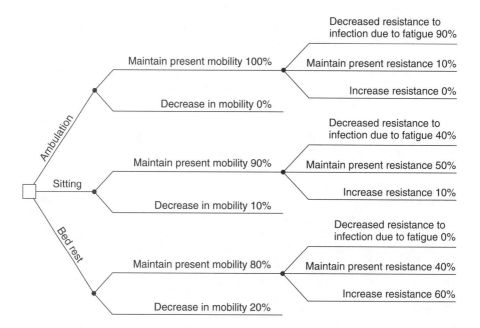

Figure 15–3. Decision tree for Mrs. Jackson (example described in text). At the square node, the choice is in the hands of the decision maker and at the circular nodes, the outcome is dictated by probability. The probabilities of each outcome as estimated by the author are shown on each branch. The tree has been pruned to remove outcomes relating to resistance to infection for the decreased mobility outcomes.

strictly hypothetical. Based on these probabilities, however, bed rest would appear to be the best decision because short-term bed rest carries a minimal risk of decrease in mobility and a high probability of preventing worsening infection caused by fatigue.

When patient values are also considered, however, sitting may be a preferred choice because Mrs. Jackson can still keep her husband company and work on her dolls. The problem is that she may still tend to overdo and become more ill as a result of a decrease in resistance to infection. Because Mrs. Jackson values her activities, she must be helped to weigh the relative impact on her long-term function of submitting to a short period of bed rest or limiting her activities to those that can be performed while sitting for short periods. If the latter is preferred, then she must be made aware of the risks of overdoing, namely, that if her respiratory infection worsens, she may need to spend a longer period in bed to recover. Placement of a temporary home health aide to assist in care of her husband or exploration of family resources to help out (eg, an adult child living nearby) could alleviate some of her concerns for her husband's care, thus reducing the value of ambulation to Mrs. Jackson by assuring that Mr. Jackson's needs would be met. A similar analytical process would be applied to each of the three choices in regard to the other seven outcomes and the choice that leads to optimal status on the most outcomes would be selected.

Decision theory could be considered a way of formalizing common sense. Although it offers no magical formulae for correct decisions, it provides a logical framework for analyzing clinical decision problems, from the simplest to the most complex, based on clinical preferences and knowledge. As medical and nursing care become more complex, such a framework for organizing available knowledge for the purpose of reaching optimally effective decisions becomes necessary. It also provides a framework that clinicians can use to help patients understand the various treatment options available to them; in the process of discussing the options, clinicians become familiar with patient priorities. Since compliance with a treatment plan is greater when patient priorities are met, tailoring treatment to patient preferences is likely to be more successful.

CLINICAL PRACTICE GUIDELINES

Variability in clinical practice has long been a fact of care delivery. Regional differences have been documented in use of hospital stay, hysterectomy rates, use of estrogen replacement therapy, and many other clinical interventions. Individual clinicians have long prided themselves on individualizing care. However, the increasing emphasis on cost and quality of care has focused discussion on clinical practice guidelines as a way of reducing variablity and improving quality, to the dismay of many clinicians.

The Institute of Medicine has defined *practice guidelines* as systematically developed statements to assist clinical practitioner and patient decisions about appropriate health care for specific clinical circumstances (Field & Lohr, 1992). Five major purposes for guidelines are: (1) assisting clinical decision making by patients and practitioners; (2) educating individuals or groups; (3) assessing and assuring the quality of care; (4) guiding allocation of resources for health care; and (5) reducing the risk of legal liability for negligent care. In addition to providing assistance in clinical decisions, guidelines can be used for quality improvement and payment policy making (Field & Lohr, 1992). Guidelines in one form or another have been promulgated by professional organizations for many years. What is new is both the emphasis on guidelines being systematically developed, based on evidence, and the use of processes, structures, and incentives to support the effective use and evaluation of guidelines. How guidelines are implemented can have major impact on their acceptability to clinicians. Within managed care organizations, there is wide variation in how guidelines are used. In not-for-profit managed care organizations, guidelines are usually established to provide support to the clinicians and patients in making care decisions; they are guides, not restrictions. Given the rapid advancements in care, it is difficult for many clinicians to keep up with the literature. Having access to guidelines that are periodically updated on the basis of new findings can be very helpful. However, in some managed care organizations the guidelines are used to limit treatment options; care outside of the approaches detailed in the guidelines require special approval by the organization (Edmunds et al, 1997). These types of guidelines are much less acceptable to clinicians.

Epidemiological research and clinical trials provide the evidence that supports guidelines development. A thorough and critical review and analysis of the literature can be time consuming and expensive. Thus it may not be practical for individual health care organizations to develop guidelines for the broad array of conditions seen by clinicians on a daily basis. As a result, national organizations, ranging from governmental agencies such as the National Cancer Institute and the Agency for Health Care Policy and Research (AHCPR) to professional organizations, are increasing their guidelines' development activities. The AHCPR has convened expert panels and published clinical practice guidelines for numerous health conditions. These guidelines are published in three parts: (1) complete rationale for the guidelines; (2) an abbreviated version for clinicians that simply lists the guidelines, without extensive documentation of rationale; and (3) a summary for patients. In Chapter 14 and in others, specific guidelines put forth by organizations such as the American Cancer Society (eg, breast and cervical cancer screening guidelines) and professional organizations (eg, the colorectal cancer screening guidelines of the American Gastroenterological Association) were mentioned. Guidelines for preventive care published by the U.S. Preventive Services Task Force, established by the U.S. Public Health Service in 1984, but comprised of a nongovernmental panel of experts, were included in Chapters 8 through 11. The experience of this body offers lessons of use to others interested in guidelines development and includes the need for expanded input from nonphysician providers such as more systematic topic selection; development of rules for extrapolating from relevant evidence; more systematic use of tools like meta-analysis, decision analysis, and cost-effectiveness studies; improved consistency in judging evidence for benefits and harms; and an ongoing mechanism for updating recommendations (Woolf et al, 1996).

The involvement of such diverse groups sometimes leads to conflicting guidelines being promulgated, eg, the different positions the National Institutes of Health and the American Cancer Society maintain on breast cancer screening for women between 40 and 49 years of age. Quality of the methods and procedures of review, and thus of the published guidelines varies widely. Little has been done to date to evaluate the impact of guidelines.

Criteria for Evaluating Practice Guidelines

Since practice guidelines are likely here to stay, criteria for evaluating them may be helpful. The Institute of Medicine has specified eight attributes of practice guidelines that, if used, may help achieve desired health outcomes (Field & Lohr, 1992). These are: validity, reliability, clinical applicability, clinical flexibility, clarity, multidisciplinary process, scheduled review, and documentation. The first four relate to substantive content of the guidelines, the last four to process or presentation of the guidelines. Guidelines are valid if they lead to the health and cost outcomes projected when followed. This implies that use is evaluated on the basis of prespecified health and cost outcomes. Also accompanying the guidelines should be documentation of the strength of the evidence and judgments made in developing the guidelines. Reliability here refers to reproducibility of conclusions from the evidence and process used to develop the guidelines and to consistency of application of the guidelines in similar clinical circumstances. Clinical applicability refers to broad inclusion of appropriate patient populations in the guidelines and to clear statements as to which populations the guidelines are applicable. Clinical flexibility relates to specification of which populations are excepted from the guidelines and how patient preferences should be identified and considered.

In order to achieve clarity, practice guidelines must use unambiguous language, define terms precisely, and be presented in a logical and easy-to-follow style. There should be thorough documentation of the process of development, including participants, evidence used, assumptions and rationales accepted, and the analytical methods employed. If the process of guideline development includes participation by representatives of key stakeholder groups, then the guidelines will be applicable to use by a broad range of clinical professions. Because new research is constantly being published and evaluation of guideline use may influence professional consensus about the usefulness of the guideline, review of the guidelines should be scheduled when use is implemented (Field & Lohr, 1992).

Guidelines developed by national groups may be adapted by local organizations to meet their unique circumstances. Such adaptation should be evidence-based, and effectiveness will need to be evaluated. Ensuring adoption of the guidelines will require a range of supportive conditions and strategies. Use of local clinicians who champion the guidelines, a focus on desired outcomes, and feedback loops that provide clinicians with information about patient outcomes and frequency with which they are deviating from the guidelines and under what circumstances are often helpful in ensuring that guidelines will be followed. Integration of the guidelines into clinical information systems also supports their use.

It is likely that accreditation bodies will increasingly look at use of guidelines. While in the past, accreditation has considered whether guidelines are in place, the accreditation review has paid little attention to the quality of the guidelines and extent to which care is monitored (Edmunds et al, 1997). This is likely to change in the future.

READING THE CLINICAL LITERATURE

It should be clear by now that clinicians, whether physicians, physician's assistants, nurse practitioners, nurses, physical therapists, or other clinical professionals, rely heavily on epidemiology for building the knowledge base necessary for clinical decision making. In Chapter 4, suggestions were provided in regard to how to read critically epidemiological articles investigating disease etiology. A few hints on what to look for in articles introducing new therapies and modifications or evaluations of previous therapies may be helpful. As stated earlier, the best way to investigate efficacy of therapies is through randomized controlled trials. However, a randomized trial does not guarantee that results will be valid. How the trial was conducted needs to be evaluated. Also, new therapies are often tested using quasi-experimental, rather than randomized designs making critical reading of the literature crucial. Table 15–3 lists important points to consider when reading reports of studies investigating new therapies. Each of these points is briefly discussed in the following paragraphs.

Randomization

Random assignment to treatment is intended to assure that every subject has an equal probability of receiving one or the other treatment. The method of random assignment should be described in the article. Usually random assignment is based on use of a table of random numbers. Evidence that random assignment accomplished its task and produced comparable groups of experimental and control patients should be provided. This usually takes the form of a table comparing entry characteristics for the two groups and a statement about their similarity.

When random assignment is not used, it is important to assess the process by which study groups are constituted to determine whether composition of study groups could contain some inherent bias that would contribute to the findings of the study. Consider the following example. A retrospective study identified patients who received a new surgical procedure and compared their outcomes with those of a group of patients with the same diagnosis, seen at the same hospital during the same year, and who received the usual medical treatment, which had been standard treatment for some time. It would not be surprising if the study results showed the new surgical procedure to have a better outcome. The reason is that the two study groups were probably quite different. It is likely that patients who underwent the surgical procedure were generally younger and healthier (better surgical risks) than the patients who received the medical treatment. Unless the study controlled in analysis for age, severity of illness, and comorbidities, one would expect *a priori* that the surgical patients would be shown to do better.

TABLE 15–3. QUESTIONS FOR EVALUATING NEW THERAPIES

1. Were patients randomly assigned to treatment groups?
2. What are the characteristics of patients in the study?
   a. Are study patients representative of patients with the condition, ie, do they represent a spectrum of disease severity, age, race, and so on?
   b. Are they similar to my patients?
3. Were all clinically relevant outcomes included?
4. Were treatments administered according to protocol?
5. Is the therapeutic intervention feasible in my practice?
6. How was significance of findings determined?
   a. Were both statistical and clinical significance assessed?
   b. If study findings were negative, was the trial large enough to show a clinically important effect if it occurred?
7. Were all patients entering the study accounted for at its conclusion?

Generalizability

Characteristics of study patients are an important factor in determining whether the study results can be generalized to other populations. Thus, criteria for cases entered into the study should be clearly stated. Many studies use only patients with advanced illness. Results of such studies provide little or no information about effectiveness of the treatment for patients at other stages of the disease. When a representative cross-section of patients is studied, results should be compared for various subgroups (eg, different age groups) to establish that treatment efficacy is equivalent for all types of patients. This information also provides a basis for each clinician to evaluate the relevance for their own practice. The importance of a clear statement of case definition and that all cases met these criteria cannot be overemphasized.

Interventions

Treatment protocols for all treatment groups should be described. The intervention ought to be one that makes sense, both clinically and biologically. It should be acceptable to patients and clinicians, and something that could be administered by clinicians. Cost and accessibility of the intervention will be important considerations for clinicians in making decisions about whether to adopt the intervention.

The description of study methods should include a description of the intervention in sufficient detail for readers to replicate it. The description should, therefore, include formulation and dose, circumstances that trigger administration, conditions under which the intended dose or formulation was modified, what side effects were monitored and what action taken when they were present, and so on. What safeguards assured that treatment was given as intended? With many people involved in the care of a single patient, there are numerous opportunities for interference with the prescribed protocol. In a study of infection rates associated with different frequencies of changing dressings, for example, a temporary nurse on a unit might change a dressing that appeared soiled or loose unless she had been notified about the study protocol and instructed to leave it alone. When trials involve outpatients, patient compliance becomes an operative factor. In addition, some patients may be intolerant to an assigned treatment and may be getting worse or experiencing life-threatening complications. The design should specify how such cases are to be handled. Many intervention trials use an intention to treat design. In these trials, subjects who are noncompliant or unable to tolerate a therapy are included in their assigned study group for analysis, since in clinical settings these problems will be part of a clinician's experience. Any bias introduced by this approach increases the likelihood of finding no difference between groups. Thus, a finding that a new treatment compared with the old is significantly better or a finding that the treated group does significantly better than a control group argues that the intervention is worthwhile.

Ideally, in a randomized clinical trial, neither the investigators nor the patients should know which patients are receiving the treatment. This is called *blinding*. In a single-blind trial the patients are unaware of what treatment they are receiving.

In double-blind trials, the investigator is also unaware of treatment assignment. In triple-blind trials, the individuals analyzing the data are also unaware as to which group received which treatment. Blinding is intended to reduce bias. Blinding can be effected with relative ease in studies where the treatment involves administration of medication because placebos can be given to those not receiving the treatment. In contrast, when the treatments under study involve clearly different approaches (eg, surgery versus medical treatment or audiovisual versus written patient teaching programs), blinding is not possible.

Specific interferences with study protocols have been termed *contamination* and *cointervention* (Sackett et al, 1991). Contamination occurs when control patients accidentally receive the experimental treatment. Cointervention is the performance of additional diagnostic or therapeutic acts on experimental, but not control, patients. The likelihood of such interferences occurring in a systematic manner is reduced when blinding can be used. Whenever possible, such interferences should be recorded so their effect can be assessed in analysis.

The question of whether all patients entering the study were accounted for at the conclusion of the study is related to the previous issue, in that final status of each subject must be accounted for, whether they changed treatments, dropped out of the study, died, or were lost to followup. If 142 patients began the study, then 142 should be accounted for at the end. Be suspicious when the final analysis is based on a smaller sample than began the study, particularly when no explanation is given. More often than not, loss of subjects is related in some way to poor outcomes, including inability to tolerate a treatment, unwillingness to comply with the treatment, or severe effects, such as death. Particularly when such losses occur from the group receiving a new, experimental treatment, results should be viewed cautiously.

Outcomes

In caring for your patients, what outcomes, good or bad, are you concerned about? Outcomes related to quality of life may be as relevant as 5-year survival rates, infection rates, or other purely physiological criteria. Differences in frequency of clinical disease are probably more important than frequencies or levels of risk factors. All the relevant outcomes should be examined by the study.

Criteria for assessing outcomes should be clearly described and similar means of assessing the outcome should be used for intervention and comparison groups. Suppose a study was testing whether nurses in a nurse-managed hypertension clinic could manage hypertensive patients as effectively as physicians. Patients referred to a particular outpatient facility because of high blood pressure who meet criteria for nurse management will be randomized to nurse management versus physician management. To prepare the nurses to manage hypertensive patients, the nurses received training in hypertension management, were given protocols to follow, and were trained in American Heart Association procedures for taking blood pressures. The outcome of interest is whether the patient's hypertension is controlled 1 year later. Control is defined as a systolic pressure less than 140 and a diastolic pressure less than or equal to 90. Charts will be reviewed to determine the outcome. What is the issue? Using chart data to assess blood pressure outcomes of the two groups may be like comparing apples and oranges. The nurses have received training in a standard approach to taking blood pressure. However, in many outpatient clinics and medical offices, there is no standard way of taking blood pressure. Readings can be affected by a variety of factors such as whether the patient has sat quietly for at least 5 minutes before having the blood pressure taken, cuff size, and positioning of patient. It is therefore likely that reliability of readings in the standard physician care setting is low. Standards of blood pressure measurement being different in the two settings will necessarily affect study results, most likely in the direction of finding that the blood pressure of a greater percentage of patients in the nurse-managed clinic is controlled than in the physician clinic.

Two measures of outcome may be used in clinical trials: statistical significance of results and clinical significance. *Statistical significance* deals with whether the findings are real (ie, whether differences in outcome between treatment groups are likely chance phenomena or can be attributed to treatment). A P value of 0.05 means that the risk of concluding erroneously that treatment A is better than treatment B is only 5 in 100. Ninety-five times in 100, a conclusion that treatment A is better, would be correct. Clinical significance refers to clinical importance. Statistically significant effects may be too small from a clinical viewpoint to justify changing clinical practice. Suppose that a randomized, controlled trial of the effects on infant birth weight of high-protein food supplements for pregnant women found an increase of 15 g in birth weight in the supplemented group compared with the non-supplemented and that this difference was statistically significant at $P = 0.01$. Is this statistically significant difference clinically important? Should pregnant women be given protein supplements on the basis of these findings? Obstetricians and clinical nurse specialists in maternal–child health might argue that at least a 50- to 100-g change in birth weight is needed to have any impact on infant morbidity or mortality. Thus, 15 g would not be considered clinically important and resources would not be diverted to supplementation programs for pregnant women. A related question, however, is whether the sample size in the trial was sufficiently large to show a clinically significant difference if it had occurred. A well-designed study will set in advance what is considered to represent a clinically significant effect. The power of the study to detect such an effect should be stated.

Feasibility

Finally, if the study design is deemed adequate and conclusions valid, clinicians must judge whether the new therapeutic intervention is feasible for their practice. Feasibility may depend on the nature of the therapeutic maneuver and availability of personnel and technological resources. For example, individualized self-hypnosis relaxation training has been demonstrated in a randomized controlled trial to be an effective form of antiemetic therapy in children (Cotanch et al, 1985). Training the children in the procedure requires a trained nurse-therapist who will spend 30 to 40 minutes with each child as well as a quiet setting. Such an intervention is probably not feasible in a busy outpatient pediatric chemotherapy clinic with a single nurse, because of both environmental and personnel limitations.

Literature in the health care field is growing rapidly as new information becomes available and new treatments are tested. Critical assessment of the literature is necessary if clinicians are to do more good than harm to patients and to aid in containing health care costs. Knowledge of the natural history of diseases and principles for applying epidemiological thinking to planning patient care can contribute to quality care for patients.

REFERENCES

Anderson D. R., Staufacker M. J. (1996) The impact of worksite-based health risk appraisal on health-related outcomes: A review of the literature. *American Journal of Health Promotion, 10*(6), 499–508.

Antrobus S. (1997) Developing the nurse as a knowledge worker in health—learning the artistry of practice. *Journal of Advanced Nursing, 25,* 829–835.

Benner P., Tanner C. (1987) Clinical judgement: How expert nurses use intuition. *American Journal of Nursing, 87,* 23–31.

Birkmeyer J. D., Welch H. G. (1997) A reader's guide to surgical decision analysis. *Journal of the American College of Surgeons, 184*(6), 589–595.

Breslow L., Beck J. C., Morgenstern H., Fielding J. E., Moore A. A., Carmel M., Higa J. (1997) Development of a health risk appraisal for the elderly (HRA-E). *American Journal of Health Promotion, 11*(5), 337–343.

Cotanch P., Hockenberry M., Herman S. (1985) Self-hypnosis as antiemetic therapy in children receiving chemotherapy. *Oncology Nursing Forum, 12*(4), 41–46.

D'Agostino R. B., Belanger A. J., Markson E. W., Kelly-Hayes M., Wolf P. A. (1995) Development of health risk appraisal functions in the presence of multiple indicators: The Framingham Study nursing home institutionalization model. *Statistical Medicine, 14*(16), 1757–1770.

Detsky A. S., Naglie G., Krahn M. D., Naimark D., Redelmeier D. A. (1997) Primer on medical decision analysis: Part 1—getting started. *Medical Decision Making, 17*(2), 123–125.

Edmunds M., Frank R., Hogan M., McCarty D., Robinson-Beale R., Weisner C. (Eds.). (1997) *Managing Managed Care. Quality Improvement in Behavioral Health.* Institute of Medicine. Washington, D.C.: National Academy Press.

Elder J. P., Williams S. J., Drew J. A., Wright B. L., Boulan T. E. (1995) Longitudinal effects of preventive services on health behaviors among an elderly cohort. *American Journal of Preventive Medicine, 11*(6), 354–359.

Elvebach L. R. (1972) How high is high? A proposed alternative to the normal range. *Mayo Clinic Proceedings, 47,* 93–97.

Field M. J., Lohr K. N. (Eds.). (1992) *Guidelines for Clinical Practice.* Institute of Medicine. Washington, D.C.: National Academy Press.

Fletcher A. E, Bulpitt C. J. (1992) How far should blood pressure be lowered? *New England Journal of Medicine, 326,* 251–254.

Fletcher R. H., Fletcher S. W., Wagner E. H. (1988) *Clinical epidemiology: The essentials.* Baltimore: Williams & Wilkins.

Grier M. R. (1976) Decision-making about patient care. *Nursing Research, 25*(2), 105–110.

Hagen M. D. (1992) Decision analysis: A review. *Family Medicine, 24*(5), 349–354.

Krahn M. D., Naglie G., Naimark D., Redelmeier D. A., Detsky A. S. (1997) Primer on medical decision analysis: Part 4—analyzing the model and interpreting the results. *Medical Decision Making, 17*(2), 142–151.

Kreuter M. W., Strecher V. J. (1996) Results from a randomized trial. *Health Education Research, 11*(1), 97–105.

Last J. M. (Ed.). (1988) *A dictionary of epidemiology.* New York: Oxford University Press.

Lawler F. H. (1995) Clinical use of decision analysis. *Primary Care, 22*(2), 281–293.

Rizzoli R., Bonjour J. P. (1997) Hormones and bones. *Lancet, 349,* sI20–sI23.

Sackett D. L., Haynes R. B., Guyatt G. H., Tugwell P. (1991) *Clinical epidemiology: A basic science for clinical medicine.* Boston: Little, Brown.

Scharbo-Dehaan M. (1996) Hormone replacement therapy. *Nurse Practitioner, 21*(12) (Pt 2):1–13.

Simpson K. N. (1994) Problems and perspectives on the use of decision-analysis models for prostate cancer. *Journal of Urology, 152*(5) (Pt. 2), 1889–1893.

Ursu S. C. (1992) Legal considerations in clinical decision making. *Journal of Dental Education, 56*(12), 808–811.

Wilson M. G., Holman P. B., Hammock A. (1996) A comprehensive review of the effects of worksite health promotion on health-related outcomes. *American Journal of Health Promotion, 10*(6), 429–435.

Woolf S. H. (1990) Practice Guidelines: A New Reality in Medicine. *Archives of Internal Medicine, 150:*1811–1818.

Health Planning and Evaluation

*t*his chapter focuses on epidemiological considerations for the planning and evaluation of health activities, services, or programs. During the process of planning and evaluating health activities, excess or unusual morbidity and mortality and excessive use of services may be considered problems. Defining these patterns as problems allows for a thorough assessment of the problem, its causes, likely solutions, and the best solution. The problem-solving approach to planning is conducive to integrating evaluation into the process of planning health care activities. This chapter provides a discussion of the cyclical nature of planning and evaluation, a brief overview of the planning and evaluation process, followed by a more thorough discussion of community assessment, the problem-solving process, and other aspects of planning and evaluation that should incorporate epidemiological principles and methods. Examples illustrate the process and issues in both public health community settings and in managed care settings.

CYCLICAL AND CONTINUOUS NATURE OF PLANNING AND EVALUATION

Implementation of a new program or activity is one step in a dynamic, cyclical, continuous process that begins with planning, then progresses through implementation, performance, and evaluation. *Process evaluation* represents one component of evaluation. It begins concurrently with implementation and monitors ongoing performance of a new program or activity. Its purpose is to determine whether implementation and performance are progressing on schedule and in the way required to achieve objectives. *Outcome evaluation* occurs after some defined period of performance to determine whether the program or activity has achieved its purpose. This process of planning, action, and evaluation represent one cycle of a total process for eliminating a health problem or service delivery problem (Fig. 16–1). Several aspects of the process may occur simultaneously in an existing program, but emphasis on any one aspect of the process will vary from week to week, month to month, and year to year.

As one planning-evaluation cycle is completed, a second planning effort should begin. Planning at this stage considers any problems that were identified during the evaluation of the previous cycle. New information that becomes available during evaluation may lead to major or minor program changes. Additional research may be required to verify or determine the causes of any new problems that become apparent as a result of evaluation. Feedback into the next phase of planning allows an administrator to make better choices and refine the plan on the basis of indications derived from the new information. This, then, starts a new cycle. With ongoing process evaluation data collected as the modified activities are initiated, the modified activities can subsequently be evaluated. Such planning and evaluation becomes a process that may be likened to an upward spiral, where each cycle is one level on the spiral (Fig. 16–1). Each time the cycle is completed, the planner continues moving up the spiral until all goals are met.

Cervical cancer serves as an example of this process. This example is simplified in the interest of brevity and is for illustrative purposes only. It is not meant to imply that the decisions made or the evaluation methods used were the best or ideal. For this example, we move back in time to the approximate beginning of the spiral. A review of data on cervical cancer mortality in community X demonstrates that

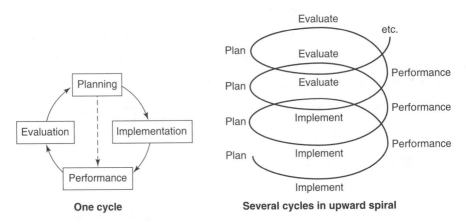

One cycle   **Several cycles in upward spiral**

Figure 16–1. Relationship of planning and evaluation.

cervical cancer mortality rates seem to be increasing over a period of years. A community assessment is conducted in which both cervical cancer mortality patterns in the community and current Pap smear rates are measured and described by neighborhood. The increase in mortality is concentrated in a fast-growing area of the city. This community has not had any recent outreach activities to encourage Pap screening, an approach that research has demonstrated can (theoretically) reduce cervical cancer mortality. The public health administrator develops a public education program to encourage women to see their physician or to come to the public health center for a Pap smear. The initial public education effort is made through newspaper and television advertisements and reports. During the first year, Pap smear screening rates and the rate at which cervical cancers are being identified among screened women are monitored. In this program, Pap smear screening rates were found to be within those specified in program objectives. As called for in the evaluation plan, the administrator reviews data on cervical cancer detection rates at the end of the first year, when it is likely that a sufficient number of cases will have accumulated to allow detection of changes in rates among screenees. Cycle 1 is now complete. It is too early to expect to detect changes in cervical cancer mortality; estimates based on existing rates of mortality and projected screening rates suggested that 3 to 5 years might be needed to detect changes in mortality.

Before proceeding with this discussion, it is important to point out that public education is only one of several possible actions that might have been taken to address this problem. Public screening programs could have been set up rather than relying on private physicians to do screening. A law could have been passed to require that all women entering hospitals be screened for cervical cancer or that all women examined by a physician must be screened. Workplace screening programs might also have been set up. The administrator, however, made the choice to implement the public education program as the preferred approach, deciding that this choice would produce a substantial public response at a lower cost than other action alternatives.

Continuing with the example, after the first cycle of planning, action, and evaluation, the first-year evaluation shows that while there are substantial increases in screening participation, rates of detection are not changing; current actions are not effective in meeting the short-term program objective of increasing detection rates. The planner suspects that some modifications are needed in the public education effort, so a descriptive study is conducted to identify who is being screened. It is found that the women who received Pap smears were women who previously had undergone the procedure. The women who did not get the procedure were primarily those who either never had a Pap smear or had not had one for quite some time. Many of these women did not know about Pap smears because they do not read newspapers or watch television. These women, when interviewed, say they would be willing to have a Pap smear. The planner decides to continue previous efforts but in order to reach those who are not reached through the newspapers and television also sends information to mothers through schools, puts up informational posters around the community, and lectures in churches, worksites, shopping centers, and women's clubs. These efforts produce some further increase in Pap smear rates and detection rates, but considerably less than projected. Program objectives are not being met. Further investigation shows that women who did not seek screening are less educated and lower income women who cannot afford preventive screening. Many of these are young women who moved to the rapidly growing areas of the community, are not linked to a private physician, and have no public screening facility easily accessible. This is also a population at high risk for cervical cancer. As a result, a public screening program is planned and implemented in these neighborhoods. The next cycle begins. The process continues as new information allows planners to refine the program to meet needs and achieve objectives.

PLANNING ACTIVITIES: AN OVERVIEW

As described in this chapter, planning includes the whole sequence of activities necessary to develop a sound, data-based program to meet a community's need. The sequence includes a community assessment, identification and description of the problem, determining the problem's causes, identifying possible methods for solving the problem, establishing goals and objectives, determining costs for the various methods, estimating the likely feasibility and effectiveness of each potential method, and documenting likely risks versus benefits for each method. Next, after comparing for each method the costs, effectiveness, risks, time requirements, and feasibility, methods for solving the problem should be prioritized. Finally, an evaluation plan must be developed. Other activities of planning are preparation of budget, formulation of detailed time plans, allocation of resources (personnel, financial, and materials), and obtaining approval and funding.

Community Assessment

Community assessment is the process of describing a community and its patterns of health and illness, often through examining rates of morbidity and mortality, then identifying which patterns are clearly in excess. Because this step provides the data for defining the problem, it is preparatory to use of the problem-solving process. The purpose of doing community assessment is to identify problems that need to be addressed and to identify those factors that may contribute to or cause the problems that have been identified. The steps in community assessment are listed in Table 16–1 and discussed later.

TABLE 16–1. STEPS IN COMMUNITY ASSESSMENT

1. Describe the population in the community
2. Describe the epidemiological characteristics of morbidity and mortality patterns in the community
3. Describe the environmental characteristics of the community
4. Collect information on other similar communities, if necessary
5. Determine which of the accidents, diseases, defects, or other pathologies may be defined as a problem
6. If desired, rank the priority for addressing each of the identified problems

Population Characteristics.   The first step in a community assessment is to describe the characteristics of the population in the community. For the hospital administrator, the population encompasses the patients, the staff, and the wider population from which the patient population is drawn. For the practitioner associated with a clinic, the community encompasses the clinic staff, the clinic patients, and the population from which the clinic patients are derived. For the public health nurse, the community is the entire population of the city, county, or state, depending on the practice area (eg, city nurse versus county nurse versus state nurse). The administrator of a health plan views the target community for planning purposes as members of the health plan, whether they have used services or not. In other words, the population to be considered in community assessment is much broader than the patients who are served during a short period of time. This information on the broader population allows for the computation of incidence, prevalence, and mortality rates, and for consideration of whether any differences of etiological significance (ie, bias or confounding factors) exist between the patient population and the population as a whole.

A description of the community population should include total population census and subcategorizations by age, sex, race, socioeconomic status, and neighborhood (or health care facility). Options for classifying socioeconomic status include average income, percentage below federal poverty guideline, and percentage on welfare. Educational attainment and occupation may be other relevant factors. Most of this information is generally available in publications from local government or the U.S. Bureau of the Census by census tract, but must be obtained by other means for members of a health plan or users of a particular hospital that draws from a broad population rather than a limited population from a geographic area.

Although health care providers may be considered a subcategory of the population as a whole, they should be described separately, because this information is necessary for considering potential factors that contribute to a problem and for formulating methods to attack the problem. The professional health care staff in hospitals, clinics, and other facilities should be characterized by professional degree (R.N., M.D., R.D.), by specialty (eg, cardiovascular, gastroenterology, oncology), and by where they practice. Within a hospital, the location of practice would be a unit. Within a city, the location of practice would be the hospital or clinic, or both. This information is necessary in formulating an etiological hypothesis, because professional staff play a role in disease transmission or in availability of services. Staff may spread infectious diseases; various specialities may obtain better or less compliance with treatment regimens; location of practice may make it prohibitive for many medical needs of the poor to be met; and inadequate numbers of some specialists may lead to unnecessary deaths. Each of these examples are of major importance in understanding some of the health care problems facing various communities today.

Community Health.   The next stage of a community assessment is to describe the epidemiological characteristics of community morbidity and mortality. Morbidity and mortality are used here in the broad sense to include birth defects, low birth weight, mental illness, accidental injury, alcohol- and drug-related pathologies, patterns of use of health services, lack of compliance with treatment regimens, pain, or ill health of any variety. The frequency count and the incidence and prevalence rates for each condition are examined by age, sex, race, and unit of care or neighborhood in the community. The amount of detail and the degree to which subdivisions or subcategorization is performed depends on the practice setting and the amount of information available. Frequency counts and rates for several years allow one to compare the present and the past. For some conditions, such as infectious diseases, daily, weekly, or monthly rates will be necessary. Other epidemiological characteristics that may be included are length or quality of survival by type of condition or both, level of function by condition, level of compliance by treatment regimen and condition, rates of side effects by condition, and rates of psychological effects by condition. The planner is cautioned about generalizing to other populations from data limited to one institution as it is based on small numbers and subject to possible biases related to who uses the facility. For instance, a university hospital may only see the worst cases of myocardial infarction (MI), and there may be any number of factors that differ between the worst cases and the less severe cases of MI in relation to an outcome of interest such as compliance with treatment regimens.

Because one of the purposes of community assessment is to identify factors that contribute to or cause the problem, it is normally necessary to include in any community assessment all diseases that may occur in the particular practice setting. In some circumstances, only one type of problem may be considered (eg, a mental health nurse considering only mental illnesses in the community or the infection control nurse considering only infectious diseases). It is generally preferable, however, to start with a broad community assessment to facilitate understanding the dynamic etiological factors involved. For instance, should a marked increase in the suicide rate be found during a study of mental illness in the community, it probably would not be recognized that a high rate of incurable cancers may be a partial explanation of excess suicides, unless data on cancer in that community were simultaneously available. An infection control nurse who does not assess overall diagnostic patterns of patients in that institution might not recognize the role that an increase in leukemia cases plays in any increase in nosocomial infections. If a limitation on the diseases to be considered is necessary, it may be better to limit the degree to which diseases are subdivided. For example, total birth defects may be reported rather than each type of birth defect, if birth defects are not the condition of primary interest. Diabetes and heart disease could be given as general categories rather than obtaining rates for all diabetic and heart pathologies such as diabetic retinopathy or mitral valve prolapse. The degree to which subdivisions are made depends on the practice setting. A neonatologist caring for infants with birth defects will definitely want to consider the various types of defects. The nurse working in the mental health area will need to know about birth defect and cancer rates in the community but may not need to know the rates for each type of birth defect and for all types of cancer. This nurse, however, will be concerned with all specific psychiatric diagnoses.

Environment.   In addition to the population characteristics of the community and the patterns of health and illness in the community, a community assessment includes a description of the community environment. Environment includes pollution, weather, geographic characteristics, industries, institutions, sanitation, food, transportation, laws and rules, and the attitudes, customs, and beliefs that prevail in the community. Which environmental factors will be considered depends on the focus of the practitioner (ie, the type of practice setting dictates the relative importance of the different environmental aspects). For instance, the environment for a hospital population encompasses the types of units within the hospital: the physical layout, including furniture arrangements within the units, arrangements of patient rooms in relation to other specialized areas (eg, treatment rooms, surgical suite, cafeteria), lighting, heating, and ventilation systems; food; clothing; housekeeping practices; safety rules and other hospital procedures; and patient and staff attitudes.

The community health nurse or public health administrator considers environment at a broader level. This broader level encompasses geographic and neighborhood characteristics, weather patterns, transportation, commerce and industry, local, state, and federal laws, health care facilities, community economics, and religious affiliations. In short, the environment encompasses all aspects of the community that may affect health either directly or indirectly. Individuals may not follow their prescribed drug treatment program because the distance to the nearest drug store is too far to walk, no one will deliver, private cars are rare, and no public transportation is available. Unemployment may be so high that suicide, violence, depression, malnutrition, and alcoholism are all increased. Teenage pregnancy rates may be high because contraceptives are unavailable to teenagers as a result of community religious mores. For the hospital practitioner, it may be that nosocomial infections have increased because of a change in housekeeping or cooking procedures. Spontaneous abortions may be above normal among staff working in operating rooms because of inadequate ventilation of waste anesthetic gases. In all these cases, knowledge of the environment is necessary to formulate the possible causes of any identified problems.

Determining Which Conditions May Be Problems.   In epidemiology, an epidemic, defined as a significant excess or unusual increase in the rate of a particular condition, is normally the criterion for a situation to be considered a problem. But health planners may define a problem more generally, as "any deviation from a standard, desired, or expected state of affairs." The comparison rate for identifying deviations can be derived in two ways: (1) in comparison with previous rates for the setting or community of interest or (2) by comparing disease rates for various settings or communities. The important issue is choosing an appropriate comparison population. An annual emergency room usage rate of 1 per 1,000 people in the community would not be seen as a problem if it were compared with a national rate of 4 per 1,000. If, however, the rate of 1 per 1,000 were compared with that of a similar health plan with a rate of 0.02 per 1,000, it may be considered a problem. Some administrators may view any use of the emergency room for conditions that could be adequately served in another setting as a problem, both because of the high cost of emergency room visits and because in the emergency room a patient's problem is dealt with out of context, with inadequate information about the individual and their history. In this latter case, a comparison population is unnecessary. When an external comparison population is needed, the community should be compared with similar communities to draw valid inferences. National or state rates tend to be relatively insensitive for comparison purposes.

Caution should be used in interpreting comparisons of rates for present and past conditions in a single community when substantial changes in the population composition or in the community structure and services available have occurred. A health plan that recently targeted recruitment of new members toward an elderly Medicare population, should expect to see an increase in visits for treatment of chronic diseases. A hospital that hires a recognized specialist in heart disease may begin seeing more of the worst MI cases and may show an increase in MI mortality rates. Such an increase may appear to be an epidemic if the change in case severity is not recognized. This mortality rate may be undesirable and may be a problem, but it is not an epidemic of MI deaths, and therefore approaches to dealing with the change will be different from those needed if this represented an epidemic. A change in diagnostic or treatment practices may also falsely suggest the presence of an epidemic. In general health care, many situations that are endemic may be considered undesirable and thus a problem. Lack of use of available services also may be unexpected and, as a result, may be considered a problem.

The individual planner or administrator must decide during a particular community assessment whether to use the all-encompassing definition of a problem as any deviation from a standard, desired, or expected state of affairs or whether to consider only epidemics and significant upward trends as problems. Scarcity of staff and financial resources may influence the definition of a problem. Because there are generally more problems than there are resources to solve them, it is often necessary to assign a priority to each of the identified problems. Efforts to solve the problems are then directed by this priority ranking. Problems with high mortality rates or substantial effects on quality of life are usually addressed first. Criteria that might be used to rank problems could include severity of health effect (eg, death, disability, defect, illness), number or rate of those suffering from the problem, cost to the individual and society, and ability of the health care practitioner to impact on the problem.

Problem Solving

Preparation of Problem Definition.   Table 16–2 provides a summary of steps for effective problem solving. The first step in the problem-solving approach is to describe and define the word *problem* for the specific problem statement being prepared, identifying whether it is a problem because of deviation from a standard situation, an undesirable situation, or an unexpected situation. This information will be relevant to evaluating when a problem is solved. A problem statement or definition includes the:

- Specific type of problem
- Extent of the problem
- Time period covered by the problem

TABLE 16–2. SUMMARY OF STEPS TO EFFECTIVE PROBLEM SOLVING

- Identify and describe problem
- List potential causes of the problem
- Determine or verify causes
- Rank causes of problem (relative to how much of the problem has been caused by each causative factor)
- Depict problem hierarchy and interrelationships of causative factors
- Determine target group(s)
- Determine potential methods and activities to attack each cause
- Determine feasibility of each method and probability of success for each method
- Determine resources needed for each method
- Prioritize methods based on target group characteristics, target group accessibility, feasibility, probability of success, potential impact on the overall problem, and required resources
- Choose or recommend a program (which may include several methods or activities) to attack the problem

- Trend for the problem over time
- Standards by which the situation is judged to be a problem
- Evidence that is available, illustrating a deviation from the standard
- Effect of the problem if it continues or if the problem becomes worse
- Relationship or relative rank of this problem to other problems for your area of practice
- Costs associated with the problem

Thus, it includes a description of the who, what, when, how much, where, relative importance, and the cost to individuals and society. If the community assessment has been completed, all the information needed for this problem statement will be in the assessment.

The description of the problem incorporates several aspects of epidemiology. The problem is usually a disease state or a less than optimal state of health (eg, hypertension, cervical cancer deaths, birth defects, or diabetic acidosis). Extensiveness of the problem is stated in terms of the overall incidence, prevalence, attack rate, and the age-, sex-, and race-specific rates for this problem, whichever is appropriate. Incidence rates, for instance, would more often be used for infectious diseases because each case is usually of short duration and quick elimination of the problem is desirable and possible. For chronic diseases of noninfectious origin such as hypertension, prevalence rates would be more useful. Whether the condition has decreased, increased, or remained the same over time is described by trends over time. The time frame for observing trends will depend on the condition or the problem of interest. Cancers and other chronic health problems require observation of rates over the longest periods. Acute health problems may be assessed over a shorter time frame, but a minimum of 3 to 5 years is usually necessary because many acute diseases are cyclical or seasonal and some fluctuation of rates may always be present. Once it is clear how the author defines a problem, data consistent with that problem definition should be presented in the problem description as supporting evidence. If any efforts were made to rule out changes in reporting habits, screening, diagnostic, or treatment practices as the cause of this problem, appropriate data should be reported as evidence that this is a real problem rather than an artifact of such changes.

The problem statement should also include probable effects that would be observed if the problem continues or becomes worse, for example, projected future disease rates or costs. Table 16–3 lists examples of three categories of costs associated with ill health: costs to individuals, costs to society, and costs to employers. The relationship of this problem to other problems within the practice setting or the community should be described; ranking where this problem falls relative to the other problems may be useful. Any criteria used to rank the problems should be clearly defined. Current costs associated with the problem should also be reported in the problem statement.

Potential Causes of the Problem.   The next step after preparation of the problem statement is to determine the likely causes of the problem. Causes can be determined by reviewing the literature for previously identified factors associated with the problem, listing all likely causes, and investigating whether any of these suspected causes can be ruled out.

Causes may be of four different types: (1) predisposing factors, (2) enabling factors, (3) precipitating factors, and (4) reinforcing factors. *Predisposing factors,*

TABLE 16–3. TYPES OF COSTS ASSOCIATED WITH ILL HEALTH

Costs to the Individual
- Lost work time
- Out-of-pocket expense
- Health insurance cost
- Cost associated with number of years lost, a theoretical value usually based on earning power if the individual had lived life the average length of time
- Survival time
- Value associated with diminished quality of life

Costs to Society
- Public health programs
- Institutional care
- Welfare
- Disability
- Unpaid medical bills
- Excess insurance costs that are absorbed by the community as a whole (eg, nonsmokers' health insurance rates reflect the cost of treating the health problems of smokers)

Costs to the Employer
- Health insurance
- Training of replacement employees
- Decreased productivity
- Equipment down time
- Workmen's compensation (for occupation-related problems)
- Possible government fines (for violation of occupational health laws)

such as age, sex, race, state of susceptibility, or attitudes toward health services, in some way condition, prepare, or sensitize the individual so that the individual reacts in a specific way to a disease agent. *Enabling factors* include climate, personal support systems, income, nutrition, health insurance coverage, housing, and availability of medical care. *A Dictionary of Epidemiology* (Last, 1988) defines enabling factors as "those that facilitate the manifestation of disease, disability, ill health, or the use of services or conversely, those that facilitate recovery from illness, maintenance or enhancement of health status, or more appropriate use of health services." *Precipitating factors* are the types of causes that are "associated with the definitive onset of a disease, illness, accident, behavioral response, or course of action" (Last, 1988). Examples of precipitating factors are exposure to a drug, a noxious agent, a specific disease, an occupational stimulus, a physical trauma, or new knowledge or information. The last type of cause, *reinforcing factors,* includes repeated exposure to the same noxious agent, presence of financial incentive or disincentive, and deprivation of personal satisfaction. Reinforcing factors tend to aggravate or perpetuate the presence of the particular health problem. They tend to be persistent, recurrent, and repetitive. Such factors may or may not be the same as the precipitating, enabling, or predisposing factors.

Within these categories (predisposing, enabling, precipitating, and reinforcing factors) of causal or precipitating factors, further categorization of factors as biological, procedural, environmental, educational/counseling, or administrative can be useful in identifying the types of activities that may help to solve the problem. Examples are given below for each category in this classification:

- Biological
  Age, sex, susceptibility to infectious agent, allergies
- Procedural
  Screening tests; drug, surgical, radiation, or other treatment modality
- Environmental
  Exposures: sanitation; air, water, soil contamination; work; food additives; infectious agent
  Sociological: family support; number of people living together; peer influence; etc
  Physical stressors: lifting; heavy labor; etc
  Economic: income; insurance
  Community: access to medical services; adequacy of medical services; location of services; transportation
- Educational/counseling
  Habits: smoking; drinking; nutrition; sedentary lifestyle
  Education: lack of knowledge; lack of awareness
  Psychological: motivation; fear; belief patterns
- Administrative
  Lack of quality control; lack of followup; inadequate, insufficient, or untrained staff; insufficient funds; poor quality of provided services; service hours; location of services

Determination of Causative Factors and Ranking of Causes.   When reviewing the literature on causality of any disease condition, the concepts presented in Chapter 4 in the section "Criteria for Evaluating Causality in the Literature" should be used. A list of all possible causes should be formulated using the information gained both from the literature and from the community assessment. Attention should be paid to all the different types of causes that may play a role in the development, presence, or continuation of the problem under consideration, recognizing that it is not necessary to understand the specific cause of a disease to be able to solve or reduce the problem. For instance, although it is still not known what causes breast cancer, breast cancer mortality has been greatly reduced in recent years through early detection with mammography and improved treatment. The different types of factors that may cause or contribute to onset of or death from breast cancer include exposure to a precipitating agent (currently not known except for possibly estrogen replacement therapy), sex (female), age (rates are higher in postmenopausal women than prior to menopause), high fat diet, upper socioeconomic status, late age at first pregnancy, not breast feeding, mammography services inaccessible or too expensive, or service hours inadequate, fear, failure to followup on positive mammograms, false-negative mammogram because of technician error, failure to follow recommended treatment, or time delays in receiving treatment. This is a list of *possible* causes of the problem.

The next step, documentation of a causal role for each of the potential causal factors, is critical. Lack of such documentation is the major reason why many planners go wrong and why many problems have not been solved. *Never assume causation.* Many activities and programs have failed merely because someone assumed what the cause of the problem was. For example, suppose the overall problem is the need to reduce mortality from cervical cancer. Most individuals today view the cause of this problem as a lack of a Pap smear. *This is an assumption.* It is possible that all or a major portion of the women who died from cervical cancer have had Pap smears. They may be dying not because they did not have a Pap smear but because they did not have enough money for treatment or the laboratory report of the test was a false-negative. In other cases, physicians may not have followed up on a positive report. Any one or a combination of factors may have contributed to the deaths, even though the women had had a Pap smear. Unless research is available on this factor for the community of interest, it is totally inappropriate to assume that the problem is lack of Pap smears. The role (or lack thereof) for each of the potential causative agents in contributing to the problem should be documented. Existing research from other settings may suggest a role for many agents, but it is necessary to assess whether they are operating in the current setting. The data used must be timely; prior data from this community may not be applicable. When a screening test is new on the market, the major reason that it is not used is lack of public and professional knowledge. Five to 10 years later, cost, fear, or accessibility may be more important factors. Opening a local neighborhood clinic with an income-adjustable fee structure could change the subsequent relationship of income to the problem. In other words, the factors that contribute to the problem vary in their relative magnitude to each other at different points in time.

The relative rank of a cause also varies by area of the community, so the planner needs some estimate of the current relative rank of each of the contributing factors to attack the problem with any efficiency. Income may play no role in failure to obtain Pap smears in an affluent neighborhood, whereas it may play a major role in a lower class neighborhood with income above eligibility for government support but insufficient incomes to cover the additional cost. Because of these differences in relative rank of the causative factors in time and place, the planner must be extra careful not to assume that today's problem is the same as yesterday's and that the problem in neighborhood A is the same as that in neighborhood B. Although the same factors may be involved, a difference in the relative rank of a contributing factor could make the difference of whether a problem-solving effort is successful as program efforts go forward in time. A substantial amount of time, cost, and effort has probably gone into programs that are unlikely to have much impact on the problem because these factors were not assessed.

Causes or contributing factors, in addition to varying in their relative rank in time, are frequently interdependent. Seldom do each of these potential causative factors exist in isolation. Usually causes are interdependent. As a result of this interdependence, a plan directed at one cause may not be sufficient to reduce the problem significantly. In some cases, if activities and methods are directed at a minor cause or if the only cause or factor under attack is highly interdependent on another factor, no impact on the problem will be observed. For example, distance to medical services (access) may be a risk factor associated with not having a periodic Pap smear. In a particular Hispanic community, distances to such services are long. In addition, peer group pressure against having a Pap smear may be strong in a Hispanic community. In such a case, it is unlikely that a program using a mobile screening unit (attacking the access problem) will have much impact. Therefore, it is important that the planner recognize the interrelationship or the interdependence of the various contributing factors.

Problem Hierarchy.   As the potential causes are studied, it becomes apparent that each cause is a problem with its own causes. The original problem can be depicted as a problem hierarchy. Cervical cancer may, again, serve as an example. We shall assume for this example that Pap smear screening is efficacious. Suppose that an epidemiological study of women who died of cervical cancer (compared with women who did not die of cervical cancer) has been done as part of the problem-solving process and suppose that, as in the study previously mentioned, a large proportion of the women who were dying from cervical cancer previously had a Pap smear. The overall problem is unnecessary cervical cancer mortality. But there are now two other problems: (1) a lack of Pap smears (demonstrated by women who die without having had Pap smears) and (2) ineffective Pap smear programs (demonstrated by women who have died despite having had Pap smears). Both of these problems have causes. Lack of knowledge may be one cause of failure to have a Pap smear. Lack of knowledge then becomes a problem with its own causes. Lack of public education on the subject may be one cause for this lack of knowledge, so lack of public education becomes a problem. Lack of funds may be a cause of the lack of public education. The same cause or contributing factor may exist for several problems. Lack of funds, lack of education, and lack of services are frequently contributing to several different problems. Attitudes and fears are also contributing factors at the root of many problems. Although the contributing factors may be interrelated and interdependent in some cases, they may be unrelated in other cases. For instance, if lack of quality control is the major cause of laboratory error, then a quality control program may significantly impact on the problem of laboratory error. But a laboratory quality control program will have no impact on why a physician does not choose to follow up on a suspicious smear (when the report is accurate). The causation/problem hierarchy should be graphically illustrated with appropriate patterns of interrelationships among significant contributing factors.

Determination of Target Groups.   At this point, the planner should have completed a problem statement, have listed potential causes of the problem, determined or verified the role of the contributing factors, determined the rank of the contributing factors relative to others in contributing to the problem, and depicted the problem hierarchy and the interrelationships of the contributing factors. The next step is to determine the potential target groups for the intervention activities. The target group is dependent on which part of the problem hierarchy is to be addressed. For laboratory errors, the target would be those laboratories without a quality control program or with an inadequate quality control program. For women who have not had a Pap smear, the target group should be those women who have not had a Pap smear and who are at high risk of developing the disease (ie, low income, multiple sexual partners, early age at first intercourse, multiple pregnancies, and of low educational attainment). Such women might be found through venereal disease or government family planning programs in particular neighborhoods, or through screening records of a health care organization. When the target group is the group of individuals most at risk of developing the disease, the scientific literature is the best place to identify the characteristics of high-risk individuals. The target group should be described in terms of their age, sex, race, socioeconomic, and neighborhood (or unit) characteristics and numbers, both for the target group as a whole and for the particular units or neighborhoods.

Selecting Methods to Resolve the Problem.   The information on the causation/problem hierarchy and on the target groups is then used to identify potential methods for attacking or resolving each level of causation. A thorough understanding of the causation/problem hierarchy frequently makes these methods quite obvious. Frequently used methods are education, counseling, quality control program, behavioral modification, isolation, immunization, screening, drug or surgical therapy, and rehabilitation.

Probability of success should be estimated for each method relative to each identified contributing factor for each problem in the hierarchy. The methods are prioritized by the following criteria: target group characteristics, target group accessibility, feasibility, probability of success, potential impact on the overall problem, and required resources to carry out the activity. Ideally, the method with the lowest cost, the largest impact, and the highest probability of success should be chosen.

This results in a list of preferred methods for attacking each of the problems within the problem hierarchy. Because it is usually not possible to implement a program that will attack all the contributing factors for the overall program, the total problem hierarchy must be reviewed to further prioritize which methods among those selected for each part of the problem will most likely meet with success and which will have the largest impact on the overall problem. With the cervical cancer example, this is exemplified by the findings that a major reason why women are still dying is associated with problems of screening. Once most women who will respond to a screening program have already been screened, it is extremely expensive in terms of resources to significantly increase the number of screenees any further. If only 20% of those dying are nonscreenees, a program aimed at the problems associated with women who have been screened may be more successful. That is, the cost per life saved and the number of lives saved may be far greater with methods that attack a major portion of the problem and that have a greater chance of success.

For some problems, there may only be one activity or method of attack, while others may be attacked in several ways. For example, childhood immunizations could be made available through a stationary clinic within a high-risk neighborhood, private physicians, hospitals, mobile vans, or temporary clinics set up in various neighborhood locations (eg, shopping centers) or by immunizing children at their school at the start of each school year. Probability of success depends on the method used and the target group. The cost in resources and the feasibility of each method is then considered for each problem within the problem hierarchy. A simple, quick, nonthreatening, low-risk, low-cost method that is easy to explain and easy to arrange in terms of patient access is most likely to be met with success.

In general, a problem must be approached sequentially. If laboratories do not know how to do a test or if the laboratory does not have the equipment necessary to do a test, public education programs will be of little benefit until that problem has been resolved.

Program Plan

At this point the planner is ready to put together the program plan. This written document is useful in seeking resources needed to implement the plan and serves as a blueprint and rationale for both implementation and evaluation. The plan consists of a description of the recommended program, including goals and objectives, a ranked listing of contributed factors, a ranked list of potential approaches for attacking each problem in the problem hierarchy, and likely success and feasibility for each, cost estimate for each approach, potential impact of selected approaches, and the rationale for choices made. A time plan for implementation and a budget are also included. (A complete list of inclusions for the program plan is given in Table 16–4). Letters of support from any individuals or groups that volunteer to help with the program in any way should also be included. If portions of the program must be subcontracted, then it is advisable to demonstrate the availability of subcontractors and their willingness to subcontract. Sample contracts may also be necessary. Any-

TABLE 16–4. PROGRAM PLAN COMPONENTS

- Problem statement
- Program goals and objectives
- List of major contributing factors with evidence supporting their role as contributing factors
- Rank of contributing factors
- Illustration of the problem hierarchy and interrelationships
- List of potential methods of attacking each of the problems in the problem hierarchy
- Rank of each method in terms of likelihood of success and feasibility for each objective
- Cost estimates for each method (rough estimates of methods not selected for utilization in final program plan)
- Potential impact on the problem for the chosen methods
- Rationale for recommended program
- Time plan for implementation of each activity associated with each objective
- Statement of what effect the lack of any program would have
- Time plan for implementation of each objective
- Statement of program limitations and potential risks
- Indication of protection of human subject requirements and how the requirements will be met
- Informed consent statements, if needed
- Professional staff and their credentials
- Data collection instruments or program forms
- Sample subcontracts, if needed
- Letters of support
- Budget
- Evaluation plan

time the program is dependent on other groups or individuals, a demonstration of their willingness to cooperate is necessary. Any recordkeeping forms for the program should be specified, and sample forms should be developed whenever possible. The program plan must also include an evaluation plan.

The program plan should also clearly state the limitations of the plan and any potential negative consequences of the program. The parts of the problem or the contributing causes that are not addressed and the likely consequences of not addressing these should be stated. For example, such a statement might read, "It is estimated that approximately 20% of the problem will remain at the completion of this program. The prevalence rate for this problem at the end of the program in the year 2000 is projected to be approximately 2 per 100,000 women in the state." As in this example, the estimates should be as specific as possible in projecting the rate and time frame and in identifying the community for which the forecast is being made. Any potential negative consequences of program activities should also be stated. Private physicians may resent a public screening program and sabotage its efforts. Drugs may have significant side effects. A screening or diagnostic device may cause health problems (eg, a proctoscope perforating the colon). The risk of such negative effects should be stated with specification of the degree of risk and who is at risk, eg, "It is estimated that a perforated colon will occur once in every 10,000 proctoscopic examinations of the target group."

A program plan should also reflect that the program has passed all requirements of the law, the institution or agency, the community, the government, and the funding agency. Informed consent may be required for participation in the program. If informed consent is necessary, an informed consent form should be included with the program plan. This, for example, may be needed for a program testing effectiveness of an intervention.

Developing Goals and Objectives.   Goals and objectives serve as a framework for the design of the program plan and evaluation. A goal is usually stated in rather global terms, for example,

1. Cervical cancer mortality will be reduced, or
2. Diabetic complications will be reduced, or
3. Compliance with prescripted treatment will be improved

Notice that these goals are not specific, do not quantitate the degree to which the problem will be reduced, and do not include a time frame for accomplishment of the goal. This overall goal usually reflects the original problem that was in need of resolution.

Objectives specify the outcomes to be achieved for each of the problems to be addressed within the problem hierarchy. Objectives should be specific to the activities to be carried out and should state the outcome to be expected, a time period in which the objectives should be accomplished, a quantitated measure of success, the target group, the location of the activity or the target group, and any qualitative aspects necessary to the objective. One way to do this is to approach the objective in a segmented way—first, a general statement of the specific objective may be made, then a sentence relative to qualitative aspects of the objective may be stated, followed by a quantitative statement. The activities associated with each objective should be listed. An example of objectives handled in this manner is provided in Table 16–5.

Program outcomes that are specified in the objectives may be of several types, including patient outcomes, process outcomes, administrative outcomes, and economic outcomes. The main focus of interest for health professionals is one or more health outcomes. These outcomes may be at the primary, secondary, or tertiary levels of prevention (see Chap. 2). Examples of *patient outcomes* are length and quality of survival, death rates, level of function, rates of psychological or physical illness, birth defects, and birth weight. Patient satisfaction, disease understanding, medical regimen compliance, and alteration of risk are *process outcomes.* Alteration of risk is usually accomplished through lifestyle changes or changes in exposure such as smoking cessation, exercise, nutrition, and use of protective equipment in the workplace. Service utilization, waiting time for service, length of time to notification of test results, and distance to services are types of *administrative outcomes.* Ordinarily, meeting objectives for patient outcomes is dependent on meeting process, administrative, and economic outcomes. The type of outcome for a given objective depends on which contributing factor is being addressed by the activities of the program. That is, different problems within the problem hierarchy have different types of outcomes associated with their objectives.

TABLE 16–5. CERVICAL CANCER PROGRAM OBJECTIVES

Ultimate goal: To reduce morbidity and, thereby, mortality from invasive cervical cancer.

Primary objective: To reach, screen, and diagnose those most at risk for cancer *in situ* of the uterine cervix (5–10 years).

Secondary objective: To reach, screen, and diagnose those most at risk for invasive cervical cancer (5–10 years).

Rationale: Future morbidity and mortality will be most affected by preventing the occurrence of invasive stages. At the same time, alteration in the present mortality may be brought about by screening directed to those now at high risk for invasive cervical cancer.

Service and Financial Assistance: All women presenting themselves for screening who are at high risk of cervical cancer will receive quality screening and followup (3-year).

SUBOBJECTIVES	QUALITATIVE	QUANTITATIVE (YEAR 1)	ACTIVITIES
1. Medically indigent women will have been screened for cervical cancer.	Medically indigent women older than age 20 years will have had a Pap smear. Emphasis on 25 to 55 year olds.	There will have been a 15% increase in the number of medically indigent women who will have received a Pap smear in the past 12 months.	Screening will be carried out at the County Hospital, Family Planning, Planned Parenthood clinics, VD clinics, and selected industries.
2. The screened population represented a group of women at high risk.	Screened women were 25 to 55 years of age, low socioeconomic, early first coitus, and poor Pap history.	80% of those screened were at high risk.	Screenee enumeration by age, socioeconomic, first coitus, and Pap history.
3. The services were sufficient to serve the needs of the target population.	Women who are at high risk were able to get a screening appointment.	90% of high-risk women calling for an appointment were able to get a screening appointment.	Record of women who did not get appointments who were at high risk.
4. The services were available to and accepted by the target population.	The high-risk population did report for screening.	15% of the population in need in areas served reported for screening.	Need level will be compared with those responding to screening.
5. The services were acceptable to the target population.	Women screened felt that services were acceptable.	90% of women screened felt that services were acceptable.	Random sample of those served. Test instrument to be developed. Including: reasonable wait time, courteous staff, questions answered, etc.
6. The screening test as administered provided results that were acceptable.	Screening test was acceptable in terms of sensitivity, specificity, underreferral, and overreferral.	Sensitivity plus 0.75 Specificity plus 0.99 Underreferral—1/1,000 screened Overreferral—10/1,000 screened	Screening test results to be measured.

EVALUATION

Evaluation Plan

The evaluation plan is developed during program planning as part of the program plan and should be based on objectives of the program. Evaluation includes all the activities designed to determine the value of efforts that have been made to reach the stated objective of a program. The process of evaluation includes carrying out the evaluation plan by collecting and analyzing data, reviewing findings, and stating conclusions. The result of evaluation should be plans for additional research, if needed, or a plan to vary or change the program activities to more effectively meet goals and objectives, or both. This chapter addresses only epidemiological considerations of planning and evaluation. The reader should refer to health administration texts for a thorough discussion of all aspects of planning and evaluation.

Criteria for Evaluation of Health Care Services.   The two criteria most often considered in health care evaluation are the *effectiveness* and the *efficiency* of the program. Effectiveness is defined as "the extent to which a specific intervention procedure, regimen, or service, when deployed in the field, does what it is intended to do for a defined population" (Last, 1988). In simpler terms, the effectiveness represents the proportion of the program objective that was met. For instance, if the objective is that 80% of children under 13 who are members of a health plan (or of a geographic community) will receive age-appropriate immunizations in the current year and 60% did receive them, then the program has been 75% effective in meeting its objective (60/80). Because a change in the quantitative value of the objective affects the value of the effectiveness, such measures of effectiveness must be interpreted with caution. If the objective for the previous example had been 65% and 60% had been reached, the program would have been 92% effective.

Efficiency is defined as "the effects or end results that are achieved in relation to the effort expended in terms of money, resources, and time" (Last, 1988). Maximum efficiency obtains the most effectiveness for the least possible cost in resources. Efficiency is usually reported as the planned dollar cost per case (the objective) divided by the dollars actually expended per case. In a screening program, for example, this might be evaluated in two ways: (1) as cost per patient screened and (2) as cost per case identified. If the objective is $30 per patient screened and the project spent $28, then the program is 107% efficient relative to that objective. If, however, $50 was spent per patient screened, then the program was only 60% efficient. Efficiency, when calculated by this method, is dependent on the cost specified in the project objective. The closer that a program efficiency approaches 100%, the better it is. An efficiency greater than 100% represents savings per case over what was projected as the cost per case.

Components of the Evaluation Plan.   Evaluation plans include the objectives to be evaluated, a prioritization of evaluation activities, the identification of target subjects and of activities to be evaluated, the measures of evaluation to be used, the data collection instrument(s), and the data analyses that are planned (Table 16–6). For each

TABLE 16–6. EVALUATION PLAN COMPONENTS

- Program plan or a reconstruction of the program plan and its objectives (if no plan exists for a program already in existence)
- Identification of evaluative measures, methods, and acceptability criteria
- Ordering and prioritization of objectives for evaluation
- Data collection forms and mechanisms
- Analysis plan, time frame, and frequency

program objective a method of evaluation must be described, including which activities contribute to a given objective (a single activity may contribute to more than one objective), what data will be collected and how, sources for any data that are not generated internally by the program (eg, mortality rates), the frequency of evaluation, and the analyses planned. The criteria for a judging acceptability or nonacceptability for meeting each objective should be stated. For example, if the objective is to have 250 adult women participate in a counseling program for 1 year, then has the objective been met if 175, or 70%, of the adult women have participated? A specific cutoff of acceptability may be specified or the program planner may choose to grade or rank the program's effectiveness in meeting its objective. One such scheme might be:

90% to 100%	Very good
70% to 89%	Good
50% to 69%	Questionably acceptable
49% or less	Unacceptable

Criteria for judging the acceptability of costs or efficiency should also be stated for each objective that is to be evaluated for efficiency. If an activity affects more than one objective, then the efficiency estimates should reflect only the costs for the proportion of the activity that were related to the particular objective being evaluated. For a new program, the quantity or value stated in an objective may be little more than a guess. Frequently, it will represent a value that the planner thinks will look good for the projected costs and looks realistic for the size and nature of the group. Obviously, a program planner can make the program look quite good if an underestimate is made of its ability to impact on the problem. The smart planner will choose an intermediate to low estimate. Too high or too much of an overestimate could make a program look bad. With an ongoing program, it is possible to make more realistic estimates of impact. When revising objectives, it is advisable to use findings of the data generated during evaluation and to try to project the highest goals that seem reasonable for the resources going into the activities associated with the objective.

The order for evaluating objectives should be stated in the evaluation plan and reflect the prioritization of the objectives. The evaluation time schedule should also reflect this prioritization. If, for some reason, a total evaluation cannot be completed, evaluation should be performed on the most important objectives, referring back to the ranking of the problems within the problem hierarchy for assistance in prioritization of objectives.

Data Collection Forms and Mechanisms.   All the program forms that provide data for evaluation should be included in the evaluation plan. The evaluation plan for each objective should specify all the data items and all the forms on which each item is found. The easiest way to do this is for each form to have a unique identification number and for each item within the form to have a unique identifier. Such specification of the sources of the data for evaluating each objective assures that when it comes time for evaluation, the necessary data are available.

An existing program that does not have a plan or objectives also will lack appropriate data for evaluation, forcing the evaluator to attempt to reconstruct objectives to the best extent possible, then to search for existing data that might be useful for evaluation or collect new information as part of an evaluation effort. A survey of people served by the program might be performed. Or, data describing the situation before program implementation and during program performance may be collected retrospectively. For instance, pathology laboratories could be surveyed to determine how many Pap smears were performed annually before March 1995 (when the program began) and how many Pap smears were performed annually from March 1995 until the present. Pap smear rates can then be determined for each period of time (ie, before and after the program began). If the program consisted of a public education effort, however, obtaining retrospective data on public awareness is unlikely. Thus, it will not be possible to draw conclusions about changes in Pap smear rates in relation to the public education effort. This example illustrates some of the problems that occur as a result of failure to build evaluation into the program design.

Analysis Plan, Time Frame, and Frequency.   The evaluation plan should specify the analyses that are planned for evaluating each objective. A profile of the group targeted by each objective and descriptive data on those reached should be provided to illustrate how the actual participants compare with the target group. In one cervical cancer screening program it was found that most of the participants were middle- to upper-class, well-educated white women with few pregnancies who had had Pap smears within 6 months before being screened by the program. The target group was lower socioeconomic, poorly educated minority women with multiple pregnancies who had not had a Pap smear in the past 3 years.

A time frame for evaluation should be included in the evaluation plan, specifying when each evaluation activity will begin, when it is projected to end, and how frequently each evaluation activity should occur. If different objectives require evaluation at different intervals at various points in time, the intervals and the length of time for the evaluation for each objective should be stated or illustrated. The evaluator should make sure that the time frame used in analysis is the same as the time frame specified in the objective. In other words, do not evaluate 6 months worth of data for a 12-month objective. The formulae that are to be used for determination of effectiveness, efficiency, adequacy, or other measures of program accomplishments should be included in the plan. (Although only one formula was given in this chapter for effectiveness and efficiency, there are several methods of calculating them.) Sensitivity, specificity, and predictive value should be calculated when evaluating any screening or diagnostic procedures (see Chap. 14).

Potential Biases and Limitations of Evaluation Plan.   The last item to be included in the evaluation plan is a statement of any biases or limitations of the evaluation. This is always important, but it is especially important for programs that have never had a program plan or specific objectives.

Program or Method Efficacy.   The question of program efficacy is sometimes raised during program evaluation. Efficacy is defined in *A Dictionary of Epidemiology* as "the extent to which a specific intervention, procedure, regimen, or service produces a beneficial result under ideal conditions. Ideally, the determination of efficacy is based on the results of a randomized controlled trial" (Last, 1988). It is this author's opinion that an activity should not be implemented as part of an ongoing program until efficacy has been demonstrated. If the only methods available that may be of value in resolving a problem have never been tested for efficacy, then it is advisable to do a randomized controlled trial before beginning the program. Subjects would be randomly assigned to several treatment modalities and then followed over time. In instances where efficacy has been demonstrated, it may be of value to reassess efficacy if the method will be used with a very different population from that on which it was originally tested. Further, an efficacious method under ideal conditions may not perform effectively under everyday field conditions, so monitoring effectiveness will be important. Testing of efficacy in field programs usually will be very difficult. A randomized controlled trial is not usually possible (for ethical reasons), so other methods will need to be used. Retrospective or prospective studies may be carried out for this purpose, but are not as definitive as a randomized controlled trial; they do require substantial time and resource efforts. The result is that it is rare to find a study of efficacy as part of an existing program.

The Evaluation Report

The actual evaluation leads to the preparation of an evaluation report. This report must describe the problem, the program objectives, the problem hierarchy, the methods of evaluation, the measures of evaluation used, the findings, criteria used for judging the acceptibility of the findings, the potential biases and limitations, conclusions, recommendations for program modifications or for research that is needed, and the rationale for any recommendations. Findings include all the pertinent data that are generated during analysis and the items chosen for analysis in the analysis plan previously discussed under the section on the evaluation plan.

Conclusions and inferences should be limited to those areas where evaluation has been completed. If the findings related to several objectives together appear to point to a particular conclusion, then the stated conclusion should include a discussion of which findings taken together support the conclusion and how. Pertinent literature references may be used in drawing these conclusions or in supporting the findings from the evaluation.

Recommendations for a program that is meeting its objectives within acceptable limits will most likely be to continue as is. Objectives with evaluation findings that are outside of acceptable limits should be submitted for problem solving and then a recommended plan of corrective action developed. Failure to meet the overall goal even though individual program objectives are being met should lead to a reassessment of the problem. An example of reassessment was discussed at the beginning of this chapter under the discussion of "Cyclical and Continuous Nature of Planning and Evaluation."

Sometimes the findings of evaluation lead to an identification of an unrecognized problem or factor that may contribute to the original problem. Evidence supporting the existence of such a problem should be included in the reporting of any such problem. If it is a significant problem or factor that has a significant impact on the overall problem and if there is evidence substantiating the existence of this contributing factor, then it should be incorporated into the problem hierarchy and ranked with the other contributing factors. In short, it requires a complete revision of the problem statement. If this problem prevents a program from meeting its overall goal, then a complete revision of the program plan is necessary. If a contributing factor is not significantly interfering with meeting of program objectives, then it should not be added to the problem hierarchy and should not result in revisions of the program plan.

The findings of a program evaluation may point to the need for a study of efficacy or it may point to the need to do a study of the risk associated with the suspected causes of the problem. This was the situation with cervical cancer, which was described under the cyclical nature of planning and evaluation earlier in this chapter. That is, research was needed to determine what factors were largely responsible for the deaths now occurring from cervical cancer. Any research of this type must use epidemiological methods of study. The focus of such studies, however, is on causative factors that are subject to disease control methods. In the cervical cancer screening example, factors that are subject to disease control methods are Pap smear status, time since last Pap smear, knowledge about Pap smears, socioeconomic status, laboratory error, and so forth.

SUMMARY

It must be emphasized that although cervical cancer has served as an example in much of this chapter, the described approach to planning and evaluation can and should be used for all types of health-related planning. The approach described is relatively straightforward as long as the steps are followed as specified. Most of the required information is available from government sources, scientific literature, or institution and agency records, although locating the information may take some effort. Thoughtful mental effort is required to generate a problem hierarchy, understand how all the problems and factors within the hierarchy interrelate, and to decide which methods or activities are the best choices for a given problem. It also takes considerable thought to decide the best way to collect the data necessary for evaluation. This process can be enjoyable and growth-producing. It will also lead to effective problem solving and the effective and efficient resolution of today's health care problems. With today's emphasis on cost and effectiveness of interventions, a systematic approach to providing services that monitor and document costs and effects of interventions on prespecified outcomes is essential.

REFERENCE

Last J. M. (Ed.). (1988) *A dictionary of epidemiology.* New York: Oxford University Press.

Glossary

Accuracy. The degree to which a measurement represents the true value of the attribute being measured.

Adaptation. The process by which organisms adjust to environmental conditions.

Agent. A factor whose presence, excessive presence, or relative absence is essential for the occurrence of a disease.

Antigenicity. The ability of agent(s) to produce a systemic or local immunologic reaction in a host.

Association. A relationship between two factors or events, usually expressed as the degree of statistical dependence. Factors or events are said to be associated when they occur more frequently together than one would expect by chance alone.

Attack rate. A cumulative incidence rate used in surveillance of infectious disease, usually in specified populations within limited time periods.

Attributable risk. Rate of a disease among exposed individuals that can be attributed to the exposure, derived by subtracting the rate of the outcome (incidence or mortality) among the unexposed from the rate among the exposed, thus removing disease occurrence due to other causes.

Biological plausibility. A reasonable physiological mechanism to explain how a casual factor could operate to bring about a particular disease.

Blinding. A procedure used in clinical trials in which observers or subjects, or both, are kept ignorant of the treatment to which subjects are assigned.

Carrier. A person or animal that harbors a specific infectious agent in the absence of clinical disease, thus serving as a potential source of infection to others.

Chronic carrier. A person or animal who harbors a specific infectious agent for an indefinite period of time.

Convalescent carrier. A person or animal who no longer has an acute infectious disease, but remains infectious to others because of continued shedding of the viable organism.

Inapparent carrier. A person or animal who is infected with an infectious organism and never develops clinical disease, but is a source of infection to others.

Incubating carrier. A person or animal who is infectious to others while incubating an infectious disease prior to development of clinical symptoms.

Case. Any person identified as having a particular disease based on presence of defined criteria.

Case-control study. A study that begins with the identification of persons with the disease (or other outcome variable of interest) and a suitable comparison (control) group of persons without the disease, then compares the diseased and nondiseased with regard to the frequency or level of presence of the hypothesized causal (or associated) attribute.

Case-finding. A concerted effort to search for previously unidentified cases of a disease.

Causality. The relating of causes to the effects they produce.

Cause. A stimulus that brings about an effect; usually defined operationally by determining that changing the amount or frequency of a suspected cause changes the amount or frequency of the related effect.

Necessary cause. A factor that must always be present before an event.

Sufficient cause. A factor that inevitably initiates or produces the effect.

Central tendency. A statistical term that refers to the most typical values in a frequency distribution. The most commonly used measures are mode, median, and mean.

Mean. The sum of observations in a distribution divided by the number of observations.

Median. The value of a middle score in a distribution.

Mode. The value that occurs more frequently than any other value in a distribution.

Chronic disease. All impairments or deviations from normal with one or more of the following characteristics: permanent, leaves residual disability, is caused by nonreversible pathological alterations, requires special training of the patient for rehabilitation, or may be expected to require long periods of supervision, observation, or care.

Clinical disease.   The stage in the natural history that begins when sufficient anatomic or functional changes have occurred to produce observable signs and symptoms of disease.

Clinical epidemiology.   The application of epidemiological principles and methods to the day-to-day care of patients.

Clinical horizon.   A point in the natural history when clinical disease becomes evident.

Cluster.   A closely grouped series of events or cases of a disease or other health-related phenomena with well-defined time and/or place distribution patterns.

Coherence.   A biologically plausible explanation for an association between two factors; such an explanation increases the likelihood of the association being causal.

Cohort.   Any designated group of persons who are followed or traced over a period of time.

Cohort anaylsis.   The following of a component of the population born during a particular period and identified by period of birth so that its characteristics (eg, causes of death) can be ascertained for each successive period of time and age.

Cohort study.   A study in which subsets of a defined population can be identified as exposed, not exposed, or exposed in varying degrees to a factor or factors hypothesized to cause a disease or other outcome. Subjects are then followed over time, and frequency of disease occurrence is determined.

Colonization.   *See* infection.

Comparison group.   Any group with which the index group is compared; a control group.

Community assessment.   The process of describing a community, its patterns of morbidity and mortality, and identifying those patterns which are clearly in excess of normal.

Consistency.   A criteria for inferrial causality that requires similar findings from multiple studies of the relationship between two variables regardless of study design.

Control group.   A group of subjects that is compared with those subjects having an attribute of interests to control for bias and provide comparison values for statistical tests.

Correlation coefficient.   A statistical measure of the strength of association between two variables.

Cost–benefit.   The ratio of the economic benefit of preventing an additional case to the economic cost of preventing an additional case. When the ratio is greater than 1, the benefits outweigh the costs.

Critical point.   A theoretical time representing a point in disease natural history that is crucial in determining whether there will be major or severe consequences of the disease. Intervention prior to this point can change the subsequent course and prognosis of the disease. Intervention after this point does not alter the course of the disease.

Cross-sectional study.   A study that determines for each member of a study population or a representative sample of a population the presence or absence of hypothetical causal factors and disease at a single point in time.

Decision analysis.   Application of probability theory to assist in making "best-choice" clinical decisions by breaking such decisions into smaller, more easily assimilated series of decisions; often expressed graphically in the form of a decision tree diagram which indicates alternative decision choices and eventualities in the order they are likely to occur and which assigns quantitative values to each outcome.

Detection point.   The point at which a disease is detectable by technological methods.

Disability.   Residual reduction in a person's capacity to function in society.

Dose-effect.   An increase in disease incidence related to the level or dose of exposure.

Ecological fallacy.   An error in inference caused by failure to distinguish between different levels of organization, eg, assuming that relationships between factors and diseases observed for groups can be equally applied to individuals.

Ecological study.   A study that looks for relationships between factors or events and disease frequency or level, based on aggregate data for entire populations; joint presence or absence of disease and the etiological factor for individuals is not established.

Effectiveness.   Extent to which a procedure or intervention achieves its intended effect when employed in the field.

Efficacy.   The extent to which a specific intervention, regimen, procedure, or service produces a beneficial result under ideal conditions.

Efficiency.   The effects or end results achieved in relation to the effort expended in terms of money, resources, and time.

Endemic disease.   The habitual presence of a disease or infectious agent in a defined geographic area or population.

Environment. All external conditions and influences affecting the life of living things.

Epidemic. Rates of a disease clearly in excess of normal or expected frequency in a defined geographic area.

Common source epidemic. An epidemic caused by exposure of a group of persons to the same source of an agent (eg, the same water supply) . (*syn.*: point source.)

Epidemic curve. A graphic plotting of the distribution of cases by time of onset.

Propagated epidemic. An epidemic caused by person-to-person transmission of a disease agent.

Epidemiology. The study of the distribution of states of health and of the determinants of deviations from health in populations.

Analytical epidemiology. Use of epidemiological methods to test hypotheses about causality; the second phase of epidemiological investigations.

Descriptive epidemiology. The first phase of epidemiological investigation; applying epidemiological methods to generate descriptions of the time, place, and person characteristics of disease distribution.

Experimental epidemiology. Use of experimental studies to establish disease causality.

Substantive epidemiology. The collection of epidemiological knowledge about diseases.

Etiology. Postulated causes that initiate the pathogenic process; *see also* cause.

Evaluation. An objective, systematic process for determining the relevance, effectiveness, and impact of program activities in relation to program objectives.

Experiment. A study in which subjects are randomly assigned to each experimental condition and the conditions of the study are under the control of the investigator; also called a randomized, controlled trial.

Factor. One of the elements, circumstances, or influences that contribute to produce a result.

False negative. A negative test result in a subject who possesses the attribute for which the test is conducted.

False positive. A positive test result in a subject who does not possess the attribute for which the test is conducted.

Health. Complete physical, mental, and social well-being.

Health promotion. Activities designed to optimize health.

Health risk appraisal.   A method of estimating an individual's risk of developing a disease or other outcome.

Healthy worker effect.   A bias in study design that reduces the difference in outcomes between a working population and population rates used for comparison.

Herd immunity.   Immunity of a group or community, where resistance of the group to invasion and spread of an infectious agent decreases the probability of exposure of the nonimmune.

Host.   A person or living animal that affords subsistence or lodgement to an infection.

Hypothesis.   A supposition provisionally adopted to explain observations and to guide investigation.

Immunity.   The resistance of an individual to a specific infectious agent or its products.
>   *Active immunity.*   Resistance developed in response to stimulus by an antigen (infective agent or vaccine) and usually characterized by the presence of antibody produced by the host.
>   *Natural immunity.*   Species-determined inherent resistance to a disease agent.
>   *Passive immunity.*   Immunity conferred by an antibody produced in another host and acquired naturally by an infant from its mother or artificially by administration of an antibody-containing preparation.

Immunization.   Administration of a living modified agent, a suspension of killed organisms, or an inactivated toxin to protect susceptible individuals from infectious disease.

Immunogenicity.   *See* antigenicity.

Incidence.   The frequency of newly occurring cases of a disease in a specified population during a given time period.
>   *Cumulative incidence.*   The proportion of persons who experience onset of a health-related event during a specified time interval.
>   *Incidence density.*   A person-time incidence rate.
>   *Lifetime incidence.*   A cumulative incidence rate where the time interval is a person's life span.

Incubation period.   A time interval beginning with invasion by an infectious agent and continuing until the organism multiplies to sufficient numbers to produce a host reaction and clinical symptoms.

Index case.   The first case in a defined population unit to come to the attention of the investigator.

Induction period.   The period of time from causal action of a factor (exposure) to initiation of the disease.

Infection.   The entry and establishment of an infectious agent in a host (*syn.*: colonization).
  Subclinical infection.   An infection detectable through antibody tests but not manifest in clinical signs or symptoms.

Infectivity.   The property of being able to lodge and multiply in a host, thus the ability to infect a host.

Isolation.   Separation, for the period of communicability, of infected individuals from those who are susceptible or who may spread the agent to others.

Latency.   The time between exposure to a disease-producing agent and manifestations of the disease.

Lead time.   The time gained in the natural progression of a disease through earlier diagnoses.

Lead time bias.   A systematic error arising when follow-up of two groups does not begin at strictly comparable times, eg, a group diagnosed early in the natural history through screening is compared with cases detected because of symptoms.

Length bias.   Error introduced to survival time estimates in screening studies due to the probability that a screening test may identify more of the slow-growing than fast-growing tumors or more cases of slow-progressing than fast-progressing disease.

Level of measurement.   The type of measure used to classify a value used to measure a variable.
  Interval measure.   Has both inherent order and equal distance between each adjacent value.
  Nominal or categorical measure.   Uses categorized with no inherent order.
  Ordinal measure.   Contains inherent order, but without equivalent intervals between adjacent values.

Life-expectancy.   The number of years of life a person of a given age can expect to live.

Mortality rate.   An estimation of the proportion of a population that dies during a specified time period.

Natural history.   Stages in the process of development and progression of a disease without intervention by man.

Nosocomial.   Relating to a hospital; arising while a patient is in a hospital or as a result of being in a hospital.

Odds.   Ratio of the occurrence of an event to that of a nonoccurrence.

Odds ratio.   Statistic comparing odds of having exposure to a factor among those with a disease to the odds among those without the disease.

Outcomes.   All possible results that may arise from exposure to a factor or an intervention.

Pandemic.   Epidemics that involve populations in widespread geographic areas of the world.

Parallel testing.   The simultaneous application of multiple diagnostic tests.

Pathogenesis.   The postulated mechanisms by which an etiological agent produces disease.

Pathogenicity.   The ability of an organism to produce overt disease.
   Pathogenicity rate.   A measure of the pathogenicity of an organism in a population; the percentage of all infected persons who have clinical disease.

Person–year.   A statistical measure representing one person at risk of developing a disease for 1 year.

Potential years of life lost.   A measure of the loss to society due to youthful or early deaths, calculated as the sum, over all persons dying from that cause, of the years these individuals would have lived had they experienced a normal life expectation.

Precision.   Accuracy of a test or measure.

Predictive values.   In screening and diagnostic tests, the probability with which test results represent correct identification of disease status.
   Positive predictive value.   The probability that a person with a positive test has the disease.
   Negative predictive value.   The probability that a person with a negative test does not have the disease.

Prepathogenesis.   First period in the natural history of disease, before initiation of any changes at the cellular level in the host; includes susceptibility and adaptation stages.

Presymptomatic disease.   An early stage in the natural history of disease when physiological changes have begun but no clinical signs or symptoms are present.

Prevalence.   Measure of the number of cases of a given disease in a specified population at a designated time; usually a rate measured at a point in time (*syn.*: point prevalence).
   Period prevalence.   Number of persons who had a disease or attribute during a specified period. Life time prevalence is a common period prevalence rate.

Prevention.   The act of hindering or forestalling development or progression of disease.

Primary prevention.   Actions directed toward intervening in the natural history of disease during the stage of susceptibility, before any pathological changes occur in a host. These actions seek to keep the agent away from the host or to increase host resistance.

Secondary prevention.   Actions directed toward early detection and treatment of disease.

Tertiary prevention.   Actions directed toward limiting disability from disease or restoring function.

Promotors.   Agents that enhance or speed up development of a disease.

Proportion.   A specific type of ratio in which the numerator is included in the denominator and the resultant value is expressed as a percentage.

Prospective study.   *See* cohort study

Quarantine.   Limitation of freedom of movement of well persons exposed to a communicable disease for a period of time no longer than the usual incubation period of the disease. The purpose of quarantine is to prevent contact with persons not exposed during the time the exposed individuals are infectious to others.

Randomized controlled trial.   An epidemiological experimental study design in which subjects are randomly assigned to treatment groups, the investigator controls the content of the treatment intervention, and rigorous comparison of outcomes is done.

Rate.   A special form of proportion that includes specification of time. *See also* proportion; *see text for specific rates.*

Ratio.   The relationship between two numbers expressed as a fraction; the value obtained by dividing the numerator of the fraction by the denominator.

Register, registry.   The file of data concerning all cases of a particular disease or other health-relevant condition in a defined population, so that cases can be related to a population base and incidence calculated. Regular, ongoing follow-up of cases to monitor remissions, exacerbations, prevalence, and survival is often done. The register is the actual document, the registry is the system of ongoing registration.

Relational study.   A study that uses information on presence or level of both the hypothesized causal factor or event and the health-related outcome or disease in each individual in order to examine relationships between the factor or event and the health-related outcome or disease.

Relationship.   *See* association.

Relative risk.   The ratio of the risk of death among those exposed to a factor to the risk among those not exposed (*syn.*: risk ratio).

Reliability.   The degree of stability exhibited when a measurement is repeated under identical conditions, ie, the repeatability or replicability.
> *Inter-rater reliability.*   Tests consistency of values produced by an individual rater.
> *Interrater reliability.*   Tests consistency of value obtained by two individuals rating the same phenomenon using the same method.
> *Test-retest reliability.*   Tests consistency of values across time with repeated testing.

Reporting system.   *See* registry.

Reservoir of infection.   The habitat in which a living organism lives and multiplies.

Retrospective study.   *See* case-control study.

Risk.   The probability that an unfavorable event will occur.

Risk appraisal, risk assessment.   An estimation of an individual's risk for developing an outcome, eg, a specific disease or death.

Risk factor.   This term is used in three ways:
1. An attribute or exposure associated with an increased probability of a specified outcome; a risk marker.
2. An attribute or exposure that increases the probability of occurrence of disease or other specified outcome; a determinant.
3. A determinant that can be modified by intervention, thus reducing the probability of occurrence of a disease or other specified outcome; a modifiable risk factor.

Sampling.   The selection of a subset of a population for study. Random (probability) selection is the preferred approach.

Sampling error.   The difference between the result for the sample used for a study and the population characteristics being estimated. Sources of error are biases in selection and random variation.

Screening.   The presumptive identification of unrecognized disease or defect by tests, examinations, or other procedures that can be applied rapidly.
> *Mass screening.*   Application of screening tests unselectively to entire populations or selectively to high-risk groups.
> *Multiphasic screening.*   Simultaneous application of screening tests for a variety of diseases or conditions, eg, multiple tests on single blood sample.

Segregation. Isolation of persons infected with a communicable disease or of areas with many infected persons from noninfected persons.

Sensitivity. The proportion of persons with a disease who test positive on a screening test.

Serial testing. The application of diagnostic tests consecutively, one at a time. The decision to use each subsequent test is dependent upon results of the previous test.

Specificity. The proportion of persons without a disease who has negative results on a screening test.

Stage-specific risk factor. A risk factor associated with only one stage in the natural history of a disease.

Standardization. Technique used to remove the effects of differences in age, sex, race, or other confounding variables when comparing rates for two or more populations.

Statistical power. The relative frequency with which a true difference of specified size between populations would be detected by the proposed experiment or test.

Statistical relationship. *See* association.

Statistical significance. A difference between sample evidence and the noll hypothesis too large to be attributed to chance, based on a statistical test.

Surveillance of disease. The system of keeping watch over all aspects of occurrence and spread of a disease that are relevant to effective control.

Susceptibility. State or quality of lacking resistance to an agent and therefore being likely to develop effects if exposed.

Temporality. Evidence that exposure to a causal factor occurred before initiation of the disease process (*syn.:* correctness of temporality).

Toxoid. A toxin, treated to destroy its toxicity but still able, upon injection, to stimulate antibody formation in a host.

Transmission of infection. Any mechanism by which an infectious agent is spread through the environment or to another person.
  Direct transmission. Transfer of an infectious agent from the reservoir to a receptive portal of entry through which human infection can take place.
  Indirect transmission. Transport of an organism by means of air, vehicles, or vectors from a reservoir to a receptive portal of entry through which human infection can take place.

True negative.   A negative test result for a subject who does not have the disease.

True positive.   A positive test result for a subject who has the disease.

Utilities.   Numerical values assigned in a decision-analysis to represent how outcomes would affect the patient's values.

Vaccine.   Immunobiological substance used for active immunization. By introducing into the body a live modified, attenuated, or killed infectious organism or its toxin an immune response is stimulated in the host, who is thus rendered resistant to infection.

Validity of measurement.   An expression of the degree to which a measure represents what it purports to measure.

Validity of a study.   The degree to which generalization of study results beyond the study sample is warranted when account is taken of study methods, representativeness of the study sample, and the nature of the population from which it is drawn.

Variable.   Any attribute, phenomenon, or event that can have different values.
    Confounding variable.   A factor that causes change in the frequency of a disease and also varies systematically with a third, potentially causal factor being studied. When uncontrolled, a confounding variable masks or distorts the effect of the study variable.
    Dependent variable.   A variable which is dependent on the effect of other variables; a manifestation or outcome we seek to explain through the influence of exposure variables.
    Independent variable.   The exposure or characteristic being observed or measured that is hypothesized to influence the outcome of interest.

Vector.   An insect or other living carrier that transports an infectious agent from an infected individual or its wastes to a susceptible individual or its food or immediate surroundings.

Vehicle.   An inanimate substance that transports an infectious agent to a susceptible host, eg, food or water.

Virulence.   The disease-provoking power of a microorganism, measured as a ratio of the number of cases of overt clinical infection to the total number of individuals infected, as determined by immunoassay.

Vital statistics.   Systematically tabulated data on births, deaths, marriages, divorces, or separations based on registrations of these events.

Web of causation.   The interrelationship among multiple factors that contributes to the occurrence of a disease.

Index

Page numbers followed by f and t indicate figures and tables, respectively.

N

R

LICENSE AGREEMENT AND LIMITED WARRANTY

READ THE FOLLOWING TERMS AND CONDITIONS CAREFULLY BEFORE OPENING THIS DISK PACKAGE. THIS IS AN AGREEMENT BETWEEN YOU AND APPLETON & LANGE (THE "COMPANY"). BY OPENING THIS SEALED PACKAGE, YOU ARE AGREEING TO BE BOUND BY THESE TERMS AND CONDITIONS. IF YOU DO NOT AGREE WITH THESE TERMS AND CONDTIONS, DO NOT OPEN THE DISK PACKAGE, PROMPTLY RETURN THE DISK PACKAGE AND ALL ACCOMPANYING ITEMS TO THE COMPANY.

1. GRANT OF LICENSE: In consideration of your purchase of this book and/or other materials published by the Company, and your agreement to abide by the terms and conditions of this Agreement, the Company grants to you a nonexclusive right to use and display the copy of the enclosed software program (hereinafter the "SOFTWARE") so long as you comply with the terms of this Agreement. The company reserves all rights not expressly granted to you under this Agreement. This license is not a sale of the original SOFTWARE or any copy to you.

2. USE RESTRICTIONS: You may not sell, license, transfer or distribute copies of the SOFTWARE or Documentation to others. You may not reverse engineer, disassemble, decompile, modify, adapt, translate or otherwise reproduce the SOFTWARE or any part of it, or create derivative works based on the SOFTWARE or the Documentation without the prior written consent of the Company.

3. MISCELLANEOUS: This Agreement shall be construed in accordance with the laws of the United States of America and the State of New York, except for that body of law dealing with conflicts of law, and shall benefit the Company, its affiliates and assignees. If any provision of this Agreement is found void or unenforceable, the remainder will remain valid and enforceable according to its terms. Use, duplication or disclosure of the SOFTWARE by the U.S. Government is subject to the restricted rights applicable to commercial computer software under FAR 52.227.19 and DFARS 252.277-7013.

4. LIMITED WARRANTY AND DISCLAIMER OF WARRANTY: Because this SOFTWARE is being given to you without charge, the Company makes no warranties about the SOFTWARE, which is provided "AS-IS." **THE COMPANY DISCLAIMS ALL WARRANTIES, EXPRESS OR IMPLIED, INCLUDING WITHOUT LIMITATION, THE IMPLIED WARRANTIES OF MERCHANTABILITY AND FITNESS FOR A PARTICULAR PURPOSE, THE COMPANY DOES NOT WARRANT, GUARANTEE OR MAKE ANY REPRESENTATION REGARDING THE USE OR THE RESULTS OF THE USE OF THE SOFTWARE. IN NO EVENT, SHALL THE COMPANY, ITS PARENTS, SUBSIDIARIES, AFFILIATES, LICENSORS, DIRECTORS, OFFICERS, EMPLOYEES, AGENTS, SUPPLIERS OR CONTRACTORS BE LIABLE FOR ANY INCIDENTAL, INDIRECT, SPECIAL OR CONSEQUENTIAL DAMAGES ARISING OUT OF OR IN CONNECTION WITH THE LICENSE GRANTED UNDER THIS AGREEMENT INCLUDING, WITHOUT LIMITATION, LOSS OF USE, LOSS OF DATA, LOSS OF INCOME OR PROFIT, OR OTHER LOSSES SUSTAINED AS RESULT OF INJURY TO ANY PERSON, OR LOSS OF OR DAMAGE TO PROPERTY, OR CLAIMS OF THIRD PARTIES, EVEN IF THE COMPANY OR AN AUTHORIZED REPRESENTATIVE OF THE COMPANY HAS BEEN ADVISED OF THE POSSIBILITY OF SUCH DAMAGES.**

SOME JURISDICTIONS DO NOT ALLOW THE EXCLUSION OF IMPLIED WARRANTIES OR THE LIMITATION ON LIABILITY FOR INCIDENTAL, INDIRECT, SPECIAL OR CONSEQUENTIAL DAMAGES, SO THE ABOVE LIMITATIONS MAY NOT ALWAYS APPLY. THE WARRANTIES IN THIS AGREEMENT GIVE YOU SPECIFIC LEGAL RIGHTS AND YOU MAY ALSO HAVE OTHER RIGHTS WHICH VARY IN ACCORDANCE WITH LOCAL LAW.

No sales personnel or other representative of any party involved in the distribution of the software is authorized by the Company to make any warranties with respect to the software beyond what is contained in this agreement. Oral statements do not constitute warranties, shall not be relied upon by you and are not part of this agreement. The entire agreement between you and the Company is embodied herein.

ACKNOWLEDGMENT

YOU ACKNOWLEDGE THAT YOU HAVE READ THIS AGREEMENT, UNDERSTAND IT AND AGREE TO BE BOUND BY ITS TERMS AND CONDITIONS. YOU ALSO AGREE THAT THIS AGREEMENT IS THE COMPLETE AND EXCLUSIVE AGREEMENT BETWEEN YOU AND THE COMPANY.

Should you have any questions concerning this agreement or if you wish to contact the Company for any reason, please contact in writing: Simon & Schuster, c/o StarTek, 237 22nd Street, Greeley, CO 80631. (800) 991-0077

NOTE
If you encounter difficulty using this software in a Windows®-based word processing program after having read the "README.TXT" file on the disk, please contact: Simon & Schuster, c/o StarTek, 237 22nd Street, Greeley, CO 80631. (800) 991-0077